Archaeology of Africa

Series Editor

The *Archaeology of Africa* series promotes innovative scholarship that positions African archaeological research at the leading edge of global academic dialogue. This extensive publishing platform supports in-depth studies of varying lengths, including monographs, edited volumes, and Springerbriefs (short publications between 50-120 pages), allowing authors to present their research with the depth and scope it demands. This series builds upon and expands the SpringerBriefs in Archaeology: Contributions from Africa series, now offering authors the flexibility to publish both short-form briefs, full-length monographs and edited volumes, while maintaining our commitment to accessible, high-impact scholarship on African archaeology.

Africa's archaeological record provides exceptional insights into all facets of human history, from early human evolution to complex state formations, and the evolving cultural landscapes of contemporary relevance. This series illustrates the transformative impact of African archaeological data on significant academic discussions regarding human development, technological advancement, social organization, economic systems, and cultural transformation.

The Archaeology of Africa series prioritizes original scholarship that:

- Develops novel interpretive frameworks based on African archaeological evidence.
- Establishes new methodological standards for archaeological practice.
- Reveals previously unknown aspects of Africa's deep history and cultural heritage.
- Connects archaeological findings to contemporary issues of identity, development, indigenous knowledge, and social justice.
- Fosters collaborative research approaches between African and international scholars.

Each publication exemplifies the highest standards of scholarly rigor via a timely review process that includes the series editorial team and independent experts. The goal is to publish books that significantly enhance archaeological knowledge about ancestral Africans and their present-day legacies.

The series, published in collaboration with the Society of Africanist Archaeologists (SAFA), represents a unified approach to archaeological scholarship that transcends geographical and institutional boundaries. Together, we are dedicated to elevating African voices in archaeology and ensuring that research produced on the continent receives the international recognition and engagement it merits.

Proposal Submissions

For a copy of the proposal form, please contact Christi Lue (christi.lue@springer.com). Initial proposals can be sent to the Series Editor (s), Helina S. Woldekiros (hswoldek@wustl.edu). Proposals should include:

- A short synopsis of the work or the introduction chapter
- The proposed Table of Contents
- The CV of the lead author(s)
- If available: one sample chapter

Tim Forssman

Archaeology in Africa: Why the Past Matters

Springer

Tim Forssman
University of Mpumalanga
Mbombela, South Africa

School of Archaeology
University of Oxford
Oxford, UK

ISSN 3120-4120 ISSN 3120-4139 (electronic)
Archaeology of Africa
ISBN 978-3-032-13364-9 ISBN 978-3-032-13365-6 (eBook)
https://doi.org/10.1007/978-3-032-13365-6

This Springer imprint is published by the registered company Springer Nature Switzerland AG
The registered company address is: Gewerbestrasse 11, 6330 Cham, Switzerland

Acknowledgements There were moments, many of them, that I wondered whether I was doing the right thing in attempting to write a book such as this. It is broad. Very broad. It covers an entire continent, a disparate and heterogeneous group of people that are spaced apart not only geographically but chronologically as well—and by a huge margin in some instances—and all of this was studied by an incredible number of people from all parts of the world. Their studies, the questions they asked, the determination it took to answer them, and the dedication and commitment to Africa's past are remarkable. It truly is. I am so grateful that for the many months while working on this book I was able to pour through archaeological and historical reports from the last century and more. It was a privilege. I digested what I could and found ways of communicating what was said but this time in my own way. I hope that this book does these many, varied, wonderful, and sometimes shocking studies justice. Thank you to the authors, scholars, archaeologists, historians, community members, travellers, journalists, and all manner of contributors for adding to our understanding of this continent's incredible history.

I wish to extend a heartfelt thank you to those who read sections of this book and provided comments and insights that helped me rework the text, shift the angle of the narrative, and include important works that I had missed. They include Chanté Barnard, Matt Caruana, Linell Chewins, Peter Delius, Kath Forssman, Frans Kruger, Matt Lotter, Peter Mitchell, John Parkington, Justine van Heerden, and Stephanie Wynne-Jones, along with two anonymous reviewers. I also wish to thank Peter Mitchell for his support and endless guidance. In a parking lot looking across the beautiful sandstone lowlands of Lesotho I mentioned that I felt like I was the wrong person to write this book and was out of my depth. His encouragement gave me the energy to press on, and our later conversations assisted me with pushing myself to complete this book.

My friends, colleagues, and students listened to me when I regaled them with stories about the past or archaeology in Africa. They had lengthy conversations with me or provided me with short and to the point comments on my meanderings. I greatly appreciate your support and insights. Thank you, Chanté Barnard, Ianco Coetzee, Kath Forssman, Matt Lotter, Siphesihle Kuhlase, Kholeka Makhubu, Mduduzi Maseko, Dan Parker, Chris Pottas, Sylvia Ubisse, Justine van Heerden, Jaco van der Spuy, and Jansen Vermeulen. Chanté, Justine and later Kholeka worked in the laboratory with me and more than anyone at work had to put up with me rambling about this book, topics, themes, or just my absence while I hid myself away to write. Thank you.

I am also incredibly grateful to my family. Without their support this would not have been possible. It was a challenge to write, and that burden was placed on them at times. However, they stood by and gave me the encouragement and support when I needed it the most. I often spent time away from home, not only for this book but my work more generally, and that impacts them all. Kath, I could not do any of this without your support and I am indebted to you for anything that I achieve. To my children, India and Bodhi, thank you for your understanding, support, and care throughout this process. I cannot count the number of times you asked me if my book was done, but it is now, and I hope you too will enjoy it one day.

Competing Interests The author has no competing interests to declare that are relevant to the content of this manuscript.

About This Book

The construction of archaeological pasts reflects the concerns, priorities, and ideologies of the present. Interpretations of the past have long been shaped by colonial interests, nation-building projects, and shifting scholarly paradigms, nowhere more so than in Africa. To understand how the past is constructed, in turn, requires considering the broader contexts in which archaeology is practiced—including who conducts the research, what questions are asked, and which narratives are privileged. Archaeology on the continent has closely tracked the legacies of colonialism and the complexities of local socio-political and economic histories. This book explores the practice of archaeology across Africa from the nineteenth century CE to the present, tracing how the discipline evolved in response to wider historical, intellectual, and institutional forces. By situating archaeology within periodised contexts, it becomes possible to see how African histories have been written, contested, and reimagined over time. Building on this background, the book ultimately asks why the past matters in Africa today. In answering this, it explores the relationship between archaeology and history, and argues that their integration can enhance efforts to address contemporary challenges such as inequality, identity politics, and heritage management. The concluding chapter reflects on the future of African archaeology, offering insights into how the field might adapt, collaborate, and contribute meaningfully to society in the years ahead.

History Is a Heavy Matter

By Gcina Mhlope

Originally written in Xhosa and translated into English

Umlando into enzima	*History is a heavy matter*
Isilo esimakhanda khanda	*It is a strange animal with multiple heads*
Usikhumba simabalabala eminingi	*Colours too many to ever count*
Ecishe ingabaleki	*The creature's unique colours have a way*
Imibalabala evusa usinga	*Of awakening the most indescribable pride*
Ijabulise inhliziyo ngaphakathi	*But others bring back such sad memories*
Neminye ethi ivuse umunyu nosizi	*The very worst memories*
Lapho sesikhumbula	*Of events that left our ancestors*
Izehlakalo ezashiya okhokho nokhokhose	*perplexed, speechless*
Bebambe ongezansi	

Contents

List of Figures

Chapter 1
Introduction

Abstract This chapter frames the book's central project: Situating African archaeology within the historical forces that have shaped how Africa has been imagined, researched, and represented. It opens by clarifying what "Africa" is, its geography, histories, and a plurality of lived worlds, and considers the risk of homogenising the continent into a singular entity. The chapter then revisits earlier discussions and re-considers Africa's past as peripheral or paramount in global narratives, tracing how external gazes and internal intellectual traditions have alternately marginalised and re-centred African histories. Finally, it lays out the approach taken in the book: a periodised, continent-wide synthesis attentive to theory, method, and politics, and organised into chapters that move from received myths and the birth of archaeology to regionally grounded case studies and contemporary debates about heritage and practice. Throughout, the chapters signal the book's commitment to reading archaeological knowledge as historically produced, whether this is by empires, institutions, or scholars, and therefore revisable. This sets up the book's dual task: to recount how archaeology in Africa came to be as it is, and to show why the past matters now for identity, equity, stewardship, and public life.

> The past is not dead nor its meaning singular and decided. It is always precariously perched on the present. (Bernbeck and Pollock 1996, p. 138, quoting Arjun Singh, 1994)

> It is very much in the present, as and when it is practiced, that archaeology produces knowledge about the past; it is in the present that this past is itself appreciated and appropriated; and it is in the present that the many values and uses it presents—for the present—are recognized and pursued by its practitioners and promoters. (Schlanger 2004, p. 165)

Of all the places across the globe that humans came to settle, it is in Africa that the longest preserved sequence and most complex of human history exists (Barham and Mitchell 2008). The continent's past reaches back to the earliest traces of human cultural remains and continues into the present unbroken. Hominins, and more so humans, have always lived in Africa, and all living humans descend from these groups. After humans left Africa, developments, innovations, and change continued upon the continent. Evidence of domestication and ceramics place the appearance of these practices and technologies among the earliest in the world (Forssman et al. 2024). In many parts of the continent, and in particular in sub-Saharan Africa, stone tool technologies gradually advanced, miniaturised, and developed to include bow

T. Forssman, *Archaeology in Africa: Why the Past Matters*, Archaeology of Africa,
https://doi.org/10.1007/978-3-032-13365-6_1

and arrow technology before eventually being replaced with metal toolkits (Holl 2005, p. 21; Willoughby 2009; Lombard et al. 2022). Systems of urbanism, agricultural practices, statehood and long-distance exchange and trade emerged that was unique compared to other parts of the globe (Connah 2016; Wynne-Jones and LaViolette 2018) . During the last 500 years, Africa was burdened by European expansion that resulted in colonisation, resource and human exploitation, and various extractive practices, all the while African kingdoms flourished and crumbled (Newitt 2004; Bennett 2019). These relations played a role in shaping the world as we know it today (French 2021). The archaeology of Africa is therefore relevant to all of human society, in one way or another.

Although the discipline of archaeology is interested primarily in the past, as the opening quotes highlight, it is the present that shapes it, that forms its character, and influences its ontology (see also for Africa Shaw 1989). It must be asked, when referring to the 'past', what does it *actually* mean? Something that happened a long time ago, human experiences from a time gone by, ancestors, or socio-cultural, economic and political developments? Michel-Ralph Touillot (1995, pp. 22–23) separated the past and its consumption into four phases: making facts, making archives, making narratives, and retrospective significance. In all cases, as a concept the past is not *really* the past, but instead a reflection of contemporary values, knowledges, biographies, political interferences, and personal aspirations. Importantly, it also hinges on what we *can* know: not everything from the past has correlates in the present; put simply, not everything preserves or is represented in a physical form. Things recorded historically were also done so unevenly, which makes their comparability unsatisfactory, and much was never recorded at all (Arowosegbe 2014; Gençoğlu 2024). Moreover, building the past depends on what is knowable at the time. Far less was known about chronologies, for example, prior to the advent of radiometric dating and this influenced how the past was understood (Chirikure et al. 2012; Loftus 2023). Archaeology is also not free of the present in the types of answers that are generated to the questions asked; they are of the present context and not the period or place under study (Derricourt 2011, p. xi). As such, reflecting on the praxis of archaeology is itself an act of contemporary social, self-reflection. Rodney Harrison et al. (2014, p. 1) summarised "the archaeological past [as] fundamentally bound up with, and always remade in, the present—that archaeology is both a product and a producer of present pasts". How the past is understood, the way scholars go about examining it, and the questions that are considered important to ask, or to fund, is very much a reflection of the era in which it is practiced. Archaeology's presentness is inescapable (Rosenzweig 2020, p. 285).

South Africa serves as a useful example to illustrate this point, but there certainly are many others. Prior to 1994, when the democratic era began, there were little more than 3000 heritage sites protected by the National Monuments Act of 1969. Of these, 95% were due to a site's architectural or historical significance, and less than 1% were for its archaeological importance (Deacon 1993). In other words, the vast majority of protected sites were such because they related to the history of European descendants, whereas the much deeper history was hardly considered important. This latter history was of course that of indigenous groups, and some the broader human community as well, but the National Party in power at the time did not consider it significant. The apartheid government is well known for peddling what is now called the 'empty land myth'. Their claims circled a central premise that when Europeans arrived in the Cape and came to occupy the interior, they did so immediately prior to any African communities living in the region. In this construction of the past, their claim to the land and its ownership was legitimised (Marks 1980) and this reflected in the protection these heritage remains received. We can widen our gaze to all of Africa and consider the so-called 'scramble for Africa' as a similar rendering of the past that placed primacy on colonial experiences and appreciations (Pakenham 1991). Jane Carruthers (1989) describes this history as the administration of a 'white' South Africa; one that was moulded by European communities to suit their desires. Today, recognising and listing sites has changed, and the importance of South Africa's precolonial past is well recognised. Of the 47,307 sites listed in 2016, 92.3% are archaeological (South African Heritage Resources Agency 2016). Archaeological introspection allows for the critique of personal or national value systems, and the perceptions of not only the past but the people to which it relates.

In ex-colonies, the discipline has an undulating history that tracks political, social and economic interests and perspectives (Holl 1990, pp. 296–297; for a comparable example from India, see Chakrabarty 2003; and from Iran, see Mohammadpour and Soleimani 2022). It is also subject to individuals and their influence (Ucko 1995, p. 4). Contemporary relationships with the past and regimes has deeply influenced research approaches and topics. For example, archaeological studies across the continent focussed more on ancient history, such as the Stone Age, than the contemporary past (Shaw 1989; Cornelissen 2024). Although immensely fascinating and worthy of attention, the dominance of research into early sequences in archaeological discourse throughout the nineteenth and twentieth century CE reflects colonial perspectives, power dynamics, and justifications (Robertshaw 1990; e.g., Andah 1995; Kinahan 1995; Lane 2011). The history of the last few hundred years, which largely related to extant African communities in the midst of oppression, was for the most part overlooked. It presented an awkward impasse: people were here before colonists and they had a complex, lengthy, and significant history. Important archaeological sites such as Great Zimbabwe (Chirikure 2020), Aksum in Ethiopia (Pankhurst 1999), or Nigeria's Igbo-Ukwu (McIntosh 2022) and Nok Culture (Breunig and Rupp 2016) challenged colonial attitudes and undermined the justifications used to legitimise imperial actions. The trajectory of archaeological research in Africa is embedded with the continent's own socio-political history.

Similarly, what the global west found interesting, or relevant, drove archaeological research directions. The 'Early Man Story' received global interest for its world-wide significance leading to disproportionate growth within the field. Stone Age sequences were often compared to those in Europe, which typically lent its nomenclature as well, and formed the foundation of humankind's diaspora into the rest of the world (Gabel 1985; Shaw 1989; Mitchell and Lane 2013a; Cornelissen 2024). After independence, there was a growing investment in Iron Age studies, as nations sought to trace the roots of agriculture, metallurgy, and state formation (Odak 1980). Such research helped contextualise contemporary societies who had been the victim of historical colonialism in many instances. Nigeria witnessed an increasing emphasis on studies and retrieval strategies of cultural material deemed aesthetically exquisite by Europeans (Shaw 1989). From this developed an interest in art history in certain areas. The Ife and Benin 'art centres' contributed to the establishment of the Nigerian Antiquities Department upon recognition of their importance and the desire to conserve and protect associated cultural finds (Connah 1975). Similarly, in East Africa, post-independence archaeology began to shift focus towards Swahili settlements and urban histories, reflecting new interests in understanding indigenous complexity and long-distance trade connections once overlooked by colonial narratives (Pradines 2017; Ichumbaki and Pollard 2021). Sites like Kilwa Kisiwani (Kilwa) and Gedi became focal points for exploring African agency in global networks (Allen 1981; Spear 2000). Many studies directly challenged colonial assumptions of African primitiveness and offered new ways to narrate African histories.

It might already be apparent that the past is a tool in the present. Stefanos Geroulanos (2024, p. 8) argued this in *The Invention of Prehistory* calling it "rooted in illusions" that has "served a ferocious power". Hyperbole aside, the central tenet is that the past has been used to empower agendas, enrich specific groups or nations, and subjugate people and their cultural histories (Kohl and Fawcett 1995; e.g., Atkinson et al. 1996; Diaz-Andreu and Champion 1996; Kohl 1998) . Studying these influencing factors are tools to understand the means social groups seek in particular situations (Patterson 1995; Trigger 2006, p. 20). During the second half of the nineteenth century CE, while archaeology was still in its infancy, it became a useful discipline for controlling and forming narratives that worked appropriately for various agendas. In some instances, this was to support Biblical accounts, promote racial views of evolutionary understandings, legitimise national claims, power legitimacy, and identity building, and validate justifications made by European settlers (Trigger 2006, pp. 3–4). The reason for considering why the past is important on the African continent, other than the basic desire of knowing it, is because it has been weaponised, and still can be. The past can be wrought into a powerful instrument and worked purposefully for the gain of one over the another (Graham et al. 2004; MacMillan 2010). It can also be used to disguise interests to make success appear natural (Barnes 1974, p. 16) and create mythologies (McNeill 1986). In both colonial and post-colonial Africa, the past has been used as a tool (Holl 1990, p. 296; Graham et al. 2004). Knowing this is important. As the past has served the ill-doings of many, it can also be used to reform and repatriate history. Africa has witnessed these attempts as well. After independence, many local scholars reversed the colonial lens and manifested African histories that were fallacious but construed to tip the weight of Eurocentric perspectives (Stahl 2014, p. 6).

Perhaps one might argue that the past should not be politicised because it is objective. History, it could be argued, no matter how disagreeable it is, cannot be changed. Sayings like 'history is written in stone', 'history doesn't care how you feel', or 'we cannot rewrite history', or any number of iterations of these, are aphorisms many have heard. But, to the contrary, they are wrong. History is what we say it is, and we know about it based on what we choose to examine or what we have the capability of examining. Not all studies are impartial and objective, and all rely on contemporary discourse, frameworks, and methodologies. The ontology of the past is constrained by the epistemes of the present. If it were not so and we could report on historical sequences that were free from bias, these would likely be used nonetheless to personal, political, or institutional gain. I do not believe it is possible to avoid the use of the past, whether with good or skewed intentions. It is fallacious to claim that the discipline is objective, nor has it ever been despite archaeologists' assertions at various moments in the discipline's lifetime. As the history of archaeology shows, this is precisely what happened around the world where European or American archaeology was exported into colonised regions. South America's history was conceived through coloniser's perspectives, its research designed with the needs of western scholarship in mind, whether consciously or not, and validated against parameters established extraneously (Politis 1995). It is much the same for Africa.

1.1 Africa

So often literary sources, whether fictional or scientific, mention Africa as the birthplace of humanity; *Homo sapiens* and their ancestors have their roots in Africa and are of Africa (e.g., Connah 2004). But, what is 'Africa' and where did it come from? One of the earliest uses of the term Africa to describe the continent was by Al-Hasan ibn Muhammad al-Wazzan, baptised as Giovanni Leone, but known more commonly as Leo Africanus (1600, the year it was printed in English) in *Description of Africa,* written in 1526 CE. He was confronted with how to distinguish his readers, Italians, from the subjects of his book, Africans, as well as describing the separate land masses from which they came. As such, he drew on conversations he had with scholars in Italy and the maps produced in Ptolemy's *Geography.* He chose the collective word 'Africa' for the countries of which he spoke that were found on the mass of land south of the Mediterranean Sea; the Maghreb, Misr (Egypt), Ifriqiya (Tunis region) and Bilad al-Sudan (sub-Saharan Africa). It was not the first use of this word. Although its origins are disputed, the Romans had previously used Africa to describe what is today Tunisia when establishing their first colony in North Africa after destroying Carthage in 146 BCE. The Roman use of Africa was not to refer to the continent as a whole, but only an area known to them (Mudimbe 1988, 1994). The lands to the south of the Sahara were known as Aethiopia (Mitchell 2005, p. 2; Pope 2022) and East Africa, most agree, was referred to as Azania, with the near mythical Rhapta as its capital (Chittick 1982), as mentioned in the *Periplus of the Erythraean Sea* from the beginning of the first millennium CE (Chami 2021, p. 13). Contact along the Atlantic and later Indian Oceans' coastlines resulted in more widespread acceptance of the cultural diversity spread across Africa's landmass (Phillips 1988). The Greeks used local names for areas when referring to regions in what is today considered Africa. Herodotus, for example, spoke of Libya, Egypt and Ethiopia as distinct from one another and not bound together geographically (Fourie 2015, p. 2). Africanus (1600), however, was the first person to use the term 'Africa' in a broader, encompassing manner, much like its use today, whereas he used Europe to describe the home territories of his readers. And with this, Africa and Europe were born as a way of describing 'them' and 'us' (Davis 2014).

'Africa' as a term is often bundled with many associations. Use of this name sometimes transcends geography and invokes a myriad of attached meanings. Many are myth, some are erroneous, others are true. What becomes problematic, though, is when the term 'Africa' creates a generalised or homogenised conception of the continent: African experiences, perceptions or tragedies are shared across the region in prose, but not in reality. Kwame Appiah (1992) noted that Africans never considered themselves part of a larger whole, never mind to one that was geographically bound. Rather, "blood and power" tied people together. The Kenyan writer and scholar, Ali Mazrui (2005, p. 70), wrote: "It took European conceptualisation and cartography to turn Africa into a continent". Africa, as a defined and fixed entity, was a "European invention" (Mitchell 2005, p. 2). Henk Wesseling (1996, p. 1) summarised this by stating:

> The partition of Africa was recorded by the Europeans on their maps, but the matter rested there for the time being... In Europe conquests preceded the drawing of maps; in Africa the map was drawn, and then it was decided what was going to happen. These maps did not therefore reflect reality but helped to create it.

The notion that Africa is and indeed has been monolithic was heavily critiqued by Appiah (1992) in his seminal work titled *In My Father's House*. He argued through the writings of many Africans, their languages, and the varied historical sequences, that Africa is a mixture of pluralistic traditions, histories, and experiences. These shape a continent of great diversity. To this day, Appiah (1992) argued, those defining Africa fail to characterise authentic Africa and continue to define it on colonial and racial terms.

Scholars have organised Africa differently (Fig. 1.1). 'African studies' is a term adopted by the global north to generally refer to sub-Saharan Africa. Graham Connah (2013, p. 16) disapprovingly referred to this as the beheading of the African continent. However, there is precedence for this when one considers the deep and long-standing connections between parts of North Africa, such as Egypt, with Mediterranean and Middle Eastern history. Conceivably, the entire Mediterranean region forms a coherent whole at one level (Abulafia 2003). In this region, Islam predominated and connections across the sea with Europe took place. These relations led to Greeks, Phoenicians and Romans establishing colonies along Africa's northern coastline, a process that was repeated during the nineteenth and twentieth century colonisation of the region (Liverani 2000, pp. 17–18). Presently, the Endangered Archaeology of the Middle East and North Africa project operates within these regions due to their shared and interlocking histories, the global importance of local archaeology, and the stressors currently overshadowing heritage preservation (Bewley et al. 2016). To think about Africa with its northern territories attached separates these regions from the Middle Eastern historical sequence that in many respects are more affiliated to the region when compared to sub-Saharan Africa.

The north-south African divide has been imposed on archaeological reconstructions as well. Initially adopted in South Africa, the Earlier, Middle and Later Stone

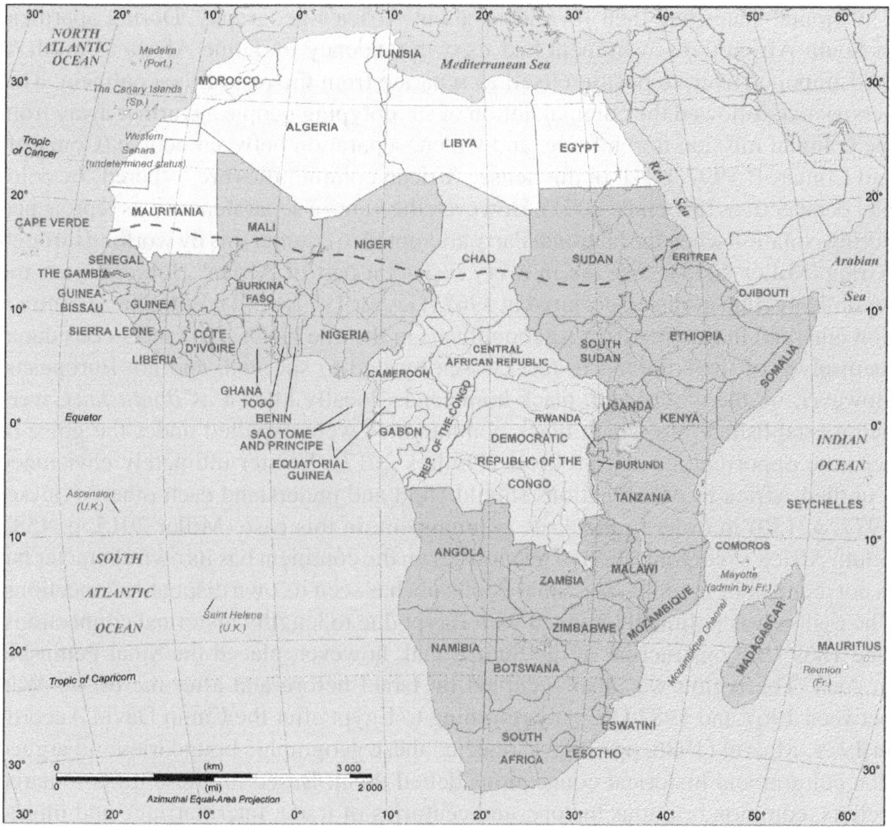

Fig. 1.1 A contemporary map of Africa showing the continent with its various nations and subregions referred to in the text, including northern, western, central, eastern, and southern Africa, as well as the separation between sub-Saharan Africa and the northern region (dashed line)

Age complexes have been inserted into much of how the Stone Age is viewed (originally used by Goodwin and Van Riet Lowe 1929; for an update see Lombard et al. 2022). These systems then 'spread' north into the rest of sub-Saharan Africa where they were adopted (Mitchell 2005), despite heterogeneity across regions (Deacon 1984; Forssman 2023). However, in northern Africa, European Palaeolithic divisions are used. Richard Klein (1999, p. 407) criticised this as reflecting "scholarly tradition and geographic distance" rather than actual archaeological distinctions. In South Africa's case this distinction was grounded in white nationalism (Schlanger 2002), but classical literature and European relations with North Africa further promoted this intra-African division (Connah 2001). Although there may also be very good reasons for this separation, notably the Sahara Desert's influence as it changed form over time, it serves to politicise Africa's past and formulate a partition based on external frameworks.

Colonial states had their own ideas about Africa's geography. During apartheid in South Africa the government had its own tendency to define Africa as north of the Limpopo River, to position itself as separate from the rest of the continent. This perspective followed the colonial notion of stereotyping people as further away from the colonial mission to reinforce, and widen, separation between people (Comaroff and Comaroff 1997, p. 4). In this sense, African communities are 'othered' by colonial perspectives (Mbembe 2001). However, the view of separateness was reproached during isolation when the National Party attempted to counter this by working through Africa (Miller 2015). "We are in every respect a part of Africa", John Vorster, the republic's prime minister, declared in 1967 (Geyser 1977, p. 74). With this, a contraction emerged in South Africa's geopolitics. On the one hand, Afrikaners considered themselves of the soil, and in fact chosen by god to succeed, and not Europeans. However, on the other hand, black homelands, locally known as *Bantustans,* were being established into which black communities were expelled under the guise of separate opportunities and progress (Phillips 2017). Vorster ultimately envisioned a unified Africa in which nations should "find and understand each other" (Geyser 1977, p. 139) in order to blockade communism, in this case (Miller 2015, p. 458). South Africa's reorganisation of geopolitics on the continent has its own character but is not alone in its attempt. The Sinai Peninsula has seen its own disputed connections. The region was politically aligned with Egypt due to lengthy historical connections. The 1869 CE construction of the Suez Canal, however, placed the Sinai Peninsula in Asia. The region was also occupied by Israel before and after the 6-Day War, between 1967 and 1982 CE, only returning to Egypt after the Camp David Accords in 1979. Mazrui (1986, pp. 28–34) rejected these geographic boundaries and argued that cultural and historical connections defied them. Based on these traits—shared beliefs, common religious history, and centuries of trade, intermarriage and migration—he argued that the peninsula should be considered as part of Africa, not Asia. These two examples show the discord between contemporary national boundaries and cultural, historical and social histories. Despite this, they shape how Africa is conceived, however temporal that may be.

What each of these systems achieves is the compartmentalisation of Africa using different, periodised systems of division, most of which are not inherently 'African' constructs. Moreover, it confines Africa to regionalised frameworks stripped of historicism; in the past, as today, the continent widely articulated through different networks with vast regions (Mitchell 2005). However, some form of categorisation is no doubt needed to frame any discussion, and it would probably be foolish to assume that *any* name given to Africa or one of the other continents would be problem-free. In the context of this book, the use of 'Africa' refers to the geographical definition of the continent. It stretches northwards from the Cape of Good Hope, in South Africa, to the Mediterranean. It bulges along its west coast but is more uniformly longitudinal in the east, until the Horn of Africa, where the continent projects north-westerly. The Suez Canal, although man-made, serves as a useable border. Finally, there are the Atlantic and Indian Ocean islands that occur along the African coastline. Africa is referred to here following its cartographic definition, but frequent historic human transgressions of this framework erode the value of a strict geographic identity when considering the past.

The African continent is vast. It is located between the latitudes 37° 21′ north and 34° 50′ south and longitudes 14° 31′ west and 51° 23′ east, and spans over 30 million square kilometres (20% of the earth's land mass). In 2024, there were 55 countries, six of which are islands, and a little under 1.4 billion people living within them (United Nations Department of Economic and Social Affairs 2024). Most of the continent's land area and population lie north of the equator, with a significant portion falling between the Tropics of Cancer and Capricorn. The continent's landscapes include open expanses of undeveloped terrain occupied by rural communities as well as large, sprawling cities, such as Cairo, Nairobi, Johannesburg and Addis Adaba, that are lived in by populations numbering in the millions.

Most of the continent consists of basins and plateaus with relatively few but nonetheless substantial mountain ranges (Fig. 1.2). Of these, those that standout are the Cape Fold Mountains in southern Africa, the Atlas Mountains in northern Africa, and the extensive Rift Valley that reaches from Botswana's Okavango Delta through Africa into Turkey via the Red Sea. Along this great rift are several large lakes, such as Malawi, Tanganyika, and largest of all Victoria (by area). Major rivers drain through these regions. The White Nile appears upstream of Lake Victoria and eventually meets the Blue Nile. It is roughly 6600 km, making it the longest river in Africa. Three other rivers are worth noting: the Congo, draining most of equatorial Africa, the Niger, which like the Congo flows into the Atlantic, and the Zambezi that ends in the Indian Ocean. Other than these, there are many other rivers that were suitably important in the past, such as the Orange/Senqu and Limpopo in southern Africa, Rufiji and Tana in East Africa, and West Africa's the Gambia, Niger, and Senegal. Common to most of these water courses are troubles navigating them. Impeding movement are cataracts, rapids, and waterfalls. In most instances, only about 500 km can be traversed in said rivers from the coastline, barring the Nile which is around three times that measure. That is not to say navigable bodies of water do not exist. To the contrary, in the Congo Basin (Eggert 1993) and Niger's Inland Delta (McIntosh 1998), there exists opportunities for more intrusive water-borne movements. Despite this, Africa's rivers offer little by way of widespread transport (Mitchell 2005).

Africa has a complex climate. Three-quarters of Africa falls between the Tropics of Cancer (northern) and Capricorn (southern). Temperatures in these areas but also those both to the north and south are high throughout the year. Cool areas exist, including areas with year-round snow and ice, such as in the high reaches of East Africa's mountains and periodically in other areas such as the Maloti-Drakensberg in Lesotho. Rainfall is variable. In some areas it is monsoonal caused by low pressure systems and higher temperatures causing warm, humid air drawn from the ocean. Two wet seasons along the equator occur and closer to the tropics, 3-month long wet episodes. In the southern Cape, winter rainfall affects the area due to the northern movement of the Inter-Tropical Convergence Zone. Droughts plague large parts of the continent, particularly in the south-western reaches where the Namib Desert is found. Other areas include extensive, low-lying swamps, inland lakes, rift valleys, and forest environments. The enduring weather systems have resulted in a

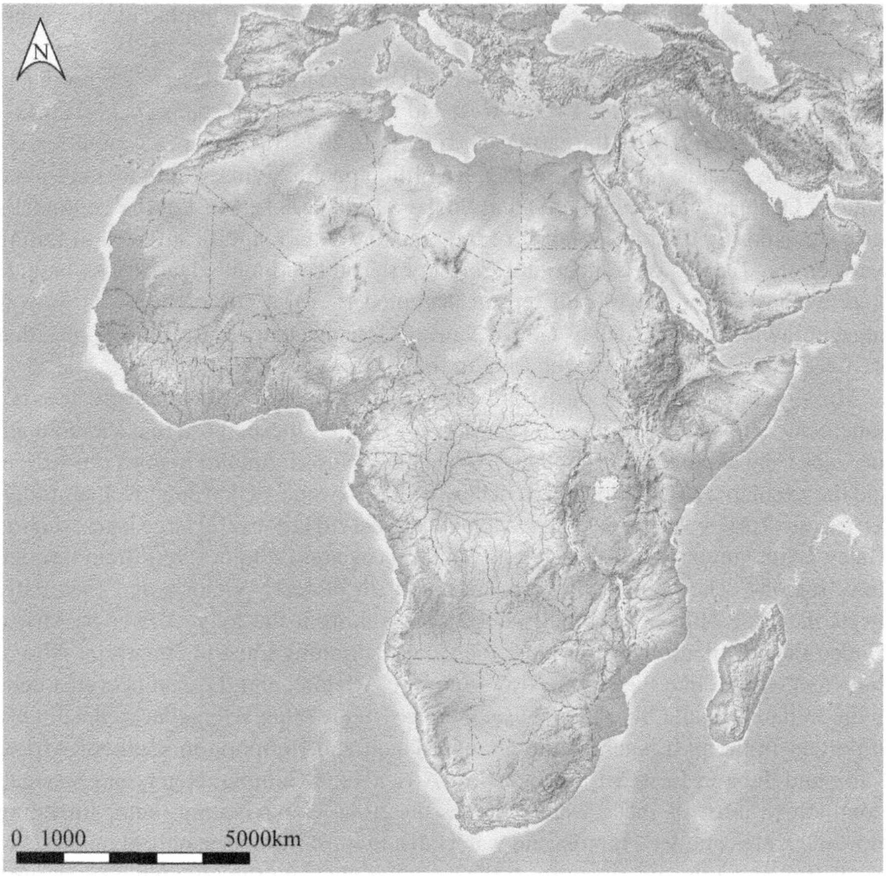

Fig. 1.2 A physical map of the African continent. *Source* https://commons.wikimedia.org/wiki/File:Africa_relief_location_map.jpg

symmetrical ecological distribution, albeit diverse (Fig. 1.3). From the northern to southern temperate zones are a range of biomes, some with high biodiversity, and several biodiversity hotspots across the continent (Lewis and Berry 2012). Africa's ecosystem diversity is under threat, with over 6400 animal and 3100 plant species at risk of extinction (UNEP-WCMC 2016). Since 1970 CE, 39% of the continent's vertebrate species have declined (McLellan 2014). The continent is also susceptible to a range environmental issues (Adams 1992; Hulme 1996; Hulme et al. 2005; Darkoh 2009; Reynolds et al. 2015; e.g., Abernethy et al. 2016). Of Africa's population, 62% depends on the natural ecosystem for energy, food, health, secure livelihoods, and water, and its decline places these people under considerable strain (Africa Center for Strategic Studies 2022). These, of course, are variable and impact nations and people in different ways. The direct human impact on the environment is also notable, and the escalation of this impact from the colonial era cannot be underestimated (Grove

1996). These issues, and others, and the economic and political context Africa finds itself in has led to the United Nations Intergovernmental Panel on Climate Change to conclude that the continent is the most vulnerable to climate change (Niang et al. 2014).

Africa faces many threats, social and natural, and is precariously placed economically and often politically. Directly as a result of climatic, environmental and social contexts in Africa, its heritage is perched on a precipice. Exacerbating this problem

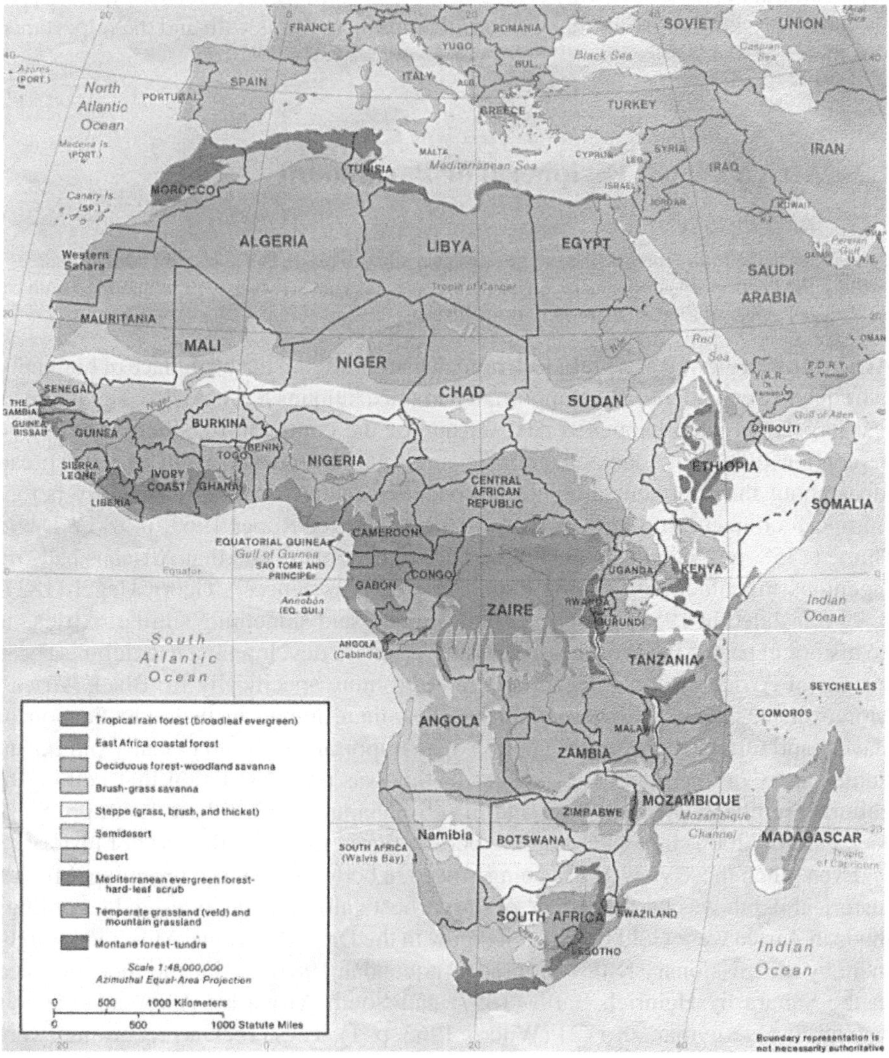

Fig. 1.3 Broad ecological zones across Africa. *Source* https://commons.wikimedia.org/wiki/File:Africa_Natural_Vegetation.jpg

is the lack of legislative strength in this sector, with most sub-Saharan countries, for example, still relying on legal frameworks gazetted in the 1970s CE (Chirikure 2013). Problematising this further is the lack of heritage inventories even when the capacity exists (Mcintosh 2013). With this broader context in mind, heritage's priority is sadly low in Africa, largely, in terms of Maslow's hierarchy of needs (Reeves and Plets 2015)—the presence of far greater challenges with more immediate impacts on peoples' lives and the difficulties they face takes precedence. Assessing cultural heritage risks presents a number of challenges, one being a lack of research on intangible cultural heritage (Crowley et al. 2022). Undermining these makes Africa's past vulnerable, risking a history that we are still coming to terms with and the importance of which is developing.

1.2 Africa's Past: Peripheral or Paramount

> Perhaps in the future there will be some African history to teach. But at present there is none; only the history of Europeans in Africa. The rest is darkness. (Mazrui 1978 quoting Hugh Trevor-Roper, an English historian, from 1963)

Africa is often viewed as a prelude to human history. Being the birthplace of humanity is frequently considered most important and once humans leave Africa, key interests rest largely on what happened next outside of the continent (cf. Stahl 2005). The perception that Africa lacks history emerged and entrenched itself in widespread ideas about the continent. Lord Dacre declared that Africa had no history before European contact but that of barbarous tribes (Trevor-Roper 1963, p. 871). David Hume (1758, p. 252), an eighteenth-century philosopher, said that Africans had "no ingenious manufacturers among them, no arts, no sciences". Georg Hegel (1837, p. 99 translated in 1956), a German philosopher, said something similar: Africa "is no historical part of the World; it has no movement or development to exhibit". These visions of Africa excluded Egypt and referred more specifically to 'Black Africa'. Moreover, enslavers viewed Africans as less than human in their justification of slavery and further repressed any notion of an important, rich and globally significant human story on the continent. As part of this was the expectation that nothing of cultural significance would be found in sub-Saharan Africa (Shaw 1989, pp. 5–6). Jack Goody (2006) in a wide-ranging book referred to this as the theft of history.

Even when these views were being voiced, a body of evidence revealing Africa's historical depth was known. Some of the earliest cultural collections and recordings made in Africa were Gold Coast 'celts' now in the Danish National Museum brought there by the missionary Ditlev Monrad (Anquandah 1981, p. 22), and rock art noted in the Sahara by Heinrich Barth (1857) and South Africa by Reverend François Valentijn, a clergyman, in 1721 (Wilcox 1963, p. 1). These rock art recordings were earlier than the discovery of similar European art (Posnansky, 1982, p. 345). In the nineteenth century CE, stone tools were recorded in Ghana (Lubbock 1870) and in South Africa (Goodwin 1946, p. 18). In what was French West Africa, monuments and tumuli were excavated and the finds were delivered to France (Desplagnes 1907, pp. 57–66). Rock art in Tanzania was discovered (Bwasiri and Smith 2015, pp. 437–438) and continued to be found in South Africa and Zimbabwe throughout the century (Breuil 1954). These finds created an awareness of an African past, but they did not convince many of the continent's important role in global history.

In 1974, J. Desmond Clark (1975) delivered a talk at the Huxley Memorial Lecture titled 'Africa in prehistory: peripheral or paramount?'. His title, and the paired presentation, challenged the notion that archaeological research in Africa, and by extension Africa's past, was peripheral. This stemmed from comments made by Cambridge University professors to scholars returning to the Alma Marta to present their research, in which they concluded Africa's past was, '[o]h, very peripheral…' (Shaw 1989, p. 12). Fast-forward to Peter Mitchell and Paul Lane's (2013b, p. 3) introduction to their edited volume where they noted that little seems to have changed in the wider appreciation of Africa's history:

> "Traditionally, however, that is also where most general textbooks—and most university archaeology courses, at least outside Africa—have tended to stop, reflecting a belief, however understated, that once *Homo sapiens* successfully exited Africa the 'real' human story developed elsewhere, leaving Africa a cultural backwater…".

A cursory examination of the most recent edition of *The Human Past* (Scarre 2024) shows that of the 20 chapters, one deals with human evolution in Africa (Toth et al. 2024) and two with the same topic globally with mention of Africa (Klein et al. 2024; Pettitt and Langley 2024), whereas one deals with Holocene Africa (Forssman et al. 2024). It would seem that at least we perceive much of Africa's past as peripheral.

Archaeology in Africa is interestingly positioned. The discipline has its roots firmly grounded in global west frameworks and histories, with its development initially in Europe but subsequent reshaping from North American scholars (Connah 2013). But interest in the past pervades most societies. It is a powerful tool that has been used in the arsenal of rulers, elites, and authorities across the globe (Schnapp 2014, p. 217). It was also mobilised in political forums to legitimise claims to authority or reinforce beliefs related to ethnicities. Settlers around the continent both foreign and local have used the past to legitimise their claim to authority or actions upon the continent. In Zimbabwe, for example, the Zimbabwe African National Union—Patriotic Front (ZANU-PF) party, while headed by Robert Mugabe, claimed a direct link to Great Zimbabwe in its bid to appropriate a history of leadership associated with the party's leader and put in place a single national identity (Ucko 1983). In Ghana, previously the Gold Coast, the nation was renamed to develop a national identity for the emerging state, and archaeological and culture resources were used by nationalists to do so (Kankpeyeng and DeCorse 2004). Outside of Africa, in Turkey, school children are taught that their forebears were the Hittites (Tekin 2019), and the Mexican flag portrays an Aztec legend, evoking a connection with a glorified past (Fowler 1987). Egypt, conversely, does not draw strongly on its Pharaonic past in national identity-making, but this is largely because of the complex role it played with regard to European coloniality and its intersectionality with paganistic values (Wood 1998). Using the past for nationalist purposes occurred in many parts of Africa, whether enacted by Europeans legitimising their activities or Africans reclaiming their past.

In 2002, at the World Summit on Sustainable Development, in front of a large audience that included all manner of specialists, and many from the field of archaeology, palaeoanthropology and primatology, Thabo Mbeki, South Africa's president at the time, fairly and accurately declared (Shepherd 2003, p. 824):

> For us to understand the significant part of the world we live in, our existence as human beings and the interdependent relations between humans and the planet, we have to scratch not just the collective mind of historians, but also most importantly, the hard surface of the African continent.

He said this in reaction to Phillip Tobias's very clear call, which although being aimed at human evolution, nevertheless transcends into very many other archaeological and historical fields (Shepherd 2003, p. 824):

> The proof is here and in other parts that this Africa was the cradle of mankind… It was Africa that perfected the hand, so that you no longer walked on it, but you had a precision tool capable of making a tool. All of this, Africa has given us and given the world…If you wanted a scientific proof of the brotherhood of man this is it.

What emerged was a trend to rewrite the past. Leaders, in particular, invoked the past to rebuild identities and think ahead. Mbeki's 'African-naissance' is a perfect example of how the past became useful in nation building after the colony (cf. Maggs 2000). Other leaders in young democracies also attempted to harness the past. Sir Seretse Khama, the first democratically elected president in Botswana, stated quite provocatively (cf. Lane 2011, p. 12):

> We should write our own history books to prove that we did have a past, and that it was a past that was just as worth writing and learning about as any other. We must do this for the simple reason that a nation without a past is a lost nation, and a people without a past are a people without a soul.

In his speech he makes very clear the link between being someone, or being human, and the past. It is a mantra that colonists flipped—undermining African humanity by denying history—and one that African nations were using equally to dig themselves out of the obscure pasts that had been created. Julius Nyerere (1968, p. 85), during his presidency of Tanzania, passionately declared that they had gathered at Dar es Salaam University College in 1965 "because we believe that a knowledge of African history is important for the growth of our continent". Against the claims by Hugh Trevor-Roper (1963) and others has emerged a large cohort of academic contributions that demonstrate a far longer African history. Along with these are books written for the public in a bid to shift the narrative around Africa's past. Books such as Patric Tariq Mellet's (2020) *The Lie of 1652*, Dipo Faloyin's (2023) *Africa is not a Country,* Howard French's (2021) *Born into Blackness,* and Zeinab Badawi's (2024) *An African History of Africa* all attempt to dispel the idea that Africa's history began with European occupation. They replace this historical void with a rich, vibrant, diverse and Afrocentric history that stretches across the continent from coast to coast.

Despite archaeology's European roots, it is a discipline better suited to the process of decolonisation than many others. Its very nature lends itself to the decolonial agenda (Lane 2011). More generally, archaeology can advance transformative views on the past and the power dynamics that interplay in its construction. Not all archaeologists may agree with this view; positivist epistemologies would argue that society and culture exerted no influence on archaeology (Wylie 1981; Atalay 2014). Instead, the discipline tests theories by assessing them against empirical data. Relativists, moderate or extreme, would be more likely to agree, at least in part. This system of thought would promote the idea that there is no singular or objective truth, and that society influences archaeological interpretations. In this framework, archaeological evidence constrains theories or speculation (Trigger 2006, p. 3). In this book, a relativist approach to the archaeological or prehistoric past is preferred, because, certainly in Africa's case, social histories and contemporary society have played a significant role in influencing archaeological thinking, approaches, interpretations, ethnic loyalties, and personal interest.

1.3 Approaching the Archaeology of Africa

This book examines the archaeology of Africa from a somewhat different perspective to those that have come before. Most books that do so consider the continent's archaeological sequence. David Phillipson's (2005) *African Archaeology* presents wide-ranging coverage of African prehistory, as does Connah (2004) in *Forgotten Africa*. These examples in English are equally met with those in other languages, such as Barbara Barich's (2010) Italian overview of Africa's prehistoric roots or François-Xaver Fauvelle-Aymar's (2018, 2020) French books covering large sections of Africa's archaeology. Mitchell and Lane's (2013a) edited *Oxford Handbook of African Archaeology* spans an incredible number of topics, including the political role of archaeology in Africa (Giblin 2013), over many regions, with a large cohort of Africanists. It serves as an incredibly detailed and in-depth examination of Africa's archaeological sequence. Similarly, Mitchell (2024) achieves the same in *The Archaeology of Southern Africa*, but for that region specifically. Other regional syntheses have appeared more regularly over time furnishing readers with great, focussed details for geographic sections of the continent (Vernet 2000; Connah 2001, 2016; Insoll 2003; Kusimba and Kusimba 2003; McIntosh 2005; Schmidt 2006; Huffman 2007; Willoughby 2007; e.g., Barham and Mitchell 2008; Beyin et al. 2023). Thinking more broadly, Mitchell's (2005) book on *African Connections* covers a multitude of archaeological sequences to illustrate the continent's global connections and its importance in world history. Peter Schmidt (2006, 2009), in various works, examined historical archaeology on the continent and advocated for post-colonial approaches, the adoption of oral histories and indigenous knowledge, and inclusive archaeological investigations while couching this all in Africa's past and present. There are no doubt many other examples. Taking a different approach in his edited book, Peter Robertshaw (1990a) in *A History of African Archaeology* coordinated contributors that examined the broader context of archaeological practice in parts of Africa covering a wide span of time.

Archaeology in Africa takes a wide perspective of archaeology on the continent, examining what Connah (2013, p. 15) referred to as the "performances and actors" in archaeology who had their own "patterns of thought behind them". It adopts a sentiment expressed by Mitchell (2024, p. 33), "[u]nderstanding the past requires us to understand how it has been created", which entails considering "the broader socio-political framework". The book does just that. It considers archaeology as it was practiced on the continent since the nineteenth century CE, how socio-political contexts shaped enquiry and praxis, and how this fashioned interpretations. As Bruce Trigger (2006,p. 25) noted: "[a] history of archaeological thought requires knowledge not only of the social setting in which archaeological research is carried out but also of the ongoing development of archaeology as a practice".

The first aim of this book is to explore archaeology in Africa. It does so by establishing four phases, laid out in chapters: antiquarianism, collections, missionaries; the emergence of archaeology; a coming of age; and post-colonialism (Fig. 1.4). There are other systems of dividing archaeological thoughts, such as Trigger's (1989) five phases: antiquarian, typological, culture history, processual, and post-processual. Thurston Shaw (1989, p. 4) also defined five phases beginning in the nineteenth century, with imperial expansion, and ended in the decade of his paper titled *African archaeology: looking back and looking forward*. Before him, Creighton Gabel (1985) divided continental archaeological research into a pioneer phase, World War I to II period, and the early post-war years. From a local perspective, Nick Shepherd (2003) ascribed South Africa's archaeological history to eight phases. The four phases used here largely follow these systems but instead organises themselves around the global west's impact across Africa, much like Francis Musonda's (2012) approach to the history of archaeology in Zambia. They are purely artificial and created as a convenient way of characterising broad archaeological phases (Shaw 1989). For example, the phases did not begin and end at the same time across the continent as a result of local geopolitics and other issues, such as conflict. They also are not precisely the same; after independence the experiences in most countries were unlike those in Namibia, South Africa and Zimbabwe, where a white-minority party ruled the countries, influencing their archaeological practices until much later (Shepherd 2003). Shaw (1989) was under no illusion that his phases were definitive, and neither am I here. If anything, they likely can very easily be picked apart, separated, refined or redefined. However, they have been created as conceptual guidelines, and should not be considered to have absolute boundaries. Many of the studies used as examples to illustrate my argument began in one phase and moved into the next with accompanying changes in approaches and interpretations. As such, the periods are relatable not in the content of research or the regions of interest, but in larger global systems or ways of thinking and themes that influenced archaeological practice in Africa during those periods, more or less. While the chapters present as chronological blocks of time, they are not dogmatic in sticking to these since many examples and themes cross these boundaries.

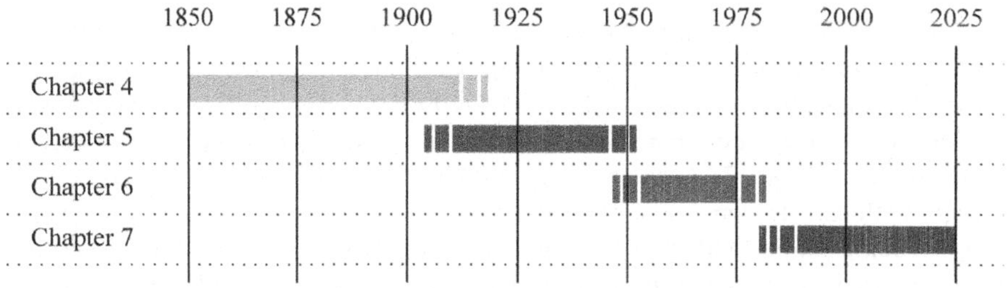

Fig. 1.4 Chapter periods: 4, antiquarianism, collections, missionaries; 5, the emergence of archaeology; 6, a coming of age; and 7, post-colonialism

Despite the arbitrariness of using phases, they have been carefully thought through. Each opens with an example, archaeological in nature, that in ways reflects the broader or a central thematic clause for that period; the birth of archaeology chapter, likewise. The first is antiquarianism, missionaries and collections (Chap. 4). Generally, this period begins not long before the mid-nineteenth century CE when the first collections of artefacts were being gathered in parts of Africa, and by which time Egyptian archaeology was growing in international recognition, albeit in an esoteric sense. Most of the renderings of the past were based on collections or observations made by amateurs or non-specialists, many of whom were not involved in academic research whatsoever. As result, the perception these accounts give are highly contentious and often problematic. During the early years of archaeology, beginning in the early twentieth century, archaeology replicated European approaches but on the African continent (Chap. 5). Importantly this was in the way sequences in Africa were divided and characterised. These early years bear great consequence on later characterisations of the past, for, although once archaeology professionalised and moved beyond these early reconstructions, they nevertheless influenced constructions of the past, and in some instances do to this day (e.g., Bank 2006). The early years stretch until about the Second World War. During this period, concerted effort was made to understand the past in a more systematic manner. It was at this time that professional archaeology began to replace amateur approaches, and the nature of archaeology shifted. Scholars and researchers began to recognise the deep antiquity of Africa and its divergent past from the rest of the world along with the richness of material cultural histories in various regions, notably those with a strong colonial presence or diligent administration. Continued growth in archaeology occurred after the Second World War when the continent entered a different phase, politically, socially, and economically. This is reflected in the next periodisation, a coming of age, so to speak, during a time of increasing independence (Chap. 6). Beginning in this phase was processual archaeology, called New Archaeology. Two major developments—the decline in colonial hegemony and the post-war global context—led to reform of archaeological approaches in Africa under the guise of science-oriented archaeological enquiry. Developments in science also led to great strides in archaeology, which significantly included the emergence of absolute chronologies for the first time. It was also a time in Africa where the dust began to settle after the European nations revised their colonial rule of African colonies, and in some instances the fleet-footed administrations abandoned the continent altogether. The final phase emerged in the 1980—1990s when scientific approaches were challenged by post-modernist thinking, stimulating the post-processual movement in archaeology (Chap. 7). Growing in volume in this period were local voices, intertwining with calls to decolonise the past. This prompted deeper reflection on whose past was being studied and why. African archaeology also expanded to engage critical theory with advanced techniques, including genetics, isotopes, and remote sensing. This blending of approaches revealed new dimensions of Africa's deep past while simultaneously raising questions about power, access, and the global circulation of knowledge.

The second aim of this book is to consider why the past matters in the African context. Archaeology remains one of the few disciplines through which Africa's deep precolonial past can be accessed and written (Mitchell 2005, p. 7). Yet, the telling of history is rarely neutral. Archaeological and historical narratives are often shaped by those in positions of power, both past and present. In such contexts, the past can serve a transformative role (Meskell 2012), particularly when freed from the constraints of Eurocentric frameworks that have long marginalised African histories (Mudimbe 1988). Reclaiming these histories, many of which were erased or distorted during colonial rule, is vital (Schmidt and Pikirayi 2018, p. 449). Since independence, community archaeology has become an important means of re-engaging with the past on African terms. Colonialism not only disrupted social and political systems but also reconfigured the past to legitimise its presence. These colonial and extractive encounters, whether European or Muslim, were deeply racialised, and archaeology was often complicit in reinforcing racial hierarchies through portrayals of Africa's past as static, primitive, or absent. Although understandings have shifted, the legacy of these narratives continues to shape archaeological practice and interpretation today. The material past, like the bodies it is often connected to, is not neutral, and questions of race remain central to how heritage is recognised, protected, and politicised across the continent. Archaeology has the potential to challenge these narratives and offer more grounded, inclusive accounts (Ogot 2009). Yet across Africa, cultural heritage remains under threat from climate change, conflict, development, looting, and tourism. These forces risk destroying the very material traces needed to question, revise, and repair the past. Without them, the capacity to confront historical misrepresentations and imagine different futures is diminished. The past matters because it enables repair, reflection, and recognition. Reviewing how it has been used reveals why it matters, but equally important is the ongoing need to show its relevance in the present (Fritz and Plog 1970). This book contextualises archaeology within Africa with the ultimate aim of considering the important role the past plays in contemporary society, and why it is crucial that it be studied from a contextualised perspective.

Problematic in this contribution is coverage. Africa is culturally, socially, economically, and geographically a diverse continent. It is as much about discontinuities as continuities across its great expanse. If you include time depth, even more so. Archaeological research, in terms of approaches, praxis, and theory, reflect this diversity. Capturing this all in a single book is impossible and it cannot in any way do justice to the variety of studies, perspectives, and developments within the field, never mind the complex historical sequences on the continent. Showing the field's developments and diversity by stringing together case studies, research agendas, and disciplinary matters is more achievable, although it no doubt overlooks many examples that readers will surely expect within these pages. Any omissions of significant archaeological histories are unintended, and it is hoped they will be received with understanding. The reality of piecing together such an incredibly complex sequence of research on a continent as varied as Africa is a challenging task. There has been a concerted attempt to include examples most pertinent to the aim of this book and which clearly demonstrate the developmental stages of archaeology in Africa. Admittedly, this comes with personal baggage and knowledge, but an attempt has been made to ensure that this does not create a parochial or colloquial perspective, which cannot be entirely stripped from the text.

The views expressed in this book are deeply embedded with my own positionality and biography—as a white male from a South African middle-class context. That is not to say the views misrepresent those of others to propagate a set of ideas, but personal interests in this topic are deeply influenced by upbringing in a democratic South Africa that is now home to a great diversity of people and a past that thrusts together different groups in various ways. It has influenced how contact, social networks, relations, and socio-historic trajectories are construed and valued. Presenting a history of any discipline is also open-ended and, moreover, can be marshalled to support any argument (Trigger 2006, p. 4). However, the aim here is to present a history of archaeology in Africa that "by its nature as part of the history of ideas, has got to be a discipline which helps actual scientists to get a deeper insight into the real nature of their own science" (Masterman 1970, p. 88). It is not a discursive account of the archaeology of Africa, but an exploration of archaeology in Africa avoiding, for the most part hopefully, presentist pitfalls (judging the past on present values). It is hoped that this book is read with this in mind, and not as an objective narrative of the history of archaeology in Africa and its importance.

Saying this leads to the final point to be made here that is of voice and representation. The views expressed herein are not those of an African collective or even a subset of archaeologists practicing on the continent. They draw from a wide spectrum of archaeological and historical practitioners, as well as others, and in this way include many voices that have been generally expressed in written scholarship. Despite synthesising these multiple perspectives and coalescing them into an argument, the narrative is none the less something fashioned by an individual from Africa, who's work experience and professional life has for the most part unfolded on the continent. It is not by any means imagined that the views contained here are representative of anyone else's, but hopefully they serve as instructive and useful in framing archaeology and thinking about its role in a post-colonial Africa. If the production of this book is an act of 'myth making', hopefully the dialogue helps guide perceptions from various readers into impactful action (McNeill 1986, p. 164). The voice here is one among a great ensemble of scholars calling from the continent, hoping to help drive change, promote growth, and ultimately learn more about, and better represent, Africa's archaeological and historical past.

The book now presents the archaeology of Africa. It first provides an overview of the perceptions of Africa, from the dark continent myth through to pan-Africanism. Following this is a history of archaeology, or archaeological thought as Trigger (2006) referred to it in his seminal work. These overviews provide the background context for understanding the unfolding practice of archaeology in Africa. Presented next are the four chapters on archaeology in Africa, as described earlier, followed by a reflective chapter on why the past matters. The concluding chapter avoids repeating what has been said in the pages before, and rather looks ahead, surveying the terrain in front of archaeology and where it might find traction moving forward.

References

Abernethy, K., F. Maisels, and L. J. T. White. 2016. Environmental issues in central Africa. *Annual Review of Environment and Resources* 41:1–33.

Abulafia, D. 2003. *The Mediterranean in history*. London: Thames & Hudson.

Adams, W. M. 1992. *Wasting the rain: Rivers, people and planning in Africa*. Minneapolis: University of Minnesota Press.

Africa Center for Strategic Studies. 2022. *African biodiversity loss raises risk to human security*. Africa Center for Strategic Studies. Washington, DC.

Africanus, L. 1600. *The history and description of Africa and of the notable things there in contained*. London: Hakluyt Society.

Allen, J. de V. 1981. Swahili culture and the nature of east coast settlement. *International Journal of African Historical Studies* 14:306–334.

Andah, B. 1995. European encumbrances to the development of relevant theory in African archaeology. In *Theory in archaeology: A world perspective*, ed. P. J. Ucko, 96–108. London: Routledge.

Anquandah, J. 1981. *Rediscovering Ghana's past*. London: Longman.

Appiah, K. A. 1992. *In my father's house: Africa in the philosophy of culture*. New York: Oxford University Press.

Arowosegbe, J. O. 2014. African studies and the bias of Eurocentricism. *Social Dynamics* 40:308–321.

Atalay, S. 2014. Engaging archaeology: Positivism, objectivity, and rigor in activist archaeology. In *Transforming archaeology*, ed. S. Atalay, L. R. Clauss, R. H. McGuire, and J. R. Welch, 45–59. London: Routledge.

Atkinson, J. A., I. Banks, and J. O'Sullivan, eds. 1996. *Nationalism and archaeology: Scottish archaeological forum*. Glasgow: Cruithne.

Badawi, Z. 2024. *An African history of Africa*. Milton Keynes: WH Allen.

Bank, A. 2006. *Bushmen in a Victorian world: The remarkable story of the Bleek-Lloyd collection of Bushmen folklore*. Cape Town: Juta and Company Ltd.

Barham, L., and P. J. Mitchell. 2008. *The first Africans: African archaeology from the earliest toolmakers to most recent foragers*. Cambridge: Cambridge University Press.

Barich, B. E. 2010. *Antica Africa: Alle origini delle società*. Rome: 'L'Erma: di Bretschneider.

Barnes, B. 1974. *Scientific knowledge and sociological theory*. London: Routledge and Kegan Paul.

Barth, H. 1857. *Travels and discoveries in northern and central Africa*. London: Longman.

Bennett, H. L. 2019. *African kings and black slaves: Sovereignty and dispossession in the early modern Atlantic*. Philadelphia: University of Pennsylvania Press.

Bernbeck, R., and S. Pollock. 1996. Ayodhya, archaeology, and identity. *Current Anthropology* 37:138–142.

Bewley, R., A. Wilson, D. Kennedy, D. Mattingly, R. Banks, M. Bishop, J. Bradbury, E. Cunliffe, M. Fradley, and R. Jennings. 2016. Endangered archaeology in the Middle East and North Africa: Introducing the EAMENA project. In *CAA2015. Keep the Revolution Going: Proceedings of the 43rd annual conference on computer applications and quantitative methods in archaeology*, ed. S. Campana, R. Scopigno, G. Carpentiero, and M. Cirillo, 919–932. Oxford: Archaeopress.

Beyin, A., D. K. Wright, J. Wilkins, and D. I. Olszewski. 2023. *Handbook of Pleistocene archaeology of Africa: Hominin behavior, geography, and chronology*. Cham: Springer Nature.

Breuil, H. 1954. Rock paintings of South Africa. *Anthropological Quarterly* 27 (2): 31–42.

Breunig, P., and N. Rupp. 2016. An outline of recent studies on the Nigerian Nok culture. *Journal of African Archaeology* 14 (3): 237–255.

Bwasiri, Emmanuel J., and Benjamin W. Smith. 2015. The rock art of Kondoa District, Tanzania. *Azania: Archaeological Research in Africa*50 (4): 437–459.

Carruthers, J. 1989. Creating a national park, 1910 to 1926. *Journal of Southern African Studies* 15 (2): 188–216.

Chakrabarty, D. K. 2003. *Archaeology in the third world: A history of Indian archaeology since 1947*. Delhi: D.K. Printworld.

Chami, F. 2021. The geographical extent of Azania. *Theoria*168 (68): 12–29.

Chirikure, S. 2013. Heritage conservation in Africa: The good, the bad, and the challenges. *South African Journal of Science* 109 (1/2): 1–3.

Chirikure, S. 2020. *Great Zimbabwe: Reclaiming a 'confiscated' past*. London: Routledge.

Chirikure, S., M. Manyanga, and A. M. Pollard. 2012. When science alone is not enough: Radiocarbon timescales, history, ethnography and elite settlements in southern Africa. *Journal of Social Archaeology* 12 (3): 356–379.

Chittick, H. N. 1982. Reconnaissance in coastal Tanzania. *Nyame Akuma*20: 65–75.

Clark, J. D. 1975. Africa in prehistory: Peripheral or paramount? *Man* 10 (2): 175–198.

Comaroff, J. L., and J. Comaroff. 1997. *Of revelation and revolution: The dialectics of modernity on a South African frontier*. Chicago: University of Chicago Press.

Connah, G. 1975. *The archaeology of Benin*. Oxford: Clarendon Press.

Connah, G. 2001. *African civilizations*. Cambridge: Cambridge University Press.

Connah, G. 2004. *Forgotten Africa: An introduction to its archaeology*. London: Routledge.

Connah, G. 2013. In *Archaeological practice in Africa: A historical perspective*, ed. P. J. Mitchell and P. J. Lane, 15–36. Oxford: Oxford University Press.

Connah, G. 2016. *African civilizations: An archaeological perspective*. Cambridge: Cambridge University Press.

Cornelissen, E. 2024. The Stone Age of the Congo basin. In *Oxford research encyclopedia of African history*, ed. T. Spear, p. 10.1093. Oxford: Oxford University Press.

Crowley, K., R. Jackson, S. O'Connell, D. Karunarthna, E. Anantasari, A. Retnowati, and D. Niemand. 2022. Cultural heritage and risk assessments: Gaps, challenges, and future research directions for the inclusion of heritage within climate change adaptation and disaster management. *Climate Resilience and Sustainability* 1 (3): e45.

Darkoh, M. B. K. 2009. An overview of environmental issues in southern Africa. *African Journal of Ecology* 47 (s1): 93–98.

Davis, N. Z. 2014. 'Leo Africanus' and his worlds of translation. In *Translators, interpreters, and cultural negotiators*, ed. F. M. Federici and D. Tessicini, 62–80. London: Palgrave Macmillan UK.

Deacon, J. 1984. *The later Stone Age of southernmost Africa*. Oxford: British Archaeological Reports.

Deacon, J. 1993. Archaeological sites as national monuments in South Africa: A review of sites declared since 1936. *South African Historical Journal* 29 (1): 118–131.

Derricourt, R. M. 2011. *Inventing Africa: History, archaeology and ideas*. New York: Pluto Press.

Desplagnes, L. 1907. *Le Plateau central Nigérien: une mission archéologique et ethnographique au Soudan Français*. Paris: E. Leroux.

Diaz-Andreu, M., and T. Champion. 1996. *Nationalism and archaeology in Europe*. Boulder: Westview.

Eggert, M. K. 1993. Central Africa and the archaeology of the equatorial rainforest: Reflections on some major topics. In *Archaeology of Africa: Food, metals and towns*, ed. T. Shaw, P. J. J. Sinclair, B. W. Andah, and A. Okpoko, 289–329. London: Routledge.

Faloyin, D. 2023. *Africa is not a country: Breaking stereotypes of modern Africa*. Dublin: Penguin Random House.

Fauvelle-Aymar, F.-X. 2018. *L'Afrique Ancienne de l'Acacus au Zimbabwe: 20 000 ans avant notre ère-xviie siècle*. Paris: Belin.

Fauvelle-Aymar, F.-X. 2020. *Leçons de l'histoire de l'Afrique*. Paris: Fayard.

Forssman, T. 2023. The end of the later stone age in the middle Limpopo valley, southern Africa. *Journal of Paleolithic Archaeology* 6:26.

Forssman, T., I. Pikirayi, and G. Connah. 2024. Holocene Africa. In *The human past: World prehistory and the development of human societies*, ed. C. Scarre, 318–353. London: Thames & Hudson.

Fourie, W. 2015. Four concepts of Africa. *HTS Teologiese Studies/Theological Studies* 71 (3): 1–10.

Fowler, D. D. 1987. Uses of the past: Archaeology in the service of the state. *American Antiquity* 52 (2): 229–248.

French, H. W. 2021. *Born in blackness: Africa, Africans, and the making of the modern world, 1471 to the second world war*. New York: WW Norton.

Fritz, John M., and Fred T. Plog. 1970. The nature of archaeological explanation. *American Antiquity* 35: 405–412.

Gabel, C. 1985. Archaeology in sub-Saharan Africa. *International Journal of African Historical Studies* 18 (2): 241–264.

Gençoğlu, H. 2024. African historiography: Reflections on rewriting the continent's past. *Chron-Africa* 1 (1): 1–10.

Geroulanos, S. 2024. *The invention of prehistory: Empire, violence, and our obsession with human origins*. New York: Liveright Publishing Corporation.

Geyser, O., ed. 1977. *B. J. Vorster: Selected speeches*. Bloemfontein: Institute of Contemporary History.

Giblin, J. 2013. Politics, ideology, and indigenous perspectives. In *The Oxford handbook of African archaeology*, ed. P. J. Mitchell and P. J. Lane, 253–265. Oxford: Oxford University Press.

Goodwin, A. J. H., and C. Van Riet Lowe. 1929. *The Stone Age cultures of South Africa*. Cape Town: AMS Press.

Goodwin, J. 1946. *The loom of prehistory*. Cape Town: South African Archaeological Society.

Goody, J. 2006. *The theft of history*. Cambridge: Cambridge University Press.

Graham, B., G. J. Ashworth, and J. E. Tunbridge. 2004. The uses and abuses of heritage. In *Heritage, museums and galleries*, ed. G. Corsane, 28–40. London: Routledge.

Grove, R. H. 1996. *Green imperialism: Colonial expansion, tropical island Edens and the origins of environmentalism, 1600–1860*. Cambridge: Cambridge University Press.

Harrison, R., L. Wilkie, A. González-Ruibal, and C. Holtorf. 2014. Editorial. *Journal of Contemporary Archaeology* 1:1–6.

Hegel, G. F. W. 1837. *The Philosophy of history*. New York: Dover Publications.

Holl, A. 2005. *The archaeology of Africa*. London: Eolss Publishers.

Holl, A. F. C. 1990. West African archaeology: Colonialism and nationalism. In *A history of African archaeology*, ed. P. Robertshaw, 296–308. Oxford: James Currey Ltd.

Huffman, T. N. 2007. *A handbook to the Iron Age: The archaeology of pre-colonial societies of southern Africa*. Pietermaritzburg: University of KwaZulu-Natal Press.

Hulme, M., ed. 1996. *Climate change and southern Africa: An exploration of some potential impacts and implications in the SADC*. Norwich: World Wildlife Fund.

Hulme, M., R. Dohery, T. Ngara, and N. New. 2005. Global warming and African climate change: A reassessment. In *Climate change and Africa*, ed. P. S. Low, 29–40. Cambridge: Cambridge University Press.

Hume, D. 1758. Of national characters. In *Essays and treatises on several subjects*, ed. D. Hume. London: A. Millar.

Ichumbaki, E. B., and E. Pollard. 2021. The Swahili civilization in eastern Africa. In *Oxford research encyclopedia of anthropology*, ed. M. S. Aldenderfer. Oxford: Oxford University Press.

Insoll, T. 2003. *The archaeology of Islam in Sub-Saharan Africa*. Cambridge: Cambridge University Press.

Kankpeyeng, B. W., and C. R. DeCorse. 2004. Ghana's vanishing past: Development, antiquities, and the destruction of the archaeological record. *African Archaeological Review* 21:89–128.

Kinahan, J. 1995. Theory, practice and criticism in the history of Namibian archaeology. In *Theory in archaeology: A world perspective*, ed. P. J. Ucko, 76–95. London: Routledge.

Klein, R. 1999. *The human career*. Chicago: Chicago University Press.

Klein, R., A. Nowell, and M. White. 2024. Hominin behaviour and dispersal in the lower and middle Pleistocene. In *The human past: World prehistory and the development of human societies*, ed. C. Scarre, 69–97. London: Thames & Hudson.

Kohl, P. L. 1998. Nationalism and archaeology: On the constructions of nations and the reconstructions of the remote past. *Annual Review of Anthropology* 27 (1): 223–246.

Kohl, P. L., and C. Fawcett, eds. 1995. *Nationalism, politics, and the practice of archaeology*. Cambridge: Cambridge University Press.

Kusimba, C. M., and S. B. Kusimba. 2003. *East African archaeology: Foragers, potters, smiths and traders*. Philadelphia: University of Pennsylvania Museum of Archaeology and Anthropology.

Lane, P. J. 2011. Possibilities for a postcolonial archaeology in sub-Saharan Africa: Indigenous and usable pasts. *World Archaeology* 43 (1): 7–25.

Lewis, L. A., and L. Berry. 2012. *African environments and resources*. London: Routledge.

Liverani, M. 2000. The Garamantes: A fresh approach. *Libyan Studies* 31:17–28.

Loftus, E. 2023. Radiocarbon dating in African archaeology. In *Handbook of Pleistocene archaeology of Africa: Hominin behavior, geography, and chronology*, ed. A. Beyin, D. K. Wright, J. Wilkins, and D. I. Olszewski, 1931–1941. Cham: Springer International Publishing.

Lombard, M., J. Bradfield, M. V. Caruana, T. V. Makhubela, G. L. Dusseldorp, J. D. Kramers, and S. Wurz. 2022. The southern African Stone Age sequence updated (II). *South African Archaeological Bulletin* 77 (217): 172–212.

Lubbock, J. 1870. Remarks on the early condition of man. *Journal of the Ethnological Society of London* 2:328–340.

MacMillan, M. 2010. *The uses and abuses of history*. London: Profile Books.

Maggs, T. 2000. African naissance: An introduction. *South African Archaeological Society Goodwin Series* 8:1–3.

Marks, S. 1980. South Africa: The myth of the empty land. *History Today* 30 (1): 7–12.

Masterman, M. 1970. The nature of a paradigm. In *Criticism and the growth of knowledge*, ed. I. Lakatos and A. Musgrave, 59–89. Cambridge: Cambridge University Press.

Mazrui, A. 1978. *Political values and the educated class in Africa*. London: Heinemann.

Mazrui, A. 1986. *The Africans: A triple heritage*. London: BBC Publications.

Mazrui, A. 2005. The re-invention of Africa: Edward Said, V. Y. Mudimbe, and beyond. *Research in African Literatures* 36:68–82.

Mbembe, A. 2001. *On the postcolony*. Berkley: University of California Press.

McIntosh, R. J. 1998. *The peoples of the middle Niger*. Oxford: Blackwells.

McIntosh, R. J. 2005. *Ancient middle Niger: Urbanism and the self-organizing landscape*. Cambridge: Cambridge University Press.

Mcintosh, S. K. 2013. Archaeological heritage management and site inventory systems in Africa. *Journal of Field Archaeology* 20 (4): 500–504.

McIntosh, S. K. 2022. Igbo-Ukwu at 50: A symposium on recent archaeological research and analysis. *African Archaeological Review* 39 (4): 369–385.

McLellan, R. 2014. *Living planet report 2014: Species and spaces, people and places*. London: World Wildlife Fund.

McNeill, W. H. 1986. *Mythistory and other essays*. Chicago: University of Chicago Press.

Mellet, P. T. 2020. *The lie of 1652: A decolonised history of land*. Cape Town: Tafelberg.
Meskell, L. 2012. *The Nature of Heritage: The new South Africa.* Malden: Wiley-Backwell.
Miller, J. 2015. Africanising apartheid: Identity, ideology, and state-building in post-independence Africa. *Journal of African History* 56:449–470.
Mitchell, P. J. 2005. *African connections: An archaeological perspective on Africa and the wider world*. Oxford: AltaMira Press.
Mitchell, P. J. 2024. *The archaeology of Southern Africa*. Cambridge: Cambridge University Press.
Mitchell, P. J., and P. J. Lane. 2013a. *The Oxford handbook of African archaeology*. Oxford: Oxford University Press.
Mitchell, P. J., and P. J. Lane. 2013b. Introducing African archaeology. In *The Oxford handbook of African archaeology*, ed. P. J. Mitchell and P. J. Lane, 3–11. Oxford: Oxford University Press.
Mohammadpour, A., and K. Soleimani. 2022. Silencing the past: Persian archaeology, race, ethnicity, and language. *Current Anthropology* 63:185–210.
Mudimbe, V. Y. 1988. *The invention of Africa: Gnosis, philosophy, and the order of knowledge*. Bloomington: Indiana University Press.
Mudimbe, V. Y. 1994. *The idea of Africa*. Bloomington: Indiana University Press.
Musonda, F. 2012. 100 years of archaeological research in Zambia: Changing historical perspectives. *South African Archaeological Bulletin* 67:88–100.
Newitt, M. 2004. *A history of Portuguese overseas expansion 1400–1668*. London: Routledge.
Niang, I., O. C. Ruppel, M. A. Abdrabo, A. Essel, C. Lennard, J. Padgham, P. Urquhart, I. Adelekan, S. Archibald, A. Barkhordarian, J. Battersby, M. Chahed, M. Chatterjee, C. T. Chidiezie, K. Descheemaeker, H. Djoudi, K. L. Ebi, P. D. Fall, R. Fuentes, R. Garland, B. Harvey, M. Hayden, A. Hemp, G. Jobbins, J. Johnson, D. Lobell, B. Locatelli, E. Ludi, L. O. Naess, M. R. Ndebele-Murisa, A. Ndiaye, A. Newsham, S. Njai, P. Pauw, E. Pramova, M.-L. Rakotondrafara, C. Raleigh, D. Roberts, M. H. Schleyer, D. Victor, K. Vincent, P. Dube, N. Leary, and L. Schulte-Uebbing. 2014. Africa. In *Climate change 2014: Impacts, adaptation, and vulnerability. Part B: Regional aspects. Contribution of working group II to the fifth assessment report of the intergovernmental panel on climate change*, ed. V. R. Barros, C. B. Field, D. J. Dokken, M. D. Mastrandrea, K. J. Mach, T. E. Bilir, M. Chatterjee, K. L. Ebi, Y. O. Estrada, R. C. Genova, B. Girma, E. S. Kissel, A. N. Levy, S. MacCracken, P. R. Mastrandrea, and L. L. White. New York: Cambridge University Press.
Nyerere, J. 1968. *Freedom and socialism/Uhuru na Ujamaa: A selection from writings and speeches 1965–1967*. Dar es Salaam: Oxford University Press.
Odak, O. 1980. Comment on D. Miller's 'archaeology and development'. *Current Anthropology* 21:721.
Ogot, B. A. 2009. Rereading the history and historiography of epistemic domination and resistance in Africa. *African Studies Review*52 (1): 1–22.
Pakenham, T. 1991. *The scramble for Africa: The white man's conquest of the dark continent from 1876 to 1912*. New York: Random House.
Pankhurst, R. 1999. Ethiopia, the Aksum obelisk, and the return of Africa's cultural heritage. *African Affairs* 98 (391): 229–239.
Patterson, T. C. 1995. *Toward a social history of archaeology in the United States*. Orlando: Harcourt Brace.
Pettitt, P., and M. C. Langley. 2024. The rise of modern humans. In *The human past: World prehistory and the development of human societies*, ed. C. Scarre, 98–128. London: Thames & Hudson.
Phillips, J. R. S. 1988. *The medieval expansion of Europe*. Oxford: Oxford University Press.
Phillips, L. 2017. History of South Africa's Bantustans. In *Oxford research encyclopedia of African history*, ed. T. Spear. Oxford: Oxford University Press.
Phillipson, D. W. 2005. *African archaeology*. Cambridge: Cambridge University Press.
Politis, G. 1995. The socio-politics of the development of archaeology in Hispanic South America. In *Social construction of the past: Representation as power*, ed. P. J. Ucko, 194–223. London: Routledge.

Pope, J. 2022. The invention of Aithiopian antecedence. *Journal of Ancient Egyptian Interconnections* 35:155–189.

Posnansky, M. 1982. African archaeology comes of age. *World Archaeology*13: 345–358.

Pradines, S. 2017. Swahili past in peril: New archaeology in east Africa. *Journal of Oriental and African Studies* 26:211–236.

Reeves, K., and G. Plets. 2015. Cultural heritage as a strategy for social needs and community identity. In *A companion to heritage studies*, ed. W. Logan, M. Nic Craith, and U. Kockel, 203–214. New York: John Wiley & Sons, Ltd.

Reynolds, T. W., S. R. Waddington, C. L. Anderson, A. Chew, Z. True, and A. Cullen. 2015. Environmental impacts and constraints associated with the production of major food crops in Sub-Saharan Africa and South Asia. *Food Security* 7:795–822.

Robertshaw, P. 1990. *A history of African archaeology*. Oxford: James Currey Ltd.

Rosenzweig, M. S. 2020. Confronting the present: Archaeology in 2019. *American Anthropologist* 122 (2): 284–305.

Scarre, C. 2024. *The human past: World prehistory and the development of human societies*. 5th ed. New York: Thames & Hudson.

Schlanger, N. 2002. Making the past for South Africa's future: The prehistory of Field-Marshal smuts (1920s–1940s). *Antiquity* 76:200–209.

Schlanger, N. 2004. The past is in the present: On the history and archives of archaeology. *Modernism/Modernity* 11:165–167.

Schmidt, P. R. 2006. *Historical archaeology in Africa: Representation, social memory, and oral traditions*. Walnut Creek: AltaMira Press.

Schmidt, P. R. 2009. *Postcolonial archaeologies in Africa*. Santa Fe: School for Advanced Research Press.

Schmidt, Peter R., and Innocent Pikirayi. 2018. Will historical archaeology escape its western prejudices to become relevant to Africa? *Archaeologies*14: 443–471.

Schnapp, A. 2014. The birth of the archaeological vision: From antiquaries to archaeologists. *West 86th: A Journal of Decorative Arts, Design History, and Material Culture* 21 (2): 216–229.

Shaw, T. 1989. African archaeology: Looking back and looking forward. *African Archaeological Review* 7 (1): 3–31.

Shepherd, N. 2003. State of the discipline: Science, culture and identity in South African archaeology, 1870–2003. *Journal of Southern African Studies* 29 (4): 823–844.

South African Heritage Resources Agency. 2016. South African heritage resources information system (SAHRIS) database. Available from https://www.sahra.org.za/sahris. 18 March 2025.

Spear, T. 2000. Early Swahili history reconsidered. *International Journal of African Historical Studies* 33 (2): 257–290.

Stahl, A. B. 2014. Africa in the world: (Re)centering African history through archaeology. *Journal of Anthropological Research* 70 (1): 5–33.

Stahl, A. B. ed. 2005. *African Archaeology: A critical introduction*. Oxford: Blackwell.

Tekin, C. 2019. *Debating Turkey in Europe: Identities and concepts*. Berlin: Walter de Gruyter GmbH & Co KG.

Toth, N., K. Schick, and A. Gidna. 2024. African origins. In *The human past: World prehistory and the development of human societies*, ed. C. Scarre, 42–68. London: Thames & Hudson.

Trevor-Roper, H. E. 1963. *The rise of Christian Europe*. Brace & World: Harcourt.

Trigger, B. G. 1989. Archaeology and anthropology: Current and future relations. *Canadian Journal of Archeology*13: 1–11.

Trigger, B. G. 2006. *A history of archaeological thought*. 2nd ed. Cambridge: Cambridge University Press.

Trouillot, M.-R. 1995. *Silencing the past: Power and the production of history*. Boston: Beacon.

Ucko, P. J. 1983. The politics of the indigenous minority. *Journal of Biosocial Science* 15 (S8): 25–40.

Ucko, P. J. 1995. Introduction: Archaeological interpretation in a world context. In *Theory in archaeology: A world perspective*, ed. P. J. Ucko, 1–28. London: Taylor & Francis.

UNEP-WCMC. 2016. *The state of biodiversity in Africa: A mid-term review of progress towards the AICHI biodiversity targets.* Cambridge: UNEP-WCMC.

United Nations Department of Economic and Social Affairs. 2024. *World population prospects 2024*, 9. New York: United Nations, No.

Vernet, R. 2000. *L'Archéologie en Afrique de l'Ouest: Sahara et Sahel.* Saint-Maur: Nouakchott.

Wesseling, H. 1996. *Divide and rule: The partition of Africa, 1880–1914.* Amsterdam: Praeger.

Wilcox, A. R. 1963. *The rock art of South Africa.* Edinburgh: Nelson.

Willoughby, P. R. 2007. *The evolution of modern humans in Africa: A comprehensive guide.* Lanham: AltaMira Press.

Willoughby, P. R. 2009. From middle to later Stone Age in eastern Africa. In *Sourcebook of Paleolithic transitions*, ed. M. Camps and P. Chauhan, 301–314. Cham: Springer.

Wood, M. 1998. The use of the pharaonic past in modern Egyptian nationalism. *Journal of the American Research Center in Egypt* 35:179–196.

Wylie, A. 1981. Positivism and the new archaeology. PhD thesis, State University of New York, Binghamton.

Wynne-Jones, S., and A. J. LaViolette, eds. 2018. *The Swahili world*. London: Routledge.

Chapter 2
From Darkness to Dawn: Dispelling the Dark Continent Myth

Abstract This chapter dismantles the long-standing "dark continent" trope that casts Africa as unknowable, static, or devoid of history. Beginning with nineteenth-century CE travelogues and popular literature that popularised darkness as metaphor and method, it shows how such narratives buttressed imperial projects and pervaded academic frameworks. It then widens the lens to earlier and parallel perspectives, including Muslim and African writers, cartographers, and travellers, whose accounts offered different geographies and historically grounded understandings of the continent. The analysis foregrounds how colonial simplifications shaped perspectives, while tracing the sustained rebuttal mounted by Africanist historiography and archaeology from the mid-twentieth century CE onward. The chapter argues that the myths about and of Africa have, in part, endured, and that confronting them requires reframing Africa as diverse, dynamic, and constitutive of global history. This reframing prepares readers to see archaeology not as a neutral science imported to reveal a blank past but as a field entangled with power, capable of both reproducing and challenging hegemonic stories.

> Africa has been the victim of generalising statements, simplifying histories and prehistories, stereotyping and imaginings from ancient times until today. The yearning to describe all or parts of the vast continent in simplified terms may be strongest in outsiders to the continent, but those living within Africa have also contributed . (Derricourt 2011, p. vi)
>
> [D]arkness is not a subject for history. (Trevor-Roper 1965, p. 9)

Paul Theroux (2004) is a twenty-first century travel writer who has produced numerous books on routes and journeys throughout the world. In his book, *Dark Star Safari,* he is the Huckleberry Finn-like character in a mythical Africa (Moolla 2013, p. 384). It details his journey from Egypt's Cairo to Cape Town in South Africa, spanning much of the length of the continent (Theroux 2004). In Chapter 1, titled *Lighting out,* Theroux (2004, p. 1) begins his book by saying: "All news out of Africa is bad". As his book unfolds, there are mentions of robbery, heat, the *bundu* (wilderness), and hunger, but he ultimately weaves his way to dismiss much of this, and instead present Africa in a romantic light – a place to escape cell phone signal and be "[o]ut of touch in Africa" (Theroux 2004, p. 4). The merging of darkness and Africa has a long history that perpetuates into the present, mostly in popular renderings of

T. Forssman, *Archaeology in Africa: Why the Past Matters*, Archaeology of Africa,
https://doi.org/10.1007/978-3-032-13365-6_2

the continent. These recurring themes are tenacious and frustrate scholars endlessly, but they have far deep historic traces.

In the latter half of the nineteenth century CE, around the time of European colonialisation, Africa was described as the 'dark continent'. Although the concept likely existed earlier, iterations of it were used by Henry Morton Stanley (1889) in his writings about his expeditions in the 1870s and 1880s. He used terms such as "the dark unknown land" or "the unopened continent" but one of his primary works carried the term in its title: *Through the Dark Continent*. Around the same period, Andrew Anderson (1888, p. vi) referred to his journey in southern Africa as adding another page to the *terra incognita* of the dark continent. In other literary accounts, Rider Haggard (1885) presented the continent as a "dark sea of barbarism, representing the dark side of the personality" (Hall 1995, p. 32) and Laurens van der Post's (1955) first book was titled *The Dark Eye of Africa*. Through these uses of the term, and others such as Joseph Conrad's (1899) *Heart of Darkness,* the phrase became popularised. The notion of a 'dark continent' held resonance, in many respects, with the views people held of Africa at the time. It was a mysterious and geographically unknown place, while appealing to racial ideologies imposed over the entire continent (Rash 2020).

The scramble for Africa followed closely on the heels of the 'dark continent's' appearance in the colonists' collective imagination. From the 1860s CE, a period of rapid colonisation began (Pakenham 1991). European powers 'scrambled' for territories in Africa with long-term plans in mind of development, growth, and exploitation (Hochschild 1998). The Industrial Revolution in Europe partly drove the scramble through its demand for new resources to supply local markets (Ocheni and Nwankwo 2012). The rapid scramble was made possible by advances in technology, including transportation and weaponry, that made it easier for European forces to conquer and control vast areas of the African continent. Rivalries between European nations led to them carving up the region to suit their resource demands and economic growth. The influence on Africa was devastating: it disrupted traditional societies, displaced populations, and exploited resources for external gains (Michalopoulos and Papaioannou 2016).

Unpacking the discourse associated with a 'dark continent' situates perceptions of Africa within a historically contingent framework. Edward Said's (1979) notion of Orientalism applies: "a way of coming to terms with the Orient that is based on the Orient's special place in European Western Experience". Much of Africa's image was created through its place relative to the global north. Even the use of the words 'Africa' or 'Africans' have implications drawn from history that continue into the present (Derricourt 2011, p. v). They may either invoke negative perceptions about social or economic conditions, or one of vast animal-filled landscapes. Complicit in these reflections of Africa are the media; the news, in stories like those from Haggard, and characters such as Tarzan. They stem, quite often, from roots burrowing into the past and dredging up old colonial views, such as the idea of a dark continent. The writings of scholars like van der Post (1958), particularly in *Venture in the Interior* (van der Post 1951) where he presented a mystical and physical dualism, fashioned an Africa and its people around what were in part romantic fabrications. The notion of 'primitive Africa' can easily be packed with these perceptions and it spills from the past into the present when we examine ecotourism and visits to wilderness areas and 'traditional' communities (such as the San or Maasai). These perceptions of Africa stem from European fantasy and imagination (Hall 1995).

These early ideas of Africa as a 'dark continent' – empty, static, and without history – were never benign. They shaped not only colonial policies and academic discourse but also came to influence how many Africans viewed their own past (Thiong'O 1986; Ndlovu 2009). While much of this thinking has been challenged and dismantled, particularly by Africanist scholars working pointedly since the 1950s to contest such views (e.g., Davidson 1959; Fage 1962; Oliver and Fage 1963; Posnansky 1966; Shaw 1977 and many others), its traces still linger in popular narratives and global archaeological frameworks, where Africa's role remains marginal or oversimplified. Too often, the continent's past is viewed as a prelude rather than an active player in world history, despite its deep and complex contributions to human development. This chapter confronts these lingering misconceptions to establish a broader global context that frames Africa. It develops a foundation for understanding how archaeology, once introduced as a tool of colonial knowledge, has been reworked as a means of challenging hegemonic narratives and becoming a critical site for rethinking Africa's past in post-colonial contexts.

2.1 Into the Gloom: The First European Gaze

At the dawn of European expansionism, Africa could not have predicted the unprecedented disruption that it was about to endure. This impact varied in character, nature, form, and brutality across the continent. Additionally, settlers were from a variety of backgrounds with different beliefs and values that influenced their attitudes and approaches (Viotti Da Costa 1985). However, in whatever way it manifested, the result was a shift in power dynamics that in most circumstances favoured the settler. In its various forms, expansionism and later colonialism set the stage for a long period of European hegemony over so many of Africa's people and places. Throughout much of this, the history of Africans and their heritage, despite its richness, was overshadowed by racialised notions of local groups and overbearingly reductionist views of their society and past. These perspectives of history and people suited European narratives and agendas.

European expansionism, which began in the late fifteenth to early sixteenth century CE, is typically distinguished from the more aggressive colonialism of the nineteenth century (Ringmar 2006). While related, these phases differed significantly. Expansionism unfolded gradually, particularly along Africa's west coast, motivated by trade, exploration, and the intellectual currents of the Enlightenment. In contrast, the later colonial period involved the formal partitioning of the continent through military and diplomatic force. During the expansionist phase, European knowledge of the continent was fragmentary, and heavily influenced by classical authorities like Ptolemy, whose maps connected Africa's southern tip to Southeast Asia, enclosing the Indian Ocean (Fig. 2.1). The Indian Ocean itself was the subject of the *Periplus of the Erythraean Sea*, a traveller's guide written in the beginning of the first millennium CE (Chami 1999), which came to inform works such as Abraham Ortelius's sixteenth century CE atlas *Teatrum Orbis Terrarum* (Seland 2022). Early thinkers, such as Aristotle and Ibn Rushd, also speculated about a southern landmass, which they felt was necessary to balance the northern world. In contrast, by the ninth century CE, Ibn Khurdadhbih developed a far more accurate understandings of African geography and described a vast ocean surrounding the landmass south of 24° latitude (Issawi 1952). Nonetheless, it was Europe's evolving engagement with Africa, through trade, theology, science, and empire, that most powerfully shaped the perceptions later embedded in archaeological discourse.

Relations between Africa and Europe did not begin uniformly across the continent. Mediterranean Africa, for instance, shared a far longer and more continuous sequence of interaction with Europe than regions such as the Gold Coast (Ghana), the Cape of Good Hope (South Africa), or Zanzibar (Tanzania). By 1100 CE, the powerful trading city-states of Venice and Genoa had established extensive networks across the Mediterranean, reaching their peak by the 1300s. Their economic dominance relied on controlling maritime trade routes that linked Europe not only to North Africa but deep into the Muslim world (Newitt 2004). The stories of Mansa Musa's extravagant pilgrimage to Cairo in the previous century, during which he spent so

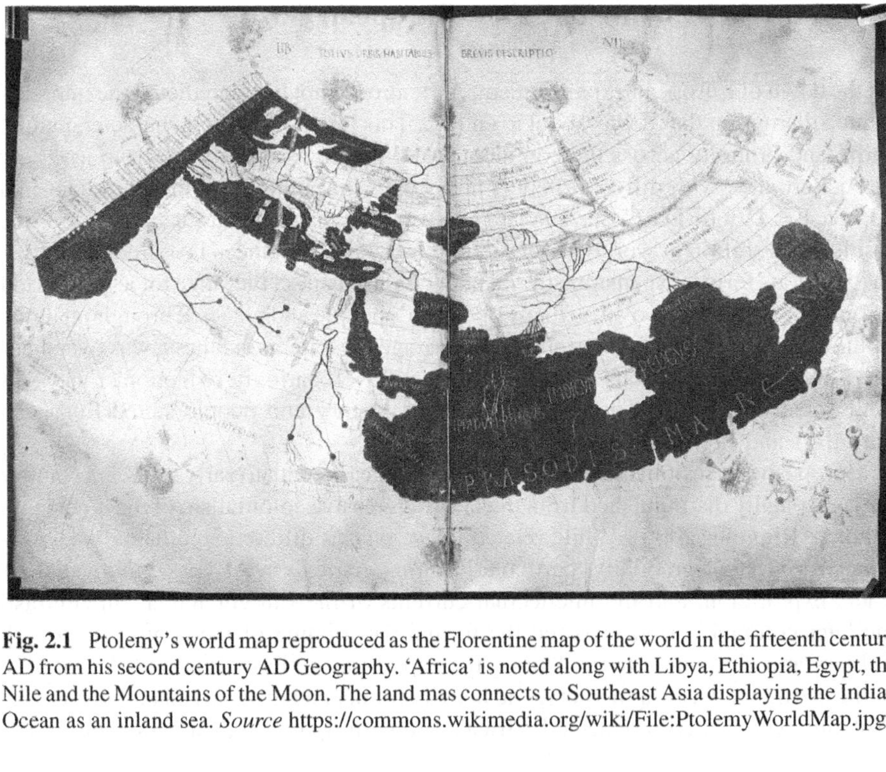

Fig. 2.1 Ptolemy's world map reproduced as the Florentine map of the world in the fifteenth century AD from his second century AD Geography. 'Africa' is noted along with Libya, Ethiopia, Egypt, the Nile and the Mountains of the Moon. The land mas connects to Southeast Asia displaying the Indian Ocean as an inland sea. *Source* https://commons.wikimedia.org/wiki/File:PtolemyWorldMap.jpg

much gold that it devalued the currency, remained vivid in European imagination (Dunn 2012, p. 290). Africa had an allure, albeit that it was shrouded in unknowns, but the prospect of great wealth was attractive.

At the opening of the fifteenth century CE, the Atlantic Ocean was still largely unknown to European mariners (Disney 2009, p. 27). By this time, various European ships, including Andalusian, Catalan, French, Genoese, and even Portuguese, and certainly fishing vessels, had ventured south along the African coastline, and possibly even beyond the Canary Islands and Morrocco. The dominant view was of a perilous and impassable ocean, a perception reinforced by misty shores, cold storms, and the strong Canary Current (Harms 2018, p. 165). The regions south of Cape Bojador were hardly known; Gomes Eanes de Zurara in his comprehensive *Chronicles of Discovery and Conquest of Guinea* commented that beyond "a cape known as Bojador… neither in writings nor memories, no man knew with any certainty the nature of the land that lay beyond the said cape" (cf. Polónia 2022, p. 171). In 1434, Gil Eanes became the first to round the northwestern coast of Africa and sailed beyond the cape and returned. This led to forays into the regions south of the cape in search of trade wealth, leading to some gains. By 1449, the Portuguese had reached the Cape Verde islands, and had likely also explored as far as Sierra Leone. After 1445, they established a trading post on the island of Argium off the Moroccan coastline (Newitt 2004, p. 24), tapping into West African gold networks via the Gambia River. The Gold Coast was reached by 1461, setting the stage for deeper commercial entrenchment. By the 1480s, the entire Atlantic African coast was charted (Disney 2009, p. 27). Finally, in 1498, Vasco da Gama rounded the Cape of Good Hope, opening the sea route to India and marking the culmination of nearly a century of Portuguese Atlantic exploration (Harms 2018, p. 166). Rounding the cape also opened Africa's eastern seaboard for explorations.

East Africa's coastline had been explored and settled by Muslim traders for more than five centuries before the Portuguese arrived (Pouwels 2002, p. 385). Muslim trade was facilitated by monsoon winds blowing northeasterly from October to April, and blowing in the opposite direction for the months between. The southeasterly winds are difficult to navigate during May through August, and strong currents in the Mozambique channel forced vessels and ships to seek refuge along the coast until the favourable September conditions (Gilbert 2002; Pouwels 2002). Although knowledge of the monsoon winds likely predated him, Hippalus, a Greek navigator of the first century CE, is traditionally credited with introducing this system to Greco-Roman navigators, enabling more direct trade between the Red Sea and India (Hatcher 2013). During the same period, Ptolemy's *Geography* indicates an east-west nexus, and by the sixth century the Sassanians, a pre-Islamic empire, had established a monopoly in both the Arabian and Red Seas (Pouwels 2002). The trade system operating along the eastern coastline in tandem with the trade winds is usually referred to as the Indian Ocean trading network.

By the late fourteenth century CE, Muslim influence dominated the eastern seaboard of Africa, where coastal towns from Mozambique Island northward to Kilwa Kisiwani (Kilwa) and Zanzibar flourished under the leadership of sheikhs and sultans. These towns were deeply integrated into the Indian Ocean trading network, connecting East Africa to Arabia, India, and beyond. Muslim merchants, in particular, played a central role in this commerce, facilitating the movement of goods such as perfumes, fine textiles, and ceramics (Newitt 2004). Trade operated under local rulers, who controlled harbours and markets with authority and sophistication. The prosperity of these towns and their cultural connections challenge the notion of Africa as an isolated or undeveloped continent. Rather, they exemplify a cosmopolitan and commercially vibrant region that had long been a participant in global exchanges, well before European maritime ventures arrived on the scene.

When the Portuguese began exploring Africa's coastline at the close of the fifteenth century CE, they encountered these thriving Muslim-controlled ports. Vasco da Gama's arrival in 1498 at Ilha do Moçambique (Mozambique Island) brought him face to face with established rulers like Sheikh Zacoeja, who commanded respect and presided over a bustling harbour (Theal 1899; Newitt 2004). Early Portuguese ambitions sought to tap into, rather than replace, these existing networks. Attempts to establish footholds at Kilwa and Sofala (Fig. 2.2) around 1505 proved challenging; shallow waters and the resilience of local economies limited their success. Gradually, Mozambique Island emerged as a more viable base for Portuguese operations, offering strategic advantages for repair, resupply, and trade (Fig. 2.3). Over time, fortifications like the imposing São Sebastião Fort, completed in the mid-sixteenth century, signalled a deeper Portuguese entrenchment. Yet, from the outset, Europeans entered a well-established and dynamic coastal world that was neither marginal nor waiting to be 'discovered', but already firmly embedded in regional and global networks.

It is important to recognise that European expansion into Africa was neither uniform nor static. While the focus here has been on the Portuguese as the first European power to arrive on most African coastlines, they were soon followed by others. From around 1500 CE, a growing number of European nations – including the French, Dutch, English and Danish – entered into maritime commerce with Africa, each pursuing their own interests, competing with one another, and contesting economically. Over time, these engagements intensified and became entangled with broader claims of sovereignty and control, and were accompanied by various socio-political shifts and economic interactions (Harms 2018, p. 166).

2.2 Illuminations from Within: African and Muslim Perspectives

Africa was not only subject of external perceptions of the continent, but also from those within. Notably, Egyptian perceptions of 'Africa' – or, outside of the pharaonic reach – extended back some 3000 years. Pharaonic Egypt, with its successive dynasties and royal houses, considered themselves as distinct and apart from other known regions in Africa. Egypt distinguished itself from the states to the east, with which it traded or periodically had conflict, the Nile Delta, and the western desert oases,

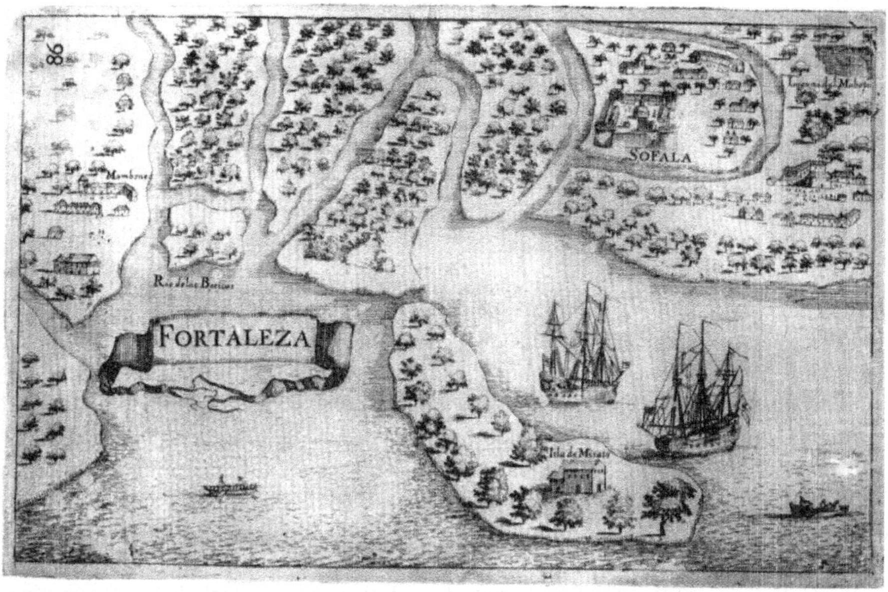

Fig. 2.2 A depiction of Sofala, Mozambique, from Manuel de Faria e Sous (1666). *Source* https://commons.wikimedia.org/wiki/File:Sofala_(1666).jpg

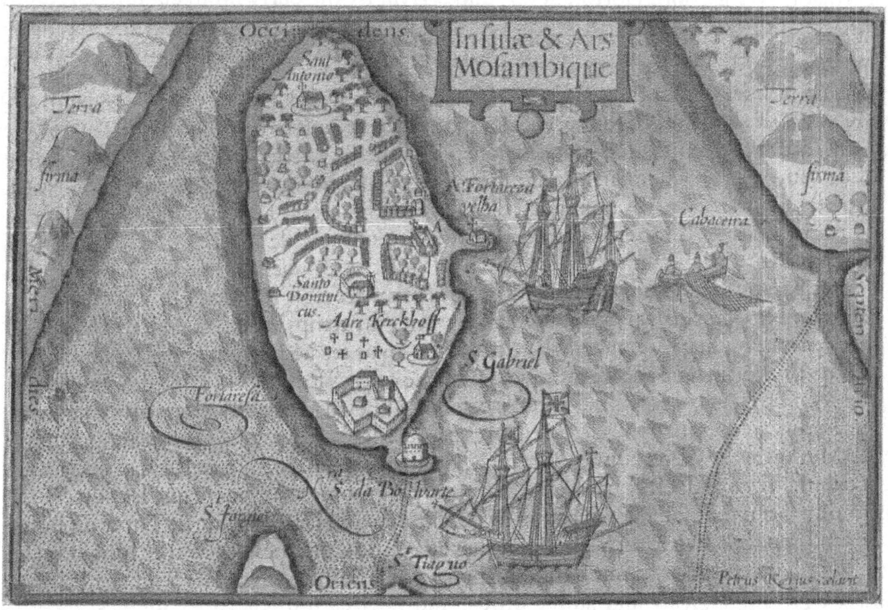

Fig. 2.3 Pieter van den Keere's 1598 CE map of Mozambique Island with Fort São Sebastião at the bottom of the island (south is orientated upwards). *Source* https://commons.wikimedia.org/wiki/File:1598_Mosambique_Kaerius.jpg

which were referred to as *khaset* (foreign lands) (Cornelius 2010). Egypt also did not geographically separate itself from the Sinai region as we do today (Mazrui 1986, p. 28–34; Derricourt 2011, p. 7). To the west were the Tjehenu and Tjemehu, used interchangeably in later times, translated as the Libyans. These generic terms were modified in the New Kingdom (1550–1070 BCE) to include groups further to the west as Libu (a Greek word from which Libya derives) and Meshwesh. Such groups would periodically enter the Egyptian territories for trade but at other times to raid (Snape 2003). South of Egypt was Ta Nehesy (Lower Nubia), followed by Kush (Middle Nubia). Beyond this was Irem (O'Connor and Reid 2016). Egypt's conception of the world, and Africa more specifically, reflected its economic and political network and its spread across the region. However, there is also the possibility that their conception of geography included vagueness. They refer to a place called Punt, from which various trade goods would come, such as ebony, myrrh, or savannah mammals, that was located further south along the Red Sea. Authors have concluded that this could be the Horn of Africa (Harvey 2003) or southern Arabia (Meeks et al. 2003), but it equally might rather refer to distant trade without a firm location. It very well might have included an undefined portion on both sides of the Red Sea that was involved in the economy.

Possibly some of the most widespread renderings of the African continent come from Muslim travellers. The influence of Muslims and Islam in Africa has shaped the continent's wider history and culture since its appearance in the seventh century CE (Insoll 2003, 2006; Horton 2005) and arrival by the early ninth century CE along Africa's east coast and almost at the same time the western Sahel (Insoll 2013, p. 168). Two notable Muslim scholars were Abu Abdullah Muhammad Ibn Battuta and Abu al-Hasan Ali ibn Husayn al-Mas'udi. Ibn Battuta was born in Tangier, modern day Morocco, in 1304 CE. At the age of 21, in 1325 CE, he left to complete his hajj, a Muslim pilgrimage to Mecca, but also to study at the various Islamic centres he came across (Mackintosh-Smith 2004, p. 99). Ibn Battuta began his journey alone, on a donkey: "having neither fellow-traveller in whose companionship I might find cheer, nor caravan whose party I might join, but swayed by an overmastering impulse within me and a desire long-cherished in my bosom to visit these illustrious sanctuaries" (Dunn 2012, p. 32). He would return to Fez some 29 years later and recount his journey to the sultan Abu 'Inan in his court and have it transcribed by Ibn Juzay (Pouwels 2019). His journeys provide incredible details about parts of Asia and Africa and immense insights into those worlds from the perspective of a Muslim traveller (Fig. 2.4).

Ibn Battuta visited continental Africa on two occasions. In the early period of his journey, he visited the Red Sea region and various African ports, including Mogadishu (Maqdashaw) and Kilwa (Kulwa), although it has been suggested that he may not have travelled there himself (Fauvelle-Aymar and Hirsch 2003). He reported that both ports were prosperous and stable cities, and he was impressed by the architecture. He was well received by the local sultans and his hosts. Additionally, he passed through Cairo roughly a year after Mansa Musa while the city was still reeling in the impact and memory of his visit (Bell 1972; Dunn 2012, p. 290). Ibn Battuta's second visit to Africa was 23 years later. On this occasion he travelled from Morocco to

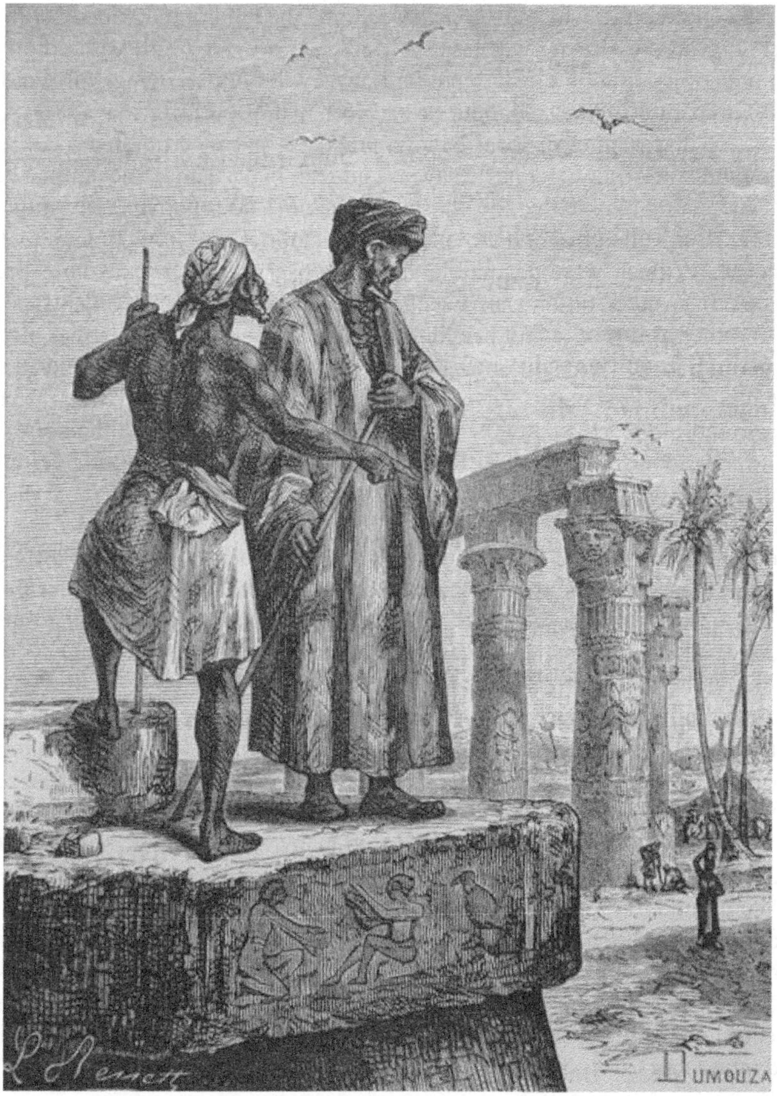

Fig. 2.4 An oil painting of Ibn Battuta drawn by Léon Benett and featured in Jules Verne's (1878) *Découverte de la Terre* (Discovery of Earth). *Source* https://commons.wikimedia.org/wiki/File:Handmade_oil_painting_reproduction_of_Ibn_Battuta_in_Egypt_a_painting_by_Hippolyte_Leon_Benett.jpg

Mali (Bilad al Sudan), which he considered to be the land of black people. In Mali, he was upset at the way he was treated. His hosts provided him with comfortable accommodation and high cuisine, but he felt they did not recognise his worth as it was not comparable to the splendour he had seen in the court (Berman 2003, p. 201). He was also disparaging of local Islamic practices that incorporated local beliefs, ways of doing, and views; some he saw as comical, in particular, the animist beliefs.

It is interesting to note that the question of identity does not vex Ibn Battuta. The world that he travelled through in Africa was one of flex and flow. Borders, whether personal or regional, were negotiable and self-observed. There was no expression that people from other cultures were seen from a essentialised or universalist perspective, but rather as different and peculiar (Moolla 2013, p. 386). What has also been noted in Ibn Battuta's account of the Africa he witnessed is a lack of similarities with a contemporary, Eurocentric version of 'Africa', namely, impoverished, primitive, mystical, and unified (Mackintosh-Smith 2004; Moolla 2013); to the contrary, he spoke of splendour and richness. Ibn Battuta's travels, therefore, provide different reflections on Africa that are not often gleaned from colonial perspectives. His views were transcribed less than a century before European expansionism and it is not clear how much Africa changed in this time, which might explain some of the differences. However, at least to some extent, these differences were likely the result of overarching incongruent attitudes towards Africa and Africans from Muslim and European perspectives. It is unlikely that these views are representative of all members of each group, but nonetheless offer valuable insight.

Prior to Ibn Battuta, there is a 400 year gap from which no considerable account of the African region has survived (Wynne-Jones and Fleisher 2021). But, in the tenth century CE, al-Mas'udi travelled widely and provided the earliest eye-witness records of pre-colonial Africa still in existence. Al-Mas'udi, born in Baghdad in 896 CE, was a geographer and historian who produced many written works, studies of Greek and Roman sources, and determined that the earth was spherical. It is estimated that he wrote around 35 books, of which two alone survive (Bennaji 2020, p. 50). He also laid the foundation for modern geomorphology with his study of landforms and the processes affecting them (Rather and Kanth 2018). Al-Mas'udi travelled from Baghdad to India through Persia, where he spent much of his time, before heading into central Asia. He then included parts of East Africa on his journey and eventually settled in modern Cairo (Fustat at the time) (Freeman-Grenville 1962; Ahmad 1987, p. 494).

Al-Mas'udi's accounts of East Africa are less detailed than some of the comments made by Ibn Battuta on his travels. He limited what he says of local communities to their adherence to Islam. However, his accounts are especially useful in understanding the importance of trade in East Africa prior to the turn of the second millennium CE (Wynne-Jones and Fleisher 2021). He described African ivory as being highly prized in China as the tusks were straight and suitable for ceremonial staffs. The easy connections from the coast to the interior, in what is largely an open country, made sourcing these valued items easy and transporting them, among other items, less troublesome (Horton 2018, p. 169).

It is also worth returning to the account of Leo Africanus in more detail. He was born in Granada around 1488 to 1490 CE and left for Morocco in 1492 after the Spanish conquest of the Iberian Peninsula. He was well schooled in law, grammar and religious doctrine in Fez, and became a young high-ranking official. He travelled extensively in North and West Africa, and parts of the Middle East, from 1506 to 1518. In the final year of his travels, while returning from a trip to the embassy in Istanbul, he was captured by Italian pirates (Davis 2014). They sent him to Pope Leo X, once they recognised him, and he was held captive for a year, during which time he received Christian instruction and was possibly schooled in Italian and Latin. After presumably 10 years in Italy, he returned to North Africa in 1528. He produced his book titled *Description of Africa* in 1526 written in Italian (Zhiri 2006). Although he wrote this from Italy, he had spent most of his life living on African soil, and so his account can certainly be considered from an insider's perspective. Africanus's (1600) book contributed immensely to perceptions of the continent that people knew very little of at the time.

Africanus' (1600) use of the term 'Africa' for his European readers resulted in a reconceptualization of the continent. The various lands he had travelled were brought together as a coherent thing, despite the great diversity he and those before him noted. He also relied on analogies to explain what he had witnessed in Africa in ways that Italian readers might understand. Doing so to explain similar clothing adornments or food types, as he did, are probably innocuous, but this became tricky when dealing with delicate issues, such as religion and sexuality. Subsequent reprints in the sixteenth century led to new renderings of the text and shifts in meaning. For example, anti-Muslim sentiments emerged in 1556 French and Latin translations and John Pory's English translation of 1600. These also portrayed the author, Leo Africanus, as more Christian than Islamic (Davis 2014). Despite these changes, his accounts of Africa, including trade, marriage, exchange, warring, and ways of living, persisted in the revised texts and translations, and continued to influence perceptions of Africa and its past.

While some records of West and East Africa exist, there are very few for southern. In the Hudud al Alam, whose author is anonymous, it states (cf. Issawi 1952, pp. 123–124):

> As regards the region lying south of the Equator some parts of it are occupied by the sea, and moreover, great heat prevails there and the people of those regions are more removed from the character of humanity. They are Zangis, Abyssinians, and the like. And farther on, down to the South Pole, no one can live on account of the excess of heat.

Marino Sanuto's map also noted the southern reaches of Africa as "uninhabitable from the heat" (ibid). Al-Mas'udi believed that south of 19° the earth was unoccupied. These views, Ibn Khaldun stated, led some philosophers to argue that no humans occupied the southern lands. However, he noted that reports of occupants exist. In Ibn Rushd's creation of the world, like Aristotle, the north and south were counterparts, and he concluded that the southern region was likely quite similar to the north climatically (Quatremère 1858; cf. Issawi 1952).

These examples serve to show the internal perceptions of Africa that were being formed. It was not only from early European travellers, explorers and merchants that an idea of Africa was assembling, but also earlier travellers on pilgrimage or otherwise explorers of various regions. These various records were not always in agreement, as Ibn Battuta's account shows, and were not widely shared between Muslims and Europeans. As such, they provide a firsthand, ahistoric glimpse into Africa from a handful of commentators but which are dispersed over a wide period (Insoll 2003, p. 448).

2.3 Dismantling the Darkness: Reclaiming Africa

> If all I knew about Africa were from popular images, I too would think that Africa was a place of beautiful landscapes, beautiful animals and incomprehensible people, fighting senseless wars, dying of poverty and AIDS, unable to speak for themselves (Adichie 2009)

Images of indigenous Africans produced in the early phases of European expansion were deeply shaped by existing European prejudices. Rooted in linear models of cultural and social evolution, such representations presumed European superiority and positioned African societies as socio-politically simple and economically undeveloped (Gronenborn 2004, p. 20). Derogatory and reductive descriptions became common tropes in colonial discourse. Yet, in parallel, a contrasting narrative developed that imagined Africa as the resting place of lost civilisations and buried treasures, obscured by time and decay (Hall 1995, p. 30). These two strands – primitivism and romanticism – coexisted, both ultimately reinforcing the idea that Africans themselves were disconnected from the grandeur of their own past.

In the independence era, African scholars and intellectuals challenged these narratives by producing emic reconstructions of Africa's history. Some of these responses, such as Cheikh Anta Diop's (1960) early work, sought to reclaim a glorious past but at times mirrored the essentialism of colonial framings in reverse. While such nationalist reconstructions may have overcorrected, they succeeded in reclaiming agency. Others offered more robust and enduring counter-narratives that destabilised Eurocentric conceptions and opened space for African-centred histories (e.g., Langley 1973; Hall 1995). Kwame Appiah (1992), for example, critiqued some forms of African constructionism, arguing that efforts to define a singular African identity risked flattening the continent's complexity. In doing so, the vast diversity of Africa's histories, languages, innovations, and internal dynamics is obscured. As he and others have pointed out (e.g., Achebe 1978), to speak of 'Africa' as one unified cultural or historical entity is to participate, even unintentionally, in the same logic that underpinned colonial myth-making. Earlier Muslim observers such as Ibn Battuta and al-Masʿudi were often more attentive to this diversity than many European commentators.

It was not only Africans that were challenging the Eurocentric trope of an African image but scholars beyond its borders that strongly contested these perceptions. An early challenge came from Basil Davidson (1959, 2014) who explored the development of African cities, such Great Zimbabwe, Swahili coastal centres, and West Sahel urban landscapes, to counter the prevailing European narrative. John Fage (1962) and then he and Roland Oliver (Oliver and Fage 1963) soon after helped establish African history as an academic field in Britain and rejected the 'tribal' lens used to characterise the continent's people and past. They did so by presenting various African kingdoms with their extensive histories, including the impact of trade and the complexities of local interactions. These examinations directly rejected the notion that Africa lacked history. Thurston Shaw (1977) similarly challenged European views of Africa through his archaeological work at Igbo-Ukwu, providing evidence of extensive trade networks and cultural developments predating the arrival of Europeans. These few examples are accompanied by a host of others (e.g., Dike 1956; Rodney 1972; Connah 1975; Ki-Zerbo 1981; Beach 1983; Vansina 1985; Thiong'O 1986; Mudimbe 1988; Robertshaw 1990; Coquéry-Vidrovitch 1991), many ironically coming from a time before Hugh Trevor-Roper's (1965) infamous remarks and when historical work in Africa boomed. All of these studies reconfigured images of Africa and cast aside reductionist perspectives.

The 'dark continent' metaphor captured this flattening of Africa into a single, unknowable identity. As colonial rule spread, such simplifications served the ideological project of domination. Colonising the past became a tool for colonising the present. As Frantz Fanon (1967, p. 169) observed, colonialism "turns to the past of the oppressed people, and distorts, disfigures and destroys it." Archaeology and history, especially in their instrumentalised forms, became central vehicles for this process, mobilised to legitimise conquest, dehumanise the colonised, and entrench coloniality (Van Dommelen 2006; Ndlovu 2009). The history of archaeology reflects these tensions. It is not only about the work of archaeologists, but also the ways in which the past has been selectively constructed, deployed, and politicised. The work of dismantling this darkness is far from complete. It is a process that continues in the hands of contemporary African scholars, archaeologists, and communities reclaiming the narratives of their pasts, which persist in the contemporary world, in media and popular texts, of romantic and backward African imaginaries.

References

Achebe, C. 1978. An image of Africa. *Research in African Literature* 9 (1): 1–15.

Adichie, C. N. 2009. *The danger of a single story*. https://jamesclear.com/great-speeches/the-danger-of-a-single-story-by-chimamanda-ngozi-adichie.Accessed on 18 August 2024.

Africanus, L. 1600. *The history and description of Africa and of the notable things therein contained*. London: Hakluyt Society.

Ahmad, K. J. 1987. *Hundred great Muslims*. Des Plaines: Library of Islam.

Anderson, A. A. 1888. *Twenty-five years in a Wagon: Sport and travel in South Africa*. London: Chapman and Hall.

Appiah, K. A. 1992. *In my father's house: Africa in the philosophy of culture*. New York: Oxford University Press.

Beach, D. 1983. *The Shona and Zimbabwe 900-1850: An outline of Shona history*. Gweru: Mambo Press.

Bell, N. M. 1972. The age of Mansa Musa of Mali: Problems in succession and chronology. *International Journal of African Historical Studies* 5 (2): 221–234.

Bennaji, Y. 2020. A critical appraisal of al-Masudi's perception of northern India: A special study on Multan. *European Journal of Language and Literature Studies* 6:50–58.

Berman, N. 2003. Questions of context: Ibn Battuta and E. W. Bovill on Africa. *Research in African Literatures* 34:199–205.

Chami, F.A., 1999. Roman beads from the Rufiji Delta, Tanzania: First incontrovertible archaeological link with the Periplus. *Current Anthropology 40*(2): 237–242.

Connah, G. 1975. *The archaeology of Benin*. Oxford: Clarendon Press.

Conrad, J. 1899. *Heart of darkness*. London: Blackwood's Magazine.

Coquéry-Vidrovitch, C. 1991. The process of urbanization in Africa (from the origins to the beginning of independence). *African Studies Review* 34 (1): 1–98.

Cornelius, S. 2010. Ancient Egypt and the other. *Scriptura: Journal for Contextual Hermeneutics in Southern Africa* 104 (1): 322–340.

Davidson, B. 1959. *Old Africa rediscovered*. London: Gollancz.

Davidson, B. 2014. *West Africa before the colonial era: A history to 1850*. London: Routledge.

Davis, N. Z. 2014. 'Leo Africanus' and his worlds of translation. In *Translators, Interpreters, and cultural negotiators*, ed. F. M. Federici and D. Tessicini, 62–80. London: Palgrave Macmillan UK.

Der Post, Van. 1955. *The dark eye in Africa*. London: Hogarth Press.

Derricourt, R. M. 2011. *Inventing Africa: History, archaeology and ideas*. New York: Pluto Press.

Dike, K. O. 1956. *Trade and politics in the Niger delta, 1830-1885*. Oxford: Clarendon Press.

Diop, C. A. 1960. *L'Afrique Noire Précoloniale: Étude comparée des systèmes politiques et sociaux de l'Europe et de l'Afrique eoire, de l'antiquité à la formation des états modernes*. Paris: Présence Africaine.

Disney, A. R. 2009. *A history of Portugal and the Portuguese empire: From beginnings to 1807*. Cambridge: Cambridge University Press.

Dunn, R. E. 2012. *The adventures of Ibn Battuta: A Muslim traveler of the 14th century*. Berkley: University of California Press.

Fage, J. D. 1962. *An introduction to the history of west Africa*. Cambridge: Cambridge University Press.

Fanon, F. 1967. *The wretched of the Earth*. Harmondsworth: Penguin Books.

Fauvelle-Aymar, F.-X., and B. Hirsch. 2003. Voyage aux frontières du monde: topologie, narration et jeux de miroir dans la Rihla de Ibn Battûta. *Afrique & Histoire* 1:75–122.

Freeman-Grenville, G. S. P. 1962. *The east African coast: Select documents from the first to the earlier nineteenth century*. Oxford University Press.

Gilbert, E. 2002. Coastal east Africa and the western Indian Ocean: Long-distance trade, empire, migration, and regional unity, 1750-1970. *The History Teacher* 36 (1): 7–34.

Gronenborn, D. 2004. Comparing contact-period archaeologies: The expansion of farming and pastoralist societies to continental temperate Europe and to southern Africa. *Before Farming* 2004 (4): 1–35.

Haggard, R. 1885. *King Solomon's Mines*. London: MacDonald.

Hall, M. 1995. Great Zimbabwe and the lost city. In *Theory in archaeology: A world perspective*, ed. P. J. Ucko, 29–46. London: Routledge.

Harms, R. 2018. *Africa in global history with sources*. London: WW Norton.

Harvey, S. P. 2003. Interpreting Punt: Geographic, cultural and artistic landscapes. In *Mysterious lands*, ed. D. O'Connor and S. Quirke, 81–92. London: Routledge.

Hatcher, S. 2013. The birth of the monsoon winds: On the existence and understanding of Hippalus, and the 'discovery' of the Apogeous trade winds. *Terrae Incognitae* 45 (1): 19–29.

Hochschild, A. 1998. *King Leopold's ghost: A story of greed, terror and heroism in colonial Africa*. London: Picador.

Horton, M. 2018. East Africa, the global gulf and the new Thalassology of the Indian Ocean. In *The gulf in world history*, ed. A. J. Fromherz, 160–181. Edinburgh: Edinburgh University Press.
Horton, M. C. 2005. The archaeology of Islam in Sub-Saharan Africa. By Timothy Insoll. *Journal of African History* 46:147–148.
Insoll, T. 2003. *The archaeology of Islam in Sub-Saharan Africa*. Cambridge: Cambridge University Press.
Insoll, T. 2006. Islamic archaeology and the Sahara. In *The Libyan desert: National resources and cultural heritage*, ed. D. J. Mattingly, S. McLaren, E. Savage, Y. al-Fasatwi, and K. Gadgood, 223–238. London: Society for Libyan studies.
Insoll, T. 2013. The archaeology of ritual and religion in Africa. In *The Oxford Handbook of African Archaeology*, ed. P. J. Mitchell and P. J. Lane, 163–175. Oxford: Oxford University Press.
Issawi, C. 1952. Arab geography and the circumnavigation of Africa. *Osiris* 10:117–128.
Ki-Zerbo, J. 1981. *General history of Africa: Methodology and African prehistory*. Paris: Heinemann.
Langley, J. A. 1973. *Pan-Africanism and nationalism in west Africa, 1900-1945: A study in ideology and social classes*. Oxford: Clarendon Press.
Mackintosh-Smith, T. 2004. *Travels with a Tangerine: From Morocco to Turkey in the footsteps of Islam's greatest traveler*. New York: Random House.
Mazrui, A. 1986. *The Africans: A triple heritage*. London: BBC Publications.
Meeks, D., D. O'Connor, and S. Quirke. 2003. Locating Punt. In *Mysterious lands*, 53–80. London: Routledge.
Michalopoulos, S., and E. Papaioannou. 2016. The long-run effects of the scramble for Africa. *American Economic Review* 106 (7): 1802–1848.
Moolla, F. F. 2013. Border crossings in the African travel narratives of Ibn Battuta, Richard Burton and Paul Theroux. *Journal of Postcolonial Writing* 49 (4): 380–390.
Mudimbe, V. Y. 1988. *The invention of Africa: Gnosis, philosophy, and the order of knowledge*. Bloomington: Indiana University Press.
Ndlovu, N. 2009. Decolonizing the mind-set: South African archaeology in a postcolonial, post-apartheid era. In *Postcolonial archaeologies in Africa*, ed. P. Schmidt, 177–192. New York: Springer.
Newitt, M. 2004. *A history of Portuguese overseas expansion 1400-1668*. London: Routledge.
O'Connor, D., and A. Reid, eds. 2016. *Ancient Egypt in Africa*. London: Routledge.
Ocheni, S., and B. C. Nwankwo. 2012. Analysis of colonialism and its impact in Africa. *Cross-Cultural Communication* 8 (3): 46–54.
Oliver, R., and J. D. Fage. 1963. *A short history of Africa*. New York: New York University Press.
Pakenham, T. 1991. *The scramble for Africa: The white Man's conquest of the dark continent from 1876 to 1912*. New York: Random House.
Polónia, A. 2022. Rounding cape Bojador: New horizons. In *The global history of Portugal: From prehistory to the modern world*, ed. C. Fiolhais, J. E. Franco, and J. P. Paiva, 170–174. Brighton: Sussex Academic Press.
Posnansky, M. 1966. Kingship, archaeology and historical myth. *Uganda Journal* 30:1–12.
Pouwels, R. L. 2002. Eastern Africa and the Indian Ocean to 1800: Reviewing relations in historical perspective. *The International Journal of African Historical Studies* 35 (2/3): 385–425.
Pouwels, R. L. 2019. Ibn Battuta in Africa and Asia. In *Oxford research encyclopedia of Asian history*, ed. D. Ludden. Oxford: Oxford University Press.https://doi.org/10.1093/acrefore/9780190277727.013.328
Quatremère, E. M. 1858. *Prolegomenes D'Ebn-Khaldoun*. Paris: La Bibliotheque Imperiale.
Rash, F. 2020. Lighting the 'dark'continent: Metaphors of darkness and light in the writings of British and German explorers and missionaries 1865–1915. In *The Discourse of British and German Colonialism*, ed. F. Rash and G. Horan, 107–127. London: Routledge. https://www.routledge.com/The-Discourse-of-British-and-German-Colonialism-Convergence-and-Competition/Rash-Horan/p/book/9780367506254

Rather, G. M., and T. A. Kanth. 2018. Contribution of Muslim scholars and its impact on development of geography. *International Journal of Movement Education and Social Science* 7:168–775.

Ringmar, E. 2006. Audience for a giraffe: European expansionism and the quest for the exotic. *Journal of World History* 17:375–397.

Robertshaw, P. 1990. *A history of African archaeology*. Oxford: James Currey Ltd.

Rodney, W. 1972. *How Europe underdeveloped Africa*. Washington: Howard University Press.

Said, E. 1979. *Orientalism*. New York: Vintage.

Seland, E. H.(2022), Spaces, places and things. *The spatial dimension of early Indian Ocean exchange*. In: Bilé, F., Mehendale, S. and Lankton, J.W. (eds) The Maritime Silk Road. Global Connectivities, Regional Nodes, Localities: 27–43.

Shaw, T. 1977. *Unearthing Igbo-Ukwu*. Ibandan: Oxford University Press.

Snape, S. 2003. The emergence of Libya on the horizon of Egypt. In *Mysterious lands*, ed. D. O'Connor and S. Quirke, 93–106. London: Routledge.

Stanley, H. M. 1889. *Through the dark continent: Or, the sources of the Nile, around the Great lakes of equatorial Africa, and down the Livingstone River to the Atlantic Ocean*. London: Sampson, Low.

Theal, G. M. 1899. *Records of south-eastern Africa: Collected in various libraries and archive departments in europe*. Cape Town: Government of the Cape Colony.

Theroux, P. 2004. *Dark star safari: Overland from Cairo to Cape Town*. Boston: Houghton Mifflin Company.

Thiong'O, N. W. 1986. *Decolonizing the mind: The politics of language in African literature*. London: James Currey Ltd.

Trevor-Roper, H. E. 1965. *The rise of Christian Europe*. Brace & World: Harcourt.

van der Post, L. 1951. *Venture in the Interior*. Harmondsworth: Penguin.

van der Post, L. 1958. *The lost world of the Kalahari*. Harmondsworth: Penguin.

Van Dommelen, P. 2006. Colonial matters: Material culture and postcolonial theory in colonial situations. In *Handbook of material culture*, ed. C. Tilley, W. Keane, S. Kuechler, M. Rowlands, and P. Spyer, 104–124. London: Sage Publications.

Vansina, J. 1985. *Oral tradition as history*. Madison: University of Wisconsin Press.

Verne, J. 1878. *Découverte de la Terre (Discovery of Earth)*. https://commons.wikimedia.org/wiki/File:Handmade_oil_painting_reproduction_of_Ibn_Battuta_in_Egypt_a_painting_by_Hippolyte_Leon_Benett.jpg. Accessed on 26 September 2024.

Viotti Da Costa, E. 1985. The Portuguese-African slave trade: A lesson in colonialism. *Latin American Perspectives* 12 (1): 41–61.

Wynne-Jones, S., and J. Fleisher. 2021. The Islamic archaeology of the eastern African coast. In *The Oxford handbook of Islamic archaeology*, ed. B. J. Walker, T. Insoll, and C. Fenwick, 377–394. Oxford: Oxford University Press.

Zhiri, O. 2006. Leo Africanus and the limits of translation. In *Travel and translation in the early modern period*, ed. C. di Biase, 175–186. Amsterdam: Rodopi.

Chapter 3
The Birth of Archaeology

Abstract Here, the book tracks archaeology's intellectual genealogy. From Egypt and Napoleonic science to the Rosetta Stone, and from nineteenth- and twentieth-century CE scholarly formations to the present, the chapter charts how antiquarian curiosity hardened into disciplinary practice. It surveys major theoretical turns—culture-historical approaches, processualism, post-processual and cognitive currents, and postcolonial critique—emphasising that archaeology's evolution is plural and non-linear. Rather than a single succession of schools, we find overlapping toolkits whose methods and assumptions shape what counts as evidence and explanation. The discussion introduces archaeology's distinctive approach—reconstructing social life from things—and its persistent debates about inference, meaning, and ethics. It closes by positioning African archaeology within, against, and beyond these global currents: deeply influenced by colonial logics and theory, yet increasingly growing self-aware and into its own identity. This historical backdrop primes the next chapters, which shift from general intellectual history to the specifically African trajectories of collecting, fieldwork, institution-building, and interpretation.

> To build their power base, kings, pharaohs, and emperors needed knowledge. Knowledge about the past—about ancient texts, traditions, and monuments—was part of the political arsenal of every ruler. (Schnapp 2014, p. 217)

At the end of the eighteenth century CE, Britain had a hold on trade through the Mediterranean to India. This was a crucial trade route that was pivotal to the nation's trading endeavours. Along this route lay Egypt, then under the control of the Mamluks, who had ruled for several centuries. Although Egypt was nominally part of the Ottoman Empire, the Mamluks operated with considerable autonomy. Their relationship with the Ottoman central authority in Istanbul (previously Constantinople) was complex; at times they aligned with the empire, but at others they engaged in skirmishes and power struggles (Flowers 2011). The Mamluk reign was turbulent and in three centuries they had approximately 250 rulers. They were also foreigners to the land with little interest in locals, other than keeping them as slaves. General Napoleon Bonaparte recognised the Mamluk instability, as well as Egypt's strategic location to potentially disrupt the trade network, and proposed an assault. In March, 1798 CE, his expedition was approved (Shortland 2022).

T. Forssman, *Archaeology in Africa: Why the Past Matters*, Archaeology of Africa,
https://doi.org/10.1007/978-3-032-13365-6_3

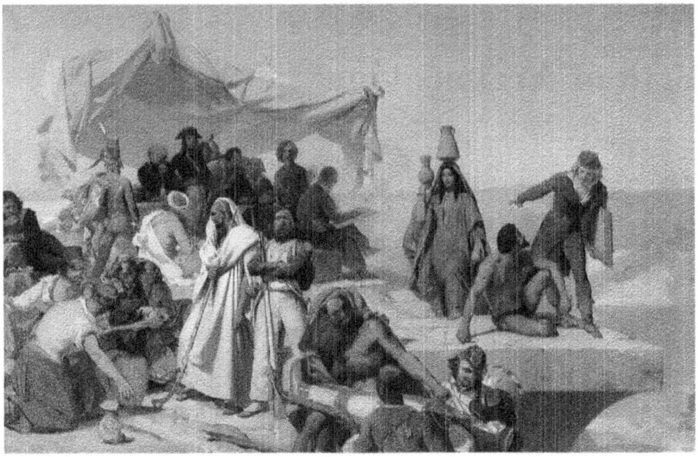

Fig. 3.1 The 1798 *L'Expédition d'Egypte* (Egyptian Expedition) under Napoleon Bonaparte. Painted by Léon Cogniet (1794–1880) in 1835 (Louvre). *Source* https://commons.wikimedia.org/wiki/File:Léon_Cogniet_-_L%27Expédition_d%27Egypte.jpg

Led by the ship *L'Orient*, Napoleon and his army sailed to Egypt to invade the African nation (Strathern 2008). The expedition included *savants* that made up the Egyptian Scientific Expeditionary group (Fig. 3.1). After first taking Malta on May 19, 1798, Napoleon and the French army reached Alexandria on July 1, taking the city and marching to Cairo 3 weeks later. They encountered the Mamluk force at the pyramids of Giza, and after a battle, they forced them to flee southwards. Victory was not to last. Admiral Horatio Nelson vanquished the French fleet on August 1, effectively cutting off supplies and forcing Napoleon to reconsider his expedition goals. He fled towards Syria. Weakened by battle and malnutrition, Napleon's army returned to Cairo, not before the Mamluk's attacked them in Abukir Bay on July 14, 1799, where they were once again beaten and forced south. Napoleon quietly sailed back to France on August 23, leaving General Jean-Baptiste Kiéber in charge of Cairo. After a defeat to the Turks in Heliopolis, the French army was left severely weakened with no signs of recovery. The British later attacked in Abukir Bay once again and were victorious on September 2, 1801, ending the French occupation of Egypt. However, the work of the *savants* was to have lasting effects. They produced *Description de l'Égypte,* a 23 volume monumental publication that was published between 1809 and 1823 (Shortland 2022, p. 51). The campaign's ultimate aims was such that "not only would the land be colonised in the present, but also the past would be colonised and exploited as well" (Shortland 2022, p. 54). Egypt's past was a commodity to France.

From the French expedition, one of the most influential archaeological finds was made. At Fort Julien, along the Egyptian coastline to the west of the Nile River and near modern el-Rashid, the French were anticipating an attack from the Ottomans or British. In their weakened and dispersed state, the Lieutenant Pierre-François

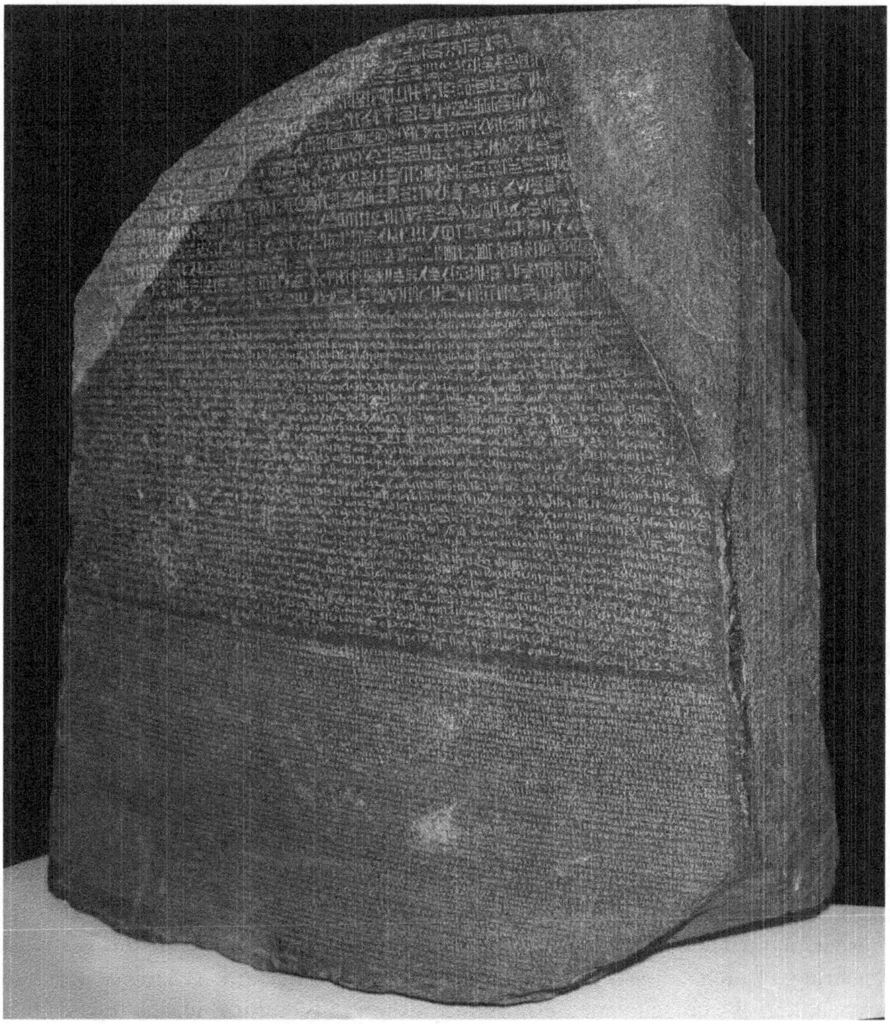

Fig. 3.2 The Rosetta Stone on display at the British museums (photograph: Awikimate). *Source* https://commons.wikimedia.org/wiki/File:Rosetta_Stone_-_front_face_-_corrected_image.jpg

Bouchard ordered troops to hastily repair the fort's defences in July of 1799. Their work led to the finding of a black grandiorite slab. Upon the slab was a decree in Ancient Greek declaring support for Ptolemy V, the new king of Egypt. Above this decree, on the same face, were two other written decrees: one in hieroglyphs and the other a Demotic script (Fig. 3.2). Although the decrees differed slightly, their similarities were such that their co-occurrence made it possible to decipher hieroglyphs for the first time. It was a monumental find with ramifications that stretched across Egypt and is vital even today (Parkinson et al. 1999).

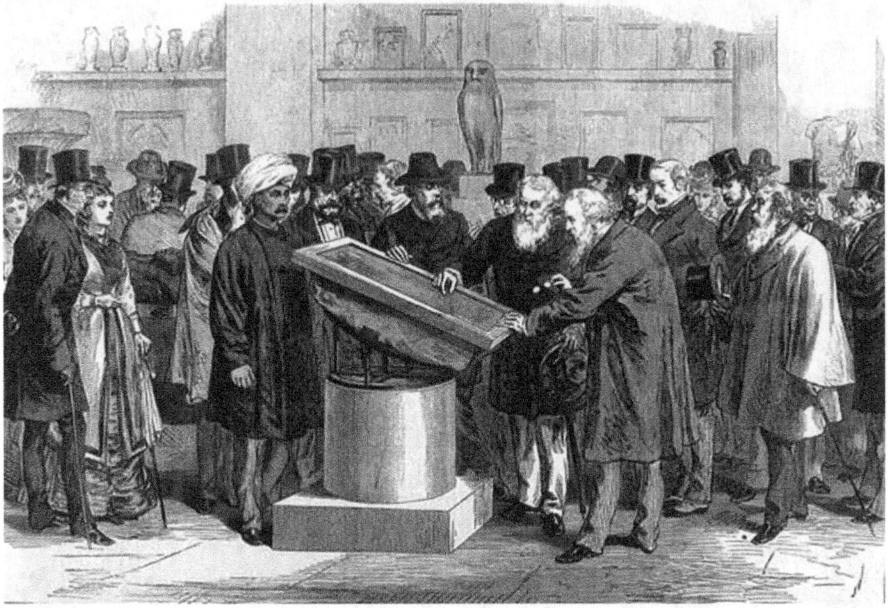

Fig. 3.3 The Rosetta Stone being investigated in 1874 at the congress of orientalists, London. *Source* https://commons.wikimedia.org/wiki/File:Rosetta_Stone_International_Congress_of_Orientalists_ILN_1874.jpg

The case of the Rosetta Stone illustrates the antiquarian birth of archaeology and its deployment in Africa. It is one of the earlier examples of interest in Africa's past from a European perspective (Fig. 3.3). Moreover, in this case, the French authorities aligned colonisation of the present with the past, evidently marking clear the power inherent in the past and its potential use to suppress people, manipulate the present, and wield its narratives in favour of one's own agenda. While this is a bleak rendering of archaeology, especially at its onset in Africa, it is largely accurate. Archaeologists and scholars are not always the guilty parties, in this regard; they mostly pursued a genuine interest in the past with the aim of learning more about past communities. However, their approaches, perspectives, attitudes, and politics coloured their reconstruction of the past. To some extent more influential was the way the past was used once it had been retrieved or reconstructed. Political parties, institutions, administrators and others took hold of these pasts and manipulated them in their present, using accepted or personal methods and theories to do so.

In Africa, archaeology occupies an intersection between a largely colonised continent, the discipline's firm roots in nationalism, and the practice's ability to amend and reproach representations of the past. Archaeology has matured from a protracted field of enquiry to a discipline with ambitious goals (Trigger 2006, p. 1). Its practice in the first half of the twentieth century CE prompted scholars to accuse the discipline of being substantially dwarfed by anthropology because of its lack of underlying theoretical frameworks and disciplinary independence (Yoffee and Sherratt 1993).

Since this critique, the discipline has overcome these challenges and demonstrated its crucial place in heritage and historical studies (Garvey 2018). Scholars now recognise the important historicism that only archaeology can bring to many research pursuits, even when interested in contemporary societies. Moreover, archaeology alone is capable of engaging pasts not written down or remembered. In regions, nations, or continents where histories are checkered by colonialism or where literate society recorded a narrow perspective of local people and their heritage, no other field can unearth lost histories in the manner that archaeology is able to. In this sense, archaeology is anti-colonial (Lane 2011), and being anti-colonial is important in contexts such as those found in Africa. However, it is important to explicitly note that the history of archaeology in Africa is inextricably linked to Europe. The role of archaeology and its impact cannot be fully understood without recognising Europe's influence on the discipline and Africa's history (Trigger 1990, p. 317).

Understanding archaeology's development as a discipline also requires considering how change is conceptualised within scientific fields more broadly. One influential way of framing disciplinary change comes from Thomas Kuhn's (1962, 1970) theory of scientific paradigms, which offers a useful lens for thinking about archaeology's shifting frameworks over time. Kuhn (1962) argued that scientific progress is not linear but shaped by dominant paradigms, which he defined as widely accepted frameworks of theories, methods, tools, and assumptions that guide what questions are asked and how knowledge is produced. These paradigms are sustained by scientific communities through teaching, publication, funding, and professional structures that reinforce shared ways of working. His ideas, influenced by Ludwik Fleck's (1981) earlier work on scientific thought collectives, emphasised that science is a social activity shaped by the beliefs and practices of its practitioners. Rather than constant incremental improvement, Kuhn (1962) described science as moving through periods of 'normal science' within a paradigm, interrupted by paradigm shifts; moments of profound change when existing frameworks can no longer accommodate new findings or ideas. In archaeology, this model helps explain why the discipline has seen distinct theoretical phases, such as culture-historical, processual, and post-processual approaches, each reflecting broader shifts in what the archaeological community considered valid knowledge. Thinking about archaeology in terms of paradigms situates its intellectual changes within larger scientific patterns of consensus, challenge, and transformation.

While Kuhn's (1962) model has been influential, scholars have also pointed out several limitations in applying paradigms too rigidly to disciplines like archaeology (Foucault 1970; Gándara 1980; Masterman 1984; Schiffer 1996; Dunnell 2001; VanPool and VanPool 2003). One concern is that Kuhn's (1962) concept of paradigms oversimplifies the complexity and diversity of research within a field, implying more consensus than often exists (Renfrew 1982; Huffman 1986). The notion that change was linear, from one paradigm to the next, has also been queried with some proposing a cyclic history of archaeological thinking (Daniel 1950; Piggott 1959), whereas others have argued that not enough change has taken place to consider developments as paradigmatic shifts (Orme 1973, p. 490; Gardin 1980, pp. 165–180). Archaeology, in particular, rarely fits neatly into a single paradigm at any one time, with competing schools of thought often coexisting (Chapman 2003, p. 14). Others argue that Kuhn's (1962) focus on revolutionary shifts neglects the slower, cumulative nature of change driven by methodological refinements, new technologies, or changing ethical considerations (Toulmin 1970). Additionally, the model risks overlooking the influence of external social, political, and economic factors that shape research directions, especially in contexts like Africa where colonial and postcolonial histories complicate disciplinary trajectories (e.g., Moro Abadía and González Morales 2003).

In considering these various perspectives, we are hardly left with a holistic concept of archaeology's philosophical development. The diverse views, approaches, recharacterizations, and dissimilar frameworks suggest a lack of philosophical specificity. What is more, the various propositions do not wholly capture the history of archaeological development across the globe. Despite the many archaeologists and social scientists that have grappled with these frameworks, no theoretical framework has emerged that neatly crosscuts contexts. In this book, the concept of schools is preferred to refer to broader canons in the field. They are not viewed as homeostatic plateaus or defined paradigms. To the contrary, they are considered heterogenous and permeable. The schools imbricate and share traits but seek out the past with sometimes cognate and other times contested interests and interpretive frameworks. They are also influenced by capitals, drawing on Pierre Bourdieu's (1986) work, which are economic, social, cultural, symbolic, but also physical (the means of doing). The influence of these capitals varies contextually and historically, and results in variable interests, topical approaches, interpretations, political aspirations, and agendas within the field. From this framework, the various changes that archaeology witnessed are viewed not as paradigm shifts but rather shifts in capital, including the tools (physical), that lead to reformations within the discipline, changing emphases, emerging and declining trends, and developments and advances in understanding. As such, archaeology and its schools of thought are historically contingent and need to be viewed alongside internal and external factors. In the context of this book, it is important to consider at least the frameworks used to understand change within archaeology. Ultimately, these factors—Intellectual, political, and economic—converge to define the discipline's basic structure, its guiding purposes, and the procedural norms that govern archaeological practice.

3.1 The Beginnings of Archaeology

Human societies have long sought to understand, commemorate, and connect with their pasts in diverse ways (Bahn 2014, p. 1; Schnapp 2014, p. 217). Whether through oral traditions, rituals, ancestor veneration, or sacred landscapes, the past has often been understood not as distant or linear, but as spiritually present, cyclical, or embodied (Matos Moctezuma 1984; Joyce 2003; Trigger 2006, p. 41). Among the Akan and Yoruba, for example, the past is accessed through libations, naming, and shrines (McCaskie 1995), while the Lakota and Navajo carry history in ceremonies and sacred sites (Deloria 1994). Similarly, the Malagasy practice Famadihana to reconnect with ancestors (Bloch 1982). These examples reflect how different world-views and cultural values shape understandings of time and history, which are often distinct from written historical traditions or material-based reconstructions associated with archaeology.

Material traces of the past – artefacts, ruins, and landscapes – were present in many societies, but their meanings were often shaped by cultural beliefs, spiritual interpretations, or mythological frameworks rather than systematic study (Schnapp 2014). In Europe, peasants once believed stone tools found in fields were 'thunderstones,' formed by lightning strikes (Heizer 1962, p. 63), while Japanese farmers attributed similar finds to supernatural armies at war (Ikawa-Smith 2001, p. 735). In North America, some Iroquoian groups viewed ancient stone tools as sacred relics left by spirits, imbuing them with power (Thwaites 1896, p. 211). Across the world, objects uncovered from the ground were often understood not as remnants of unknown ancestors, but as gifts, omens, or relics linked to divine forces. In Mesopotamia, rulers saw the past as a source of legitimacy, retrieving and copying earlier inscriptions and artefacts to connect themselves to great ancestors or mythic origins (Bahn 2014, p. 1). Likewise, Egypt's Twelfth Dynasty craftsmen deliberately reproduced Old Kingdom art and architecture as acts of reverence and political memory (Edwards 1985; Dodson 1988; Loprieno 2003; Tait 2003). Yet, in these instances, material remains were rarely studied systematically or used to build empirical histories. Instead, they were incorporated into cosmologies, ritual practices, or political narratives. There is little evidence of early societies using artefacts to 'interpret' history in a way recognisable as archaeology today. Rather, these encounters with the past reveal a broader human impulse to attribute meaning, power, and memory to ancient things.

The intellectual roots of archaeology, as a formal discipline, emerged in Europe during the Renaissance and into the fifteenth century CE (Ucko 1995). Antiquarians like Cyriacus of Ancona (Greenhalgh 2013) and later scholars such as Nicolas-Claude Fabri de Peiresc and Jacob Spon (1673) began systematically recording inscriptions and artefacts in recognition of their historical value. By the eighteenth century, figures like Anne Claude Philippe and Johann Winckelmann (1764) advanced chronological thinking and detailed recording practices, laying groundwork for archaeology's scientific turn (see Trigger 2006; Bahn 2014; Schnapp 2014; Smith 2017). Although motivated by aesthetics, nationalism, or colonial ambitions, these developments marked a gradual shift toward treating material remains as sources of knowledge about past societies, setting the stage for archaeology's formal frameworks in the centuries that followed.

By the late nineteenth and early twentieth centuries, archaeology was emerging as a formal discipline, increasingly shaped by European intellectual traditions. Early archaeological studies were chiefly interested in two aspects of the past: diffusion and migration. Both ideas hinged on the notion that cultural items moved between people, from one group to the next, or were transported by people as they moved to occupy new regions. To unpack this, the notion of culture needs some understanding. Gustaf Kossinna (1911, p. 3), who was an early propagator of these ideas, said of culture as a concept: "Sharply defined archaeological culture areas correspond at all times with the areas of particular people or tribes". He was interested in the idea of a primordial

Germanic society, romanticised by nineteenth century archaeologists, and viewed it as an idealised forerunner of national society (Mertens 2004; Puschner 2004). He studied the movement of 'barbarians' in the post-Roman migration era and focussed on the co-occurrence of cultural items within assemblages from bounded spaces, such as archaeological sites, to establish settlement areas of distinct ethnic groups. In this model, the migratory movements of specific peoples could be traced through material culture, and conversely, the presence of material culture could be used to infer the movements and identities of people in the past (Veit 1984; Shennan 1987, pp. 366–367). Kossinna (1911) drew on German diffusionists such as Friederich Ratzel (1899) and Fritz Graebner (1911) who were interested in the 'Kulturkreise', or culture area. Identifying a culture relied on assembling a canon of diagnostic traits that, in combination, signalled ethnic affiliation (Burmeister 2023, p. 50). Recognising these markers, and understanding which were significant, required a degree of cultural competence. Crucially, this entire approach hinged on the central notion of ethnic identity being materially visible. Kossinna's (1911) axiomatic approach provided archaeologists with theoretical and methodological foundations for developing culture-historical models, which shaped archaeological practice well into the twentieth century CE.

However, even before this, in the late eighteenth century, German scholars reformulated concepts of nation and culture, influenced by Charles-Louis de Secondat's (Montesquieu) belief that customs, habits and laws characterised a nation. Others felt that this was too reductionist; Johan Herder added constituent parts to this definition, such as language and poetry (Koselleck 1992, p. 30). Stefan Burmeister (2023, p. 57) describes Kossinna's (1911) use of culture, diffusion and migration as a Trojan horse; it was an attractive model that hid racial, territorial, and nationalist agendas. His major contribution to archaeology is entangled with his ethno-nationalist agenda. As time went by, he himself became more radicalised, and his ideas of the past, its useability, and the structure of archaeology were influenced by this, according to his biographer (Grünert 2002, p. 229). The approaches proposed by Kossinna (1911) were strongly aligned with Germany's own nation-forming history and unfurling nationalist agendas linked to this process (Burmeister 2023, p. 57). Playing a strong influential role in these ideas and the debate about what it means to be a nation was the French Revolution (1789–1799 CE). Specifically, it drew into contrast what it meant to be German in a space occupied by multiple political units. Unlike in France, and others nations, where common state and civil rights formed the nation, in Germany it was culture, common ancestry, and language (Burmeister 2023, p. 54). Archaeology's formation more generally was deeply entrenched in nationalism, possibly being stimulated by it in the first place (Díaz-Andreu 2018, p. 3).

V. Gordon Childe (1925, 1929, 1950) played a pivotal role in formalising early archaeological approaches to migration and diffusion, stripping them of overt political agendas and integrating them into a systematic reconstruction of European prehistory. Central to Childe's (1925, 1929) framework was the argument that archaeological cultures represented actual societies, and that migration and diffusion were primary forces driving intersocietal relations and social evolution (Anthony 1990, p. 898). His reworking of these concepts became foundational to the culture-historical approach that dominated mid-twentieth-century archaeology. In this model, recurrent material patterns, such as architectural styles, burial customs, and ceramics, were interpreted as defining features of distinct cultural groups. Migration, in particular, emerged as a principal explanatory mechanism for change and cultural transmission (Adams et al. 1978, p. 493). Culture-historical archaeology thus sought to construct large-scale sequences through which individual cultures could be traced over time and space (Daniel 1950). Within this paradigm, material culture in any given place was understood as having arrived either through the movement of people or through the gradual transfer of objects and ideas from one group to another, ultimately becoming embedded in societies distinct from their original producers (Trigger 1990, p. 311).

Discontent with traditional, culture-historical archaeology grew steadily through the mid-twentieth century, culminating in the 1960s and 1970s when the field began to fall out of favour, particularly among English-speaking archaeologists (Burmeister 2000, p. 539). A major point of critique was its reliance on diffusion and migration as primary explanatory frameworks. These models, once dominant, came to be seen as vague and reductionist, offering little insight into motivation, agency, or the complex factors that shaped past human behaviour. William Adams et al. (1978) described this shift as a "retreat from migrationism," with new approaches favouring "indigenist" or "immobilist" models that placed greater emphasis on local innovation (Chapman and Hamerow 1998; Härke 1998). Bruce Trigger (1969, p. 27), however, cautioned against discarding diffusion altogether, arguing that simplistic readings of cultural transmission ignored the agency of recipient societies and the specific conditions that enabled such processes.

Archaeology's theoretical limitations stood in sharp contrast to developments in related disciplines. While archaeologists distanced themselves from migration models, anthropologists, historians, and linguists continued to explore migration as a key mechanism for cultural and social change. Anthropologists studied it as a driver of kinship structures and population dynamics (Rapoport et al. 2020); historians traced its role in the spread of languages, religions, and trade networks (Grollemund et al. 2015, 2023; Bostoen 2020); and linguists used migration to explain major dispersals, such as the Bantu and Indo-European expansions (Renfrew 1989; Koile et al. 2022). These disciplines managed to engage with migration without relying on the racialised or essentialist assumptions that had tarnished its use in archaeology. Still, critics within archaeology grew frustrated with the discipline's descriptive bent and limited analytical reach. David Clarke (1973) urged archaeologists to confront the field's theoretical and methodological shortcomings and move beyond collecting, describing, and cataloguing artefacts. Earlier scholars such as Walter Taylor (1948) and E. Adamson Hoebel (1949) had already challenged the field's foundational assumptions, with Taylor (1948) arguing that material culture alone could not explain human life, and Hoebel (1949, p 436) asserting that archaeology was "always the lesser part of anthropology." By the 1950s, as other social sciences adopted new forms of analysis, archaeology's narrow scope appeared increasingly dated. Despite new techniques like chemical sourcing and systematic surveys (Posnansky 1976; Merrick and Brown 1984), the discipline remained anchored in typologies and polarising explanations of change (Trigger 1984), rarely grounded in empirical critique

(Binford and Sabloff 1982, p. 148). Clarke's (1973) notion of a "loss of innocence" captured this disciplinary reckoning – an end to the belief that objective knowledge of the past could be produced through data collection alone.

3.2 New Archaeology: Processualism

> The loss of disciplinary innocence is the price of expanding consciousness; certainly the price is high but the loss is irreversible and the prize substantial (Clarke 1973, p. 6)

Advances in science and technology, spurred in part by the Second World War, introduced new techniques, data processing methods, and analytical tools, pushing archaeologists to rethink the discipline's aims. The emerging 'New Archaeology', or processualism, rejected simple descriptions of the past, as scholars grew frustrated with the field's inability to explain human behaviour or social change (Binford 1977). Influenced by scientific models, this approach sought to uncover broad patterns in human history through systems thinking—treating societies and material culture as components within dynamic cultural and natural processes (Shanks and Hodder 2013). Human history, it was argued, could be modelled by identifying the rules and interactions that produced specific outcomes within these systems. Yet, archaeology faced a fundamental challenge; it could not observe past human behaviour or thought directly (Trigger 1989). As a result, archaeologists turned towards anthropological science rather than history, aligning the discipline more closely with scientific reasoning, generalisation, and theoretical modelling (Willey and Phillips 1958, p. 2). This turn in approaches used logical positivism to solve philosophical problems (Earle and Preucel 1987). The shift ushered in a period of greater self-critique and methodological sophistication, marking a significant departure from earlier approaches (Clarke 1973).

Processualism's dawn in the 1960s brought with it access to a wide range of methods and approaches, as well as data-processing capabilities, co-opted from other scientific disciplines. Some subject fields were more influential than others, such as anthropology, ecology, environmental science, or geography, but they all contributed to build archaeology's new character. Processual archaeology, despite this, was anthropological in nature with its interest in reconstructing social pasts (Shanks and Hodder 2013). The dominant theoretical framework at the time was that society was composed of patterned behaviour. This view is often described as systems thinking in which different sets of organisations, requirements, and necessities sit in tension with one another. These typically include economic strategies, resources, subsistence, trade and exchange, and technology, and later ritual and symbolism. As one changes or is adjusted the equilibrium between them realigns, influencing human society. Society is the human adaptation to these interlocked systems. Material remains are the product of patterned behaviour, and as such they reflect human society (Binford 1962). However, they might also be the result of natural processes, such as decay or post-depositional movements, but these can be defined scientifically

(Ascher 1961). Due to the predictability of these systems, society can be typed, and, as such, cultural evolution schemes are discernible. Crucial to processual approaches was the search for universal truths. These views were in contrast to early notions of change, and Lewis Binford (1962, p. 217) rejected whimsical approaches that viewed change as the result of "'influences', 'stimuli,' or even 'migrations' between and among geographically defined units". A major focus of processual archaeology was to develop an objective reading of the past, which could be achieved by relying on scientific procedures (Binford and Sabloff 1982).

Processual archaeology's emphasis on scientific reasoning led to significant methodological advancements (Willey and Phillips 1958). Archaeologists sought to reconstruct past human behaviour by applying rigorous field and laboratory techniques, and later middle-range theory, such as experimental archaeology and ethnoarchaeology (Binford 1983). Settlement pattern studies, for example, allowed archaeologists to model how societies were structured in relation to their environment, while statistical methods helped identify trends in artefact distributions (Clarke 1978). These approaches strengthened archaeology's claim to be an explanatory science rather than a descriptive pursuit. However, while processualists aimed for objectivity, later scholars, including Binford (1983) himself, acknowledged that interpretation inevitably involved some level of inference. Middle-range theory was developed as a bridge between static material remains and dynamic human behaviour, using modern analogies to infer past processes. Despite its scientific ambitions, processualism was later critiqued for assuming universal laws of cultural change and underestimating the role of human agency (Hodder 2001) and that it shifted the field towards science at the expense of humanism (Hawkes 1968; Clarke 1978). Nevertheless, it laid the foundation for archaeology as a discipline grounded in systematic methodologies and testable hypotheses, shifting the field from a largely descriptive to an analytical science.

3.3 Post-Processual Frameworks

By the late 1970s, growing dissatisfaction with the scientific ambitions of processual archaeology gave rise to what became known as post-processual archaeology. Processualism's critics argued that this focus often reduced human societies to predictable systems, failing to adequately address meaning, symbolism, power, and individual agency (Hodder 1982; Shanks and Tilley 1987). These critiques were not purely theoretical; they reflected broader intellectual shifts influenced by post-structuralism, Marxism, and interpretive social science (Johnson, 2010). However, unlike processualism, post-processual archaeology did not emerge as a single, coherent movement but as a loose collection of approaches united by their critique of positivism and cultural evolutionary thinking. Ian Hodder (1982), one of the leading figures, rejected the idea that archaeology could, or should, seek universal laws of cultural change. Instead, post-processualists advocated for a more nuanced, context-specific understanding of the past, placing emphasis on human intentionality, meaning, and the historically situated nature of social life (Shanks and Tilley 1992). As Michael Rowlands (1989) noted, this required moving away from the generalising tendencies of processual archaeology towards recognising local histories, unique trajectories, and the complexity of social change.

Central to this shift was the concept of agency – the capacity of individuals and groups to act within, resist, or reshape the structures of their societies. Drawing from social theorists such asBourdieu (1972) and Anthony Giddens (1984), post-processualists viewed human action as neither fully determined by cultural systems nor entirely free. Instead, society was understood as a dynamic interplay between enduring structures and the creative practices of individuals. Archaeology, therefore, could no longer treat material culture as passive reflections of social organisation but needed to explore how objects were implicated in power relations, identity formation, and social reproduction (Miller and Tilley 1984). This new focus opened archaeology to a range of interpretive questions about embodiment, memory, ritual, and place. Scholars examined how material culture shaped and was shaped by human experience, with particular attention paid to how people engaged with landscapes, monuments, and artefacts (Shanks 1999; Meskell and Joyce 2003). Phenomenological approaches to landscape, for instance, sought to explore how places were experienced bodily and emotionally, rather than simply mapped or measured (Tilley 1994). This attention to lived experience challenged the processual focus on external environmental factors and economic rationality.

Another major strand of post-processual thought was its critique of normative cultural models and Eurocentric assumptions that had long structured archaeological interpretation. Models that categorised societies into types – for example, Elman Service's (1960) bands, tribes, chiefdoms, and states, an influential concept even today – were seen as overly rigid and deeply entangled with colonial histories (Burmeister 2000, 2023). Archaeologists increasingly recognised that such typologies, especially when applied outside Europe, risked essentialising cultural groups and naturalising power imbalances. Antoine Lema (1993), for instance, critiqued the concept of the "tribe" as a colonial construct designed to categorise and control non-Western societies. Referencing Frantz Fanon (1967), he argued that such frameworks forced colonised people to grapple with distorted identities imposed upon them by outsiders. Post-processualism thus called for an archaeology attentive to local knowledge systems, social dynamics, and power relations. It rejected deterministic models of culture and emphasised the importance of historicism, being the understanding that all societies develop through unique historical processes embedded within specific social and environmental contexts (Pluciennik 2005). Grand narratives, such as the inevitable rise of complex society or the universal path to agriculture, were critically examined. Instead, scholars asked how these developments unfolded differently across time and space and how they were experienced by people on the ground (Shanks 2008, p. 137).

However, post-processual archaeology was not without its critics. A major concern was that its rejection of scientific generalisation left it vulnerable to subjectivity and relativism. Critics argued that without clear methodologies, post-processual approaches risked producing speculative narratives rather than testable knowledge

(Watson 1990; Yoffee and Sherratt 1993). Binford (2009) accused the movement of abandoning science altogether, suggesting that post-processualism's emphasis on meaning and symbolism could never generate the kinds of secure knowledge archaeology required. Michael Shanks (2008, p. 133) himself acknowledged that post-processualism was sometimes caricatured as "an extreme and politically motivated relativism," though he argued that this was a misrepresentation of its aims.

The tension between science and interpretation became a defining feature of the debate, often framed as a polarisation between processual and post-processual camps. Yet, as Trigger (1989) pointed out, this binary obscured the fact that archaeology, as a discipline, is inherently interpretive, even when employing scientific methods. All archaeological reconstructions, he argued, rely on inference and are shaped by contemporary concerns. For example, global perspectives complicated what was in fact an Anglo-American debate between schools of thought. Archaeologists working outside dominant academic centres, particularly in Australia, Africa, and parts of Latin America, highlighted the Eurocentrism of both processual and post-processual approaches (Huffman 2004; Jones 2024). In these contexts, archaeology was entangled with local political struggles, heritage concerns, and indigenous knowledge systems. Scholars called for greater reflexivity, inclusivity, and attention to how archaeological narratives were produced and by whom (Smith 2000; LeBlanc and Watson 2014). They critiqued both the universalising attempts of processualism and the tendency of post-processualism to remain confined within Euro-American academic discourse. From this perspective, considerable emphasis was placed on recognising the inherent subjectivity of archaeological interpretation. It was argued that all knowledge of the past was mediated by the contemporary perspectives, values, and experiences of researchers (Shanks and Tilley 1987; Hodder 1991). Rather than seeing subjectivity as a flaw, post-processual archaeologists viewed it as unavoidable and something to be reflected upon critically. Shanks and Christopher Tilley (1992) proposed that by embracing reflexivity and acknowledging how archaeologists shape the narratives they produce, the discipline could develop richer, more meaningful interpretations of the past. This stance challenged processual claims to neutrality and underscored the need to understand archaeology as both a scientific and inherently interpretive endeavour (Trigger 2006).

Ultimately, post-processual archaeology expanded the intellectual horizons of the discipline. It forced archaeologists to grapple with questions of meaning, identity, and power, issues that had long been marginalised in favour of materialist explanations. Its emphasis on interpretation, historicism, and local context opened new avenues for understanding the past as a product of human creativity, agency, and experience. Its legacy is evident in contemporary archaeology's greater theoretical diversity, its attention to ethics and reflexivity, and its willingness to engage with complex social questions. These shifts laid the foundation for later developments in archaeology, particularly the growth of post-colonial and indigenous archaeologies that further interrogate power, identity, and knowledge production in the discipline.

3.4 Cognitive Archaeology

Despite their frequent disagreements, both processual and post-processual archaeologies shared core concerns about understanding the human past. Their differences lie in their methods and epistemologies, but each tradition sought to explain how past societies functioned and why particular cultural patterns emerged. Both were driven by theoretical engagement and critical reflection: questioning assumptions, refining methodologies, and challenging inherited models (Shanks 2008). As Margaret Blackie (2022) noted in her reflections on scientific theory, similar tensions appear in other disciplines, underscoring the productive potential of debate in refining understanding. In archaeology, this shared foundation created space for new approaches to emerge – those that grappled with the fundamental challenge of finding meaning in the material traces of past societies. Post-processual archaeologists were especially concerned with the question of meaning and how it might be accessed through archaeological data. Hodder (1986, 1987) argued that meaning is embedded in context; in the specific cultural, spatial, and social conditions in which objects were created, used, and discarded. His "contextual archaeology"sought to move beyond universalist explanations toward interpretations that accounted for the symbolic and cultural frameworks of past societies. However, others, most notably Trigger (2006), warned that archaeology often lacks sufficient evidence to reconstruct such meaning directly. Historical materialism, ethnography, and oral traditions, among other methods, became critical tools for enriching interpretations (Leone 1982). These approaches allowed archaeologists to probe questions of meaning and agency, though not without critique. Scholars working in Africa, such as Laurence Barham (1992), Lane (2004), and Benjamin Smith (2010), highlighted the dangers of projecting contemporary perspectives or over-relying on problematic written records.

Finding meaning often required bridging the gap between past and present, a challenge tackled through middle-range theory and analogy. By comparing patterns in archaeological materials with those observed ethnographically, archaeologists could generate plausible interpretations of past behaviour (Binford 1983). This approach reshaped understandings of groups such as the San of southern Africa, who, like others, were long stereotyped as timeless hunter-gatherers (Wobst 1978; Schrire 1980; Parkington 1984). Instead of seeing such groups as living fossils locked into a developmental "stage," middle-range theory illuminated the complexity and dynamism of forager societies, past and present. It also underscored the importance of historicism – recognising that contemporary groups cannot be used uncritically to reconstruct the past without accounting for the historical processes that shaped them (Wolf 1982).

Emerging from these debates was cognitive archaeology, often seen as a bridge between processualism's focus on systems and post-processualism's attention to meaning and agency. Cognitive archaeology, in its broadest sense, is concerned with exploring how past people thought, by investigating their worldviews, belief systems, and symbolic frameworks, rather than simply what they thought (Fagan and Durrani

2016, p. 235). As Kent Flannery and Joyce Marcus (1993, p. 262) defined it, cognitive archaeology studies "all those aspects of ancient culture that are the product of the ancient mind". Two overlapping strands thread through cognitive archaeology. The first is evolutionary and cognitive science, examining the emergence of modern cognitive capacities, such as language, abstract reasoning, and symbolic behaviour, often through studies of tool production, art, and early social organisation (Mithen 1996; Tomasello et al. 2005). The second strand, more aligned with interpretive approaches, focuses on later prehistoric and historic societies, investigating how worldviews, religion, cosmology, and social symbolism shaped material culture and landscapes (Huffman 1986, 2015). This includes studies of iconography, burial practices, monumental architecture, gift exchange, and the structuring of space – all aimed at reconstructing the mental worlds of past peoples. Such an approach demands robust methods and, often, rich ethnographic or ethnohistorical data.

Ultimately, cognitive archaeology extends archaeology's ambition beyond reconstructing past economies or settlement patterns. It seeks to access the mental and symbolic worlds that shaped human experience, creating space for archaeology to engage more fully with issues of belief, identity, and meaning, which are themes increasingly central to African archaeological scholarship.

3.5 Postcolonial Archaeology

The beginning of archaeology in Africa was deeply tethered to the arrival of Europeans and the colonial occupation of the continent that eventually ensued (Robertshaw 1990a; Shepherd 2002; Lane 2011). In these early renderings, and indeed long after them, the emphasis was on a "unilinear cultural evolution" in which societies were imagined to progress from simple, savage, hunter-gatherer-type societies to the industrialised global west nations (Giblin 2013, p. 253). While at first this recognised the potential for all societies to develop, it came to confine racial groups into inferior cultures based on biological unchangeability (Trigger 2006). It was in Africa that these two viewpoints emerged the most pronounced; colonialism was largely seen as bringing civilisation to 'backward' African societies, albeit informed also by superior and extractive approaches (Holl 1990, p. 297). This perspective influenced the initial value of archaeology on the African continent. At the time of European settlement, it was thought that the various cultural evolutionary stages of humankind were present in its various forms. For example, hunter-gatherers, such as the San or Ife, were considered un-evolved relics of the Stone Age (Robertshaw 1990b, p. 4). Archaeology could demonstrate how cultural evolution occurred but could teach us little more about each phase than the present could show us. These sentiments form part of the foundation of archaeological practice in the late nineteenth century CE.

From Enrique Dussel's (1996) perspective, colonial histories exploited the "underside" of modernity. Dussel's (1996) term is similar to that of Gayatri Spivak's (1988) "subaltern" and one that Paget Henry (2000) and Lewis Gordon (2000, p. 3) both referred to as "Caliban", referencing William Shakespeare's *Tempest* and Prospero's colonisation of Caliban's island. Early critiques of these notions emerged at the end of the nineteenth century by the likes of William Du Bois (1897) in his works *Conservation of the Races* and *The Study of Negro Problems* (Du Bois 1898), among others, and influenced many scholars such as Alain Locke (1925) and his study of "New Negro", and of course Fanon's (1967) search for post-racist society in a post-colonial context. These approaches influenced broader examinations of suppression and coloniality, such as Edward Said's (1979) *Orientalism* and Paulo Friere's (1990) *Pedagogy of the Oppressed*, and continue to do so in the likes of Cornel West's (1982) and Bell Hooks' (1990) work on African American humanism and pedagogical liberation, respectively. Studying Africa involves many of these anthropological approaches and frameworks, but they seldom enter archaeological thinking in a directed fashion. Perhaps this is largely the result of their impact being somewhat outside of the domain of archaeology. Given that findings do not speak for themselves, and that many are old enough that they cannot be connected to contemporary groups or that they relate to the broader human race, using them to examine African existentialism (see Gordon 2000) may not be possible. But regardless, the present is contingent on the past, and knowing the past and using it has direct impact on contemporary groups. It is necessary to think about archaeology alongside colonial thinking in the same way that we can offset it with coloniality and expansion in Africa.

Post-colonial archaeology emerged as a critique of the discipline's complicity in colonial knowledge production and the unequal power dynamics embedded in archaeological interpretations. It challenges the ways in which archaeology has historically constructed narratives about others, particularly indigenous and colonised peoples, and questions whose voices, values, and knowledge systems shape our understanding of the past (Shepherd 2002; Atalay 2006). Central to this critique is the idea that archaeology was never a neutral science. Instead, it was, and often still is, entangled with political agendas, colonial projects, and the maintenance of global inequalities. One of the key concepts scrutinised by post-colonial archaeologists is the term 'culture' itself. Rather than being a neutral descriptor, 'culture' has historically served to categorise, essentialise, and confine groups of people within static, hierarchical frameworks. Scholars such as Said (1979, 1993) and Homi Bhabha (1994) argued that 'culture' was often deployed to position colonised or subaltern groups as 'other'. These notions were often coupled with a sense of unchanging, primitive, and fundamentally different from the west. This conceptualisation reinforced racial and civilisational hierarchies and justified colonial domination. As Burmeister (2023, p. 50) observed, in archaeological practice, the idea of culture frequently carried political weight, shaping who was seen as belonging to history and who was relegated to prehistory or savagery.

In African contexts, this dynamic is particularly evident. The colonial project relied on archaeological and ethnographic representations that froze African societies in time, portraying them as living examples of humanity's evolutionary past. Ethnography, which developed alongside archaeology, was instrumental in this process. Initially conceived in the mid-nineteenth century CE to study indigenous groups in the Americas, ethnography soon became a tool used globally to document 'disappearing' cultures (Trigger 1980). In the United States, it was explicitly linked to the idea of preserving indigenous cultures, while also facilitating their assimilation into Euro-American civilisation (Hinsley Jr 1985). Similar logics were applied in Africa, where archaeological and ethnographic studies often naturalised tribal divisions and presented African societies as static and incapable of change.

Post-colonial archaeology also foregrounds the politics of knowledge production. It asks, whose past is being studied, who is doing the studying, and to what ends? Nadia Abu El-Haj's (2001) study of archaeology in Israel powerfully demonstrated how archaeological practice can become entangled in nation-building, territorial claims, and identity politics. In her work, archaeology is not merely about unearthing the past; it is a field where colonial, national, and cultural imaginations are constructed and contested. Archaeology, she argued, operates at "the nexus of multiple social and political fields" (Abu El-Haj 2001, p. 2). Similar critiques have been raised in Africa, where the discipline's colonial roots have left lasting legacies. Nick Shepherd (2002, 2003) and Ndukuyakhe Ndlovu and Smith (2019) argued that African archaeology often reproduced Eurocentric scientific frameworks that marginalised local voices and knowledge systems. This is evident in debates about who controls heritage, whose narratives are prioritised, and how archaeological research relates to contemporary African identities and struggles for sovereignty. As Lane (2011) noted, post-colonial archaeology in Africa must grapple not only with the colonial past but also with the ongoing marginalisation of African scholars and communities in global archaeological discourse.

A growing body of work advocates for decolonising archaeology. It is a movement that proposes a shift in the power dynamics that have historically structured the discipline. This involves recognising indigenous knowledge systems, collaborating meaningfully with local communities, and questioning the universal applicability of Eurocentric scientific methods (Smith 2004; Atalay 2006, 2014). In Africa, this has taken the form of heritage projects that foreground local perspectives, efforts to repatriate cultural objects, and critical reflections on the discipline's role in reinforcing post-colonial inequalities (e.g., Meskell 2002; Fontein 2006; Schmidt 2009; Chirikure 2020; Hicks 2020; Lupuwana 2024). Additionally, the process of decolonising archaeology is not just a critique of the past but a call to rethink the purpose and practice of archaeology in the present. It demands that archaeologists engage with the political implications of their work, especially where the stakes of heritage, identity, and memory remain deeply contested. As the following chapters explore, this shift has profound implications for how archaeology is conducted on the continent, and whose pasts it seeks to recover.

3.6 Archaeology and the Making of the Past

Defining archaeology has never been simple, nor is there consensus. As the discipline evolved, so too did the ways in which it was described and practised. For some, like Binford (1962, 1983), archaeology sought generalisable models of cultural change; for others, it was about reconstructing the past through material traces (Gardin 1980; Klejn 2001). What most perspectives share is an emphasis on the recovery and analysis of cultural materials to explore human history (Trigger 2006). Yet archaeology is inherently interdisciplinary, borrowing techniques and theories from fields as diverse as botany, philosophy, psychology, and indigenous knowledge systems (Maggio 2018). Its distinctiveness lies in grappling with the materiality of human life, piecing together past behaviours, choices, and social structures without the benefit of direct observation (Meskell 2002; Trigger 2006). This distance forces archaeology into a space of both scientific conjecture and creative reconstruction, shaping its enduring debates and methodologies.

While this chapter has traced a broad intellectual history of archaeology, it must be stated that the discipline's change is not a neat linear progression. Theories rise, overlap, and sometimes fracture, with few offering a singular solution to the challenges of interpreting the past. Instead, archaeology today is an assemblage of approaches that are complementary, contradictory, and always evolving. The once-fiery debates between schools have cooled, replaced by a more pragmatic recognition that each framework, with its own interests and methods, contributes to a richer understanding of human history, if contested. This context is crucial for what follows. As the book turns toward archaeology in Africa, it explores how archaeology on the continent has developed within, against, and beyond these global currents. Shaped by its own histories of colonialism, nationalism, and scientific ambition, African archaeology grapples with many of the same tensions: power and knowledge, memory and material, past and present. As Angela Bond and George Gilliam (1994, p. 5) stated "[s]ocial constructions of both the past and the present are pliable, flexible and amenable to different interpretations and interests." Archaeology's role in these constructions requires close attention, particularly in Africa, where its impacts remain deeply entangled with contemporary identities, politics, and the pursuit of historical understanding.

References

Abu El-Haj, N. 2001. *Facts on the ground: Archaeological practice and territorial self-fashioning in Israeli society*. Chicago: University of Chicago Press.

Adams, W. Y., D. P. Van Gerven, and R. S. Levy. 1978. The retreat from migrationism. *Annual Review of Anthropology* 7:483–532.

Anthony, D. W. 1990. Migration in archeology: The baby and the bathwater. *American Anthropologist* 92 (4): 895–914.

Ascher, R. 1961. Analogy in archaeological interpretation. *Southwestern Journal of Anthropology* 17:317–325.

Atalay, S. 2006. Guest editor's remarks: Decolonising archaeology. *American Indian Quarterly* 30:269–279.
Atalay, S. 2014. Engaging archaeology: Positivism, objectivity, and rigor in activist archaeology. In *Transforming archaeology*, ed. S. Atalay, L. R. Clauss, R. H. McGuire, and J. R. Welch, 45–59. London: Routledge.
Bahn, P. 2014. The archaeology of archaeology: Pre-modern views of the past. In *The history of archaeology: An introduction*, ed. P. Bahn, 1–14. London: Routledge.
Barham, L. 1992. Let's walk before we run: An appraisal of historical materialist approaches to the later Stone Age. *South African Archaeological Bulletin* 47:44–51.
Bhabha, H. K. 1994. *The location of culture*. London: Routledge.
Binford, L. R. 1962. *Archaeology as anthropology. American antiquity* 28 (2): 217–225.
Binford, L. R., ed. 1977. *For theory building in archaeology*. New York: Academic.
Binford, L. R. 1983. *In pursuit of the past: Decoding the archaeological record*. London: Thames & Hudson.
Binford, L. R. 2009. Science to seance, or processual to "post-processual" archaeology. In *Debating archaeology*, ed. L. R. Binford, 27–40. New York: Routledge.
Binford, L. R., and J. A. Sabloff. 1982. Paradigms, systematics, and archaeology. *Journal of Anthropological Research* 38:137–153.
Blackie, M. A. L. 2022. An examination of the practice of chemistry through the lens of critical realism. *Journal of Critical Realism* 21 (4): 401–415.
Bloch, M. 1982. *Death, women and power: Anthropology of mortuary rituals*. London: Free Association Books.
Bond, G. C., and A. Gilliam. 1994. Introduction. In *Social construction of the past: representation as power*, ed. G. C. Bond and A. Gilliam, 1–22. London: Routledge.
Bostoen, K. 2020. The Bantu expansion: Some facts and fiction. In *Language dispersal, diversification, and contact*, ed. M. Crevels and P. Muysken. Oxford: Oxford University Press. https://doi.org/10.1093/oso/9780198723813.003.0013
Bourdieu, P. 1972. *Outline of a theory of practice*. Cambridge: Cambridge University Press.
Bourdieu, P. 1986. The forms of capital. In *Handbook of theory and research for the sociology of education*, ed. J. Richardson, 241–258. Greenwood: Westport.
Burmeister, S. 2000. Archaeology and migration: Approaches to an archaeological proof of migration. *Current Anthropology* 41 (4): 539–567.
Burmeister, S. 2023. Gustaf Kossinna's nationalistic agenda as Trojan horse in the archaeological concept of culture. *CAS Sofia Working Paper Series* 2 (14): 48–59.
Chapman, J., and H. Hamerow, eds. 1998. *Migrations and invasions in archaeological perspective*. Oxford: British Archaeological Reports.
Chapman, R. 2003. *Archaeologies of complexity*. London: Routledge.
Childe, V. G. 1925. *The Aryans: A study of Indo-European origins*. London: Routledge and Kegan Paul.
Childe, V. G. 1929. *The dawn of European civilization*. London: Routledge and Kegan Paul.
Childe, V. G. 1950. *Prehistoric migrations in Europe*. Oslo: Institutet for Sammenlignende Kulturforskning.
Chirikure, S. 2020. *Great Zimbabwe: Reclaiming a 'confiscated' past*. London: Routledge.
Clarke, D. 1973. Archaeology: The loss of innocence. *Antiquity* 47 (185): 6–18.
Clarke, D. 1978. *Analytical archaeology*. London: Metheun.
Daniel, G. 1950. *A hundred years of archaeology*. London: Gerald Duckworth.
Deloria, V. 1994. *God is red: A native view of religion*. Arvada: Fulcrum Publishing.
Díaz-Andreu, M. 2018. Archaeology and imperialism: From nineteenth-century new imperialism to twentieth-century decolonization. In *Unmasking ideology in imperial and colonial archaeology: Vocabulary, symbols, and legacy*, ed. B. Effros and G. Lai, 3–28. Los Angelse: Costen Institute of Archaeology.
Dodson, A. 1988. Egypt's first antiquarians? *Antiquity* 62:513–517.

Du Bois, W. E. B. 1897. *The conservation of the races*. Washington: The America Negro Academy Occassional Papers.

Du Bois, W. E. B. 1898. *The study of the Negro problems*. Washington: The America Negro Academy Occassional Papers.

Dunnell, R. 2001. United States of America, prehistoric archaeology. In *Encyclopedia of archaeology: History and discoveries*, ed. T. Murray, 1289–1307. Santa Barbara: ABC-CLIO.

Dussel, E. 1996. *The underside of modernity: Apel, Ricoeur, Rorty, Taylor, and the philosophy of liberation*. New York: Prometheus Books/Humanity Books.

Earle, T. K., and R. W. Preucel. 1987. Processual archaeology and the radical critique. *Current Anthropology* 28 (4): 501–538.

Edwards, I. E. S. 1985. *The pyramids of Egypt*. Revised ed. Harmondsworth: Penguin.

Fagan, B. M., and N. Durrani. 2016. *A brief history of archaeology: Classical times to the twenty-first century*. London: Routledge.

Fanon, F. 1967. *The wretched of the Earth*. Harmondsworth: Penguin Books.

Flannery, K., and J. Marcus. 1993. Cognitive archaeology. *Cambridge Archaeological Journal* 3:260–267.

Fleck, L., 1981. *Genesis and development of a scientific fact*. Chicago: University of Chicago Press.

Flowers, R. 2011. *Napoleon to Nasser:The story of modern Egypt*. New Orleans: Garrett Country Press.

Fontein, J. 2006. *The silence of great Zimbabwe: Contested landscapes and the power of heritage*. London: Routledge.

Foucault, M. 1970. *The order of things: An archaeology of the human sciences*. London: Tavistock.

Friere, P. 1990. *Pedagogy of the oppressed*. New York: Continuum.

Gándara, M. 1980. La vieja "Nueva Arqueolog'ıa" (primera parte). *Antropolgia Americana* 2:7–45.

Gardin, J. C. 1980. *Archaeological constructs: An aspect of theoretical archaeology*. Cambridge: Cambridge University Press.

Garvey, R. 2018. Current and potential roles of archaeology in the development of cultural evolutionary theory. *Philosophical Transactions of the Royal Society B: Biological Sciences* 373 (1743): 20170057.

Giblin, J. 2013. Politics, ideology, and indigenous perspectives. In *The Oxford handbook of African archaeology*, ed. P. J. Mitchell and P. J. Lane, 253–265. Oxford: Oxford University Press.

Giddens, A. 1984. *The constitution of society*. Berkley: University of California Press.

Gordon, L. 2000. *Existentia Africana: Understanding Africana existential thought*. New York: Routledge.

Graebner, F. 1911. *Methode der Ethnologie*. Heidelberg: C. Winter.

Greenhalgh, M. 2013. *From the Romans to the railways: The fate of antiquities in Asia Minor*. Leiden: Brill.

Grollemund, R., S. Branford, K. Bostoen, A. Meade, C. Venditti, and M. Pagel. 2015. Bantu expansion shows that habitat alters the route and pace of human dispersals. *Proceedings of the National Academy of Sciences* 112:13296–13301.

Grollemund, R., D. Schoenbrun, and J. Vansina. 2023. Moving histories: Bantu language expansions, eclectic economies, and Mobilities. *Journal of African History* 64 (1): 13–37.

Grünert, H. 2002. *Gustaf Kossinna (1858–1931). Vom Germanisten zum Prähistoriker. Ein Wis senschaftler im Kaiserreich und in der Weimarer Republik*. Rahden/Westfalen: Leidorf.

Härke, H. 1998. Archaeologists and migrations: A problem of attitude? *Current Anthropology* 39 (1): 19–46.

Hawkes, J. 1968. The proper study of mankind. *Antiquity* 42:255–262.

Heizer, R. F., ed. 1962. *Man's discovery of his past: Literary landmarks in archaeology*. Englewood Cliffs: Prentice-Hall.

Henry, P. 2000. *Caliban's reason: Introducing in Afro-Caribbean philosophy*. New York: Routledge.

Hicks, D. 2020. *The Brutish museums: The Benin bronzes, colonial violence and cultural restitution*. London: Pluto Press.

Hinsley, C. M., Jr. 1985. From shell-heaps to stelae: Early anthropology at the Peabody Museum. In *Objects and others: Essays on museums and material culture*, ed. G. W. Stocking, 49–74. New York: Free Press.

Hodder, I. 1982. *Symbols in action*. Cambridge: Cambridge University Press.

Hodder, I. 1986. *Reading the past*. Cambridge: Cambridge University Press.

Hodder, I. 1987. *The archaeology of contextual meaning*. Cambridge: Cambridge University Press.

Hodder, I. 1991. Interpretive archaeology and its role. *American Antiquity* 56:7–18.

Hodder, I. 2001. Postprocessual archaeology and the current debate. In *Processual and post-processual archaeology: Multiple ways of knowing the past*, ed. R. W. Preucel, 30–41. Carbondale: Southern Illinois University at Carbondale.

Hoebel, E. A. 1949. *Man in the primitive world*. New York: McGraw-Hill.

Holl, A. F. C. 1990. West African archaeology: Colonialism and nationalism. In *A history of African archaeology*, ed. P. Robertshaw, 296–308. Oxford: James Currey Ltd.

Hooks, B. 1990. *Yearning: Race, gender, and cultural politics*. Boston: South End Press.

Huffman, T. N. 1986. Cognitive studies of the Iron Age in southern Africa. *World Archaeology* 18:84–95.

Huffman, T. N. 2004. Beyond data: The aim and practice of archaeology. *South African Archaeological Bulletin* 59:66–69.

Huffman, T. N. 2015. Settlements and culture: Cognitive models in African prehistory. In *Theory in Africa, Africa in theory*, ed. S. Wynne-Jones and J. Fleisher, 111–136. London: Routledge.

Ikawa-Smith, F. 2001. Japan. In *Encyclopedia of archaeology: History and discoveries*, ed. T. Murray, 734–744. Santa Barbara: ABC-CLIO.

Johnson, M.H., 2010. *Archaeological theory*. Chichester: Wiley-Blackwell.

Jones, D. S. 2024. Protecting Australian first nation's Dja: Whither cultural values assessments about country in the face of land use development pressures. In *Sacred landscapes, indigenous knowledge, and ethno-culture in natural resource management*, ed. S. C. Rai and P. K. Mishra, 227–267. Springer Nature Singapore: Singapore.

Joyce, R. A. 2003. Concrete memories: Fragments of the past in the classic Maya present (500–1000 AD). In *Archaeologies of memory*, ed. R. M. Van Dyke and S. E. Alcock, 104–125. Oxford: Blackwell Publishing.

Klejn, L. 2001. Metaarchaeology. *Acta Archaeologica* 27:1–149.

Koile, E., S. J. Greenhill, D. E. Blasi, R. Bouckaert, and R. D. Gray. 2022. Phylogeographic analysis of the Bantu language expansion supports a rainforest route. *Proceedings of the National Academy of Sciences* 119 (32): e2112853119.

Koselleck, R. 1992. Volk, nation, nationalismus, masse. In *Geschichtliche Grundbegriffe: Historisches Lexikon zur politischsozialen Sprache in Deutschland*, ed. O. Brunner, W. Conze, and R. Koselleck, 141–431. Stuttgart: Klett-Cotta.

Kossinna, G. 1911. *Die Herkunft der Germanen. Zur methode der siedlungsarchäologie*. Würzburg: Kabitzsch.

Kuhn, T. 1962. *The structure of scientific revolutions*. Chicago: University of Chicago Press.

Kuhn, T. 1970. *The structure of scientific revolutions*. Chicago: University of Chicago Press.

Lane, P. J. 2004. The 'moving frontier' and the transition to food production in Kenya. *Azania: Archaeological Research in Africa* 39 (1): 243–264.

Lane, P. J. 2011. Possibilities for a postcolonial archaeology in sub-Saharan Africa: Indigenous and usable pasts. *World Archaeology* 43 (1): 7–25.

LeBlanc, S. A., and P. J. Watson. 2014. Processualism in archaeological theory. In *Encyclopedia of global archaeology*, ed. C. Smith, 6144–6149. New York: Springer Science+Business Media.

Lema, A. 1993. *Africa divided: The creation of "ethnic groups"*. Lund: Lund University Press.

Leone, M. 1982. Some opinions about recovering mind. *American Antiquity* 47:742–760.

Locke, A. 1925. *The new Negro: An interpretation*. New York: Albert and Charles Boni.

Loprieno, A. 2003. Views of the past in Egypt during the first millennium BC. In *"Never had the like occurred": Egypt's view of its past*, ed. J. Tait, 139–154. London: UCL Press.

Lupuwana, V. 2024. Heritage and social justice in southern Africa: Rethinking spaces of community involvement in heritage Management. In *Routledge handbook of critical African heritage studies*, ed. A. Sinamai, J. Giblin, S. Chirikure, and I. Odiaua, 88–100. Oxford: Routledge.
Maggio, A. 2018. Interdisciplinarity and archaeology. In *Encyclopedia of global archaeology*, ed. C. Smith, 1–7. Cham: Springer International Publishing.
Masterman, M. 1984. The nature of a paradigm. In *Criticism and the growth of knowledge*, ed. I. Lakatos and A. Musgrave, 59–89. Cambridge: Cambridge University Press.
Matos Moctezuma, E. 1984. The templo mayor of tenochtitlan: Economics and ideology. In *Ritual Human Sacrifice in Mesoamerica*, ed. E. Boone, 133–164. Washington: Dumbarton Oaks.
McCaskie, T. C. 1995. *State and society in pre-colonial Asante*. Cambridge: Cambridge University Press.
Merrick, H. V., and F. H. Brown. 1984. Obsidian sources and patterns of source utilization in Kenya and northern Tanzania: Some initial findings. *African Archaeological Review* 2:129–152.
Mertens, D. 2004. Die Instrumentalisiserung der "Germania" des Tacitus durch die deutschen Humanisten. In *Zur Geschichte der Gleichung "germanisch-deutsch". Sprache und Namen, Geschichte und Institutionen*, ed. H. Beck, D. Geunich, H. Steuer, and D. Hakelberg, 37–102. Berlin: Walter de Gruyter.
Meskell, L. 2002. The intersections of identity and politics in archaeology. *Annual Review of Anthropology* 31:279–301.
Meskell, L., and R. A. Joyce. 2003. *Embodied lives: Figuring ancient Maya and Egyptian experience*. London: Routledge.
Miller, D., and C. Tilley, eds. 1984. *Ideology, power and prehistory*. Cambridge: Cambridge University Press.
Mithen, S. 1996. *The prehistory of the mind: A search for the origins of art, religion, and science*. London: Thames & Hudson.
Moro Abadía, O., and M. R. González Morales. 2003. L'art bourgeois de la fin du XIXe si'ecle face 'a l'art mobilier Pal'eolithique. *L'anthropologie* 107:455–470.
Ndlovu, N., and B. W. Smith. 2019. The past is a divided country: Transforming archaeology in South Africa. *African Archaeological Review* 36:172–192.
Orme, B. 1973. Archaeology and ethnology. In *The explanation of culture change: Models in prehistory*, ed. C. Renfrew, 481–492. London: Duckworth.
Parkington, J. E. 1984. Soaqua and Bushmen: Hunters and robbers. In *Past and present in hunter-gatherer studies*, ed. C. Schrire, 151–174. New York: Academic.
Parkinson, R. B., W. Diffie, M. Fischer, and R. S. Simpson. 1999. *Cracking codes: The Rosetta Stone and decipherment*. Oakland: University of California Press.
Piggott, S. 1959. *Approach to archaeology*. Cambridge: Harvard University Press.
Pluciennik, M. 2005. *Social evolution*. London: Duckworth.
Posnansky, M. 1976. Archaeology and the origins of Akan society. In *Problems in economic and social archaeology*, ed. I. H. Longworth and K. E. Wilson, 49–59. London: Duckworth.
Puschner, U. 2004. Germanenideologie und völkische Weltanschauung. In *Zur Geschichte der Gleichung "germanisch-deutsch". Sprache und Namen, Geschichte und Institutionen*, ed. H. Beck, D. Geunich, H. Steuer, and D. Hakelberg, 103–130. Berlin: Walter de Gruyter.
Rapoport, H., S. Sardoschau, and A. Silve. 2020. *Migration and cultural change*. Munich: CESifo.
Ratzel, F. 1899. *Anthropogeographie*. Stuttgart: J. Engelhorn.
Renfrew, C. 1982. *Towards an archaeology of mind*. Cambridge: Cambridge University Press.
Renfrew, C. 1989. The origins of Indo-European languages. *Scientific American* 261 (4): 106–115.
Robertshaw, P. 1990a. *A history of African archaeology*. Oxford: James Currey Ltd.
Robertshaw, P. 1990b. A history of African archaeology: An introduction. In *A history of African archaeology*, ed. P. Robertshaw, 3–12. Oxford: James Currey Ltd.
Rowlands, M. 1989. Repetition and exteriorisation in narratives of historical origins. *Critique of Anthropology* 8:43–62.
Said, E. 1979. *Orientalism*. New York: Vintage.
Said, E. 1993. *Culture and imperialism*. New York: Knopf.

Schiffer, M. 1996. Some relationships between behavioral and evolutionary archaeologies. *American Antiquity* 61:643–662.

Schmidt, P. R. 2009. *Postcolonial archaeologies in Africa*. Santa Fe: School for Advanced Research Press.

Schnapp, A. 2014. The birth of the archaeological vision: From antiquaries to archaeologists. *West 86th: A Journal of Decorative Arts, Design History, and Material Culture* 21 (2): 216–229.

Schrire, C. 1980. An inquiry into the evolutionary status and apparent identity of San hunter-gatherers. *Human Ecology* 8 (1): 9–32.

Shanks, M. 1999. *Art and the early Greek state: An interpretive archaeology*. Cambridge: Cambridge University Press.

Shanks, M. 2008. Post-processual archaeology and after. In *Handbook of archaeological theories*, ed. R. A. Bentley, H. Maschner, and C. Chippindale, 133–147. Walnut Creek: AltaMira Press.

Shanks, M., and I. Hodder. 2013. Processual, postprocessual and interpretive archaeologies. In *Interpreting archaeology*, ed. M. Shanks and I. Hodder, 3–29. London: Routledge.

Shanks, M., and C. Tilley. 1987. *Social theory and archaeology*. Cambridge: Blackwell Polity.

Shanks, M., and C. Tilley. 1992. *Reconstructing archaeology: Theory and practice*. London: Routledge.

Shennan, S. J. 1987. Treads in the study of later European prehistory. *Annual Review of Anthropology* 16:365–382.

Shepherd, N. 2002. The politics of archaeology in Africa. *Annual Review of Anthropology* 31:189–209.

Shepherd, N. 2003. State of the discipline: Science, culture and identity in South African archaeology, 1870–2003. *Journal of Southern African Studies* 29 (4): 823–844.

Shortland, A. 2022. Napoleon, savants, and the Description de l'Égypte: Capturing history. In *Cultural heritage in modern conflict*, ed. T. Clack and M. Dunkley, 51–65. London: Routledge.

Smith, A. C. 2017. Winckelmann, Greek masterpieces, and architectural sculpture. Prolegomena to a history of classical archaeology in museums. *Studies in Classical Archaeology* 1:23–45.

Smith, B. W. 2010. Envisioning San history: Problems in the reading of history in the rock art of the Maloti-Drakensberg mountains of South Africa. *African Studies* 69 (2): 345–359.

Smith, L. 2000. A history of Aboriginal heritage legislation in south-eastern Australia. *Australian Archaeology* 50:109–118.

Smith, L. 2004. *Archaeological theory and the politics of cultural heritage*. Oxford: Routledge.

Spivak, G. 1988. Can the subaltern speak? In *Marxism and the interpretation of culture*, ed. C. Nelson and L. Grossberg, 271–313. Urbana-Champaign: University of Illinois Press.

Spon, J. 1673. *Recherche des antiquités et curiosités de la ville de Lyon*. Lyon: Faeton.

Strathern, P. 2008. *Napoleon in Egypt*. London: Random House.

Tait, J. 2003. *"Never had the like occurred": Egypt's view of its past*. London: UCL Press.

Taylor, W. W. 1948. *A study of archeology*. 69th ed. Menasha: American Anthropological Association Memoir.

Thwaites, R. G. 1896. *The Jesuit relations and allied documents*. Cleveland: Burrows Brothers.

Tilley, C. Y. 1994. *A phenomenology of landscape: Places, paths, and monuments*. Oxford: Berg.

Tomasello, M., M. Carpenter, J. Call, T. Behne, and H. Moll. 2005. Understanding and sharing intentions: The origins of cultural cognition. *Behavioral and Brain Sciences* 28 (5): 675–691.

Toulmin, S. E. 1970. Does the distinction between normal and revolutionary science hold water? In *Criticism and the growth of knowledge*, ed. I. Lakatos and A. Musgrave, 39–47. Cambridge: Cambridge University Press.

Trigger, B. G. 1969. The myth of Meroe and the African Iron Age. *African Historical Studies* 2 (1): 23–50.

Trigger, B. G. 1980. Archaeology and the image of the American Indian. *American Antiquity* 45 (4): 662–676.

Trigger, B. G. 1984. Archaeology at the crossroads: What's new. *Annual Review of Anthropology* 13:275–300.

Trigger, B. G. 1989. Archaeology and anthropology: Current and future relations. *Canadian Journal of Archeology* 13:1–11.
Trigger, B. G. 1990. The history of African archaeology in world perspective. In *A history of African archaeology*, ed. P. Robertshaw, 303–319. Oxford: James Currey Ltd.
Trigger, B. G. 2006. *A History of archaeological thought*. 2nd ed. Cambridge: Cambridge University Press.
Ucko, P. J. 1995. Introduction: Archaeological interpretation in a world context. In *Theory in Archaeology: A world perspective*, ed. P. J. Ucko, 1–28. London: Taylor & Francis.
VanPool, T., and C. S. VanPool, eds. 2003. *Essential tensions in archaeological method and theory*. Salt Lake City: University of Utah Press.
Veit, U. 1984. Gustaf Kossinna und V. Gordon Childe: Ansatze zu einer theoretischen Grundlegung der Vorgeschichte. *Saeculum* 35:326–364.
Watson, R. 1990. Ozymandias, king of kings: Postprocessual radical archaeology as critique. *American Antiquity* 55:673–689.
West, C. 1982. *Prophesy, deliverance!: An Afro-American revolutionary Christianity*. Philadelphia: Westminster Press.
Willey, G. R., and P. Phillips. 1958. *Method and theory in archaeology*. Chicago: University of Chicago Press.
Winckelmann, J. J. 1764. *Geschichte der Kunst des Alterthums*. Dresden: Johann Thomas von Trattner.
Wobst, H. M. 1978. The archaeo-ethnology of hunter-gatherers or the tyranny of the ethnographic record in archaeology. *American Antiquity* 43 (2): 303–309.
Wolf, E. 1982. *Europe and the people without history*. Berkley: University of California Press.
Yoffee, N., and A. Sherratt, eds. 1993. *Archaeological theory: Who sets the agenda?* Cambridge: Cambridge University Press.

Chapter 4
Antiquarianism, Collections, Missionaries: The Early Years

Abstract This chapter examines the late nineteenth- to early twentieth-century CE, when Africa's past became an object of European fascination. Opening with the Berlin Conference and the scramble for Africa, it traces how museums, missionary networks, administrators, and travellers assembled objects and narratives that mapped neatly onto colonial priorities. Different colonial regimes, ecologies, and precolonial histories are reviewed, each producing distinct archaeological perspectives and archives. Yet a common pattern emerges: archaeology served as a technology of rule and display, simultaneously erasing and exoticising African agency. The chapter also recovers the African presence often excluded from research approaches. By the close, it is clear how the infrastructures of collecting and knowledge production laid both constraints and foundations for later scholarship, and how early interpretations sedimented into museum canons and public imaginaries that persist. Recognising these origins is essential for understanding subsequent efforts to provincialise, repatriate, and re-narrate Africa's archaeological heritage.

Twelve European nations along with the United States and the Ottoman Empire gathered in the summer of 1884 CE in Wilhelmstrasse, Germany. They were there on invitation of the German Chancellor, Otto van Bismarck. The delegates were seated in the Reich Chancellery around a horse-shoe table overlooking expansive, well-curated gardens. Not all nations represented agreed with one another at the time; the table was being shared by members of states with vastly different views to one another and attritional political histories. Yet all of these nations were there for another, more profound purpose. Hanging above the table, was a map of Africa, very dissimilar to what we find today. Their task, which took 4 months to complete, from 15 November to 26 February of the following year, was to agree on how to divide Africa and share it among themselves (Fig. 4.1). No African nation, king, or representative was invited to the meeting, although it became known as the West Africa or Congo Conference (Uzoigwe 1985, p. 15). Africans were included, apparently, as beneficiaries since Europe was to bring to them civilisation, education, religion, economy, and development. However, all of this was about to be lost to Africa along

T. Forssman, *Archaeology in Africa: Why the Past Matters*, Archaeology of Africa,
https://doi.org/10.1007/978-3-032-13365-6_4

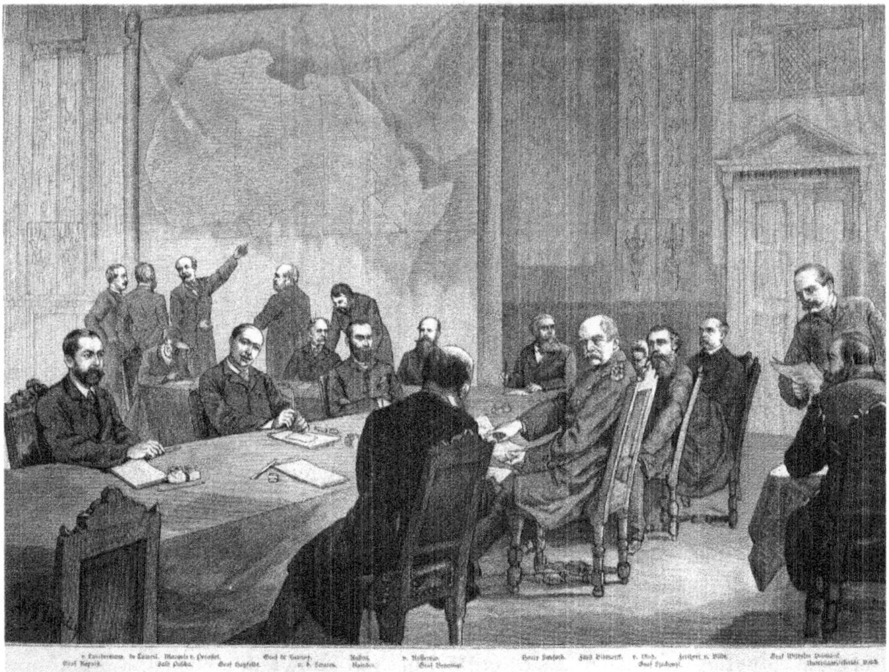

Fig. 4.1 A depiction of the Berlin congress with a map of Africa hanging above the table. *Source* https://commons.wikimedia.org/wiki/File:Kongokonferenz.jpg

with its territory as Europe furthered its imperialism over Africa and fixed it into a Western image, taming the continent and its people.

By the time the Berlin Conference was convened, the so-called Scramble for Africa was already well underway. Portuguese influence on the continent was declining, while British and French imperial ambitions were expanding rapidly (Rashid 2014). The primary purpose of the congress was not to initiate colonisation but to regulate it. In effect, it legitimised existing and future European claims by formalising the rules for Africa's partition. While one of the stated aims was to consider the interests of African people, it remains unclear what this meant in practice, if anything. Questions of African sovereignty were entirely excluded from the discussion. The agenda was unmistakably economic, focused on securing access to trade and resources. The resulting General Act, signed by 13 European powers (excluding the United States), outlawed slavery, established free trade in Central Africa, and laid out the legal basis for European occupation of African territories. In doing so, the conference sanctioned both colonisation and imperialism—overlapping processes referred to here collectively as colonisation (see Jacobs 1996, p. 16; Ypi 2013; Kohn and Reddy 2024). It also laid the foundation for what Terence Ranger (1993, p. 6) later described as the "systematic invention of African traditions" to serve colonial governance. A central motivation behind the conference was to prevent conflict between European states as they competed for territory (De Leon 1886). At the time, European control was mostly confined to coastal zones, and the Berlin Act provided a framework for expanding into Africa's interior with international backing.

Africa's coastline had become a largely accessible strip of territory and burgeoning trade increased its commercial value. The trade that it enabled made it possible for European nations to explore and settle vast regions of the New World and finance the industrial revolution (Williams 1966). The impact this had on Africa, however, was immense. Hussein Bulhan (2015) summarised at least three outcomes from trans-Atlantic trade: it depopulated the African continent, consolidated the dominated-dominant dichotomy between Africa and Europe, and the economic benefits propelled Europe forward, allowing them to conquer additional lands and people. These outcomes are further unpacked in Walter Rodney's (1972) seminal work *How Europe Underdeveloped Africa.* While history cannot be so reduced, it is far more dynamic, nuanced and regionalised, the outcome was a Europe marching towards far wider dominion leading into the nineteenth century CE. By the end of the century the partitioning of Africa would unfold in a short space of time, approximately two decades, and by its end the continent was divided with mostly new and unfamiliar boundaries (Sanderson 1975).

Africa's partitioning was a complex process and the result of a longer sequence of European expansion and occupation, as well as African responses. It is contested in many regards as the history is not straight-forward in all cases. Much of it, for example, was not recorded in great detail for various political and economic reasons. It also has roots in internal European nation-building processes and other contexts; material, strategic and social in nature (Barnhart 2016). There is also seldom agreement on all the processes driving the scramble for Africa's territories. In the context of this book, it is not feasible to fully review colonialism as it unfolded from the late nineteenth century CE onwards. For more information on these historical processes, alternate sources should be consulted (Robinson and Gallagher 1966; Chamberlain 1974; Sanderson 1975; Pakenham 1991; Mommsen 1995; e.g., Barnhart 2016; Rash and Horan 2021).

4.1 Approaching the Past at the Birth of Colonialism

> There is no novelty in the observation that history often serves to rationalise national purpose, and that archaeology is a form of historical inquiry. But the history espoused by officialdom conventionally serves to sanction present practices by arguing that they have always been thus. Colonial ventures are ruptures of what has always, or at least previously, been. In this context, archaeology has been a vehicle for explaining away the obvious, for transforming a decisive break with the past into an inconsequential moment, and it can do this because its esoteric practices uncover a past invisible to the observer. Absent approval from the deity (which, of course, many have claimed) colonialists may not be able to find a better means to justify actions illegal by any people's customary standards (Kuklick 1991, p. 165)

Henrika Kuklick's (1991) reflection captures how colonial powers relied on archaeology to reframe ruptures as continuity, and in so doing legitimise domination by manufacturing historical inevitability. This logic extended into broader narratives about Africa itself. Colonial commentators portrayed the continent as historically stagnant, devoid of independent innovation, and in need of external intervention. Africa was cast as an evolutionary backwater, its communities framed as living relics. Statements such as "Africa has never invented anything, but has only received from others" (Ankermann 1905, p. 55) were symptomatic of a wider belief in African inferiority. Instead, Africa's history was populated with wild, fantastical interpretations that squarely placed foreign and exotic origins or connections for much of its attributes (Pwiti and Ndoro 1999; Folorunso 2003; Solomon 2014). Kuklick (1991, p. 147) summarised the dominant sentiment at the time as "Africans were incapable of great achievements unless forcefully supervised by a superior race". What is often the case, the superior race that introduced transformative change in Africa were from the north (Hall 1905; e.g., Breuil 1948), including Egyptians, the so-called Hamites, Phoenicians, Semites and more (Solomon 2014, p. 120). These views ultimately considered Africa's architecture, art and culture as imports, arriving via either migration or diffusion.

During the colonial expansion into Africa, the expectation of interesting archaeology was almost absent outside of already known regions such as Egypt, Ethiopia and other parts of North Africa. The views of David Hume, Georg Hegel and Hugh Trevor-Roper are all reflections of this attitude. Hegel (1894) argued for example, that sub-Saharan Africans' migration through Africa was destructive and that local cultures were of no significance. Thomas Bowen (1857, p. 18), a missionary in 1857, who identified the first stone tools from Nigeria, opened his book, *Central Africa: Adventures and missionary labors*, by stating that "[n]o quarter of the globe is so imperfectly known as Africa", going onto note that it is "cut off from the rest of the world". He conceded shortly after that the fifteenth and sixteenth centuries CE Portuguese knew more of Africa than he and his peers did in the nineteenth century. By and large, though, people knew very little of Africa even after centuries of expansionism and the onset of colonialism. As William Du Bois (1896) commented, Africa was left without a culture or history.

The colonial period brought upon an influx of Europeans into sub-Saharan Africa. This resulted in an increase in the identification of archaeological materials. Missionaries, geologists, soldiers, mining engineers, and administrators, among others, noted various finds. Notably, none of these investigators had archaeological training. Many were inflicted by what has been dubbed the 'Egyptian disease', and because diffusion was the main explanatory source, most of these finds were attributed to places far way. During this period, Egyptians as great explorers was propagated and used to explain much of Africa's past; they brought light to a dark world (Smith 1915, 1933; Perry 1923). These ideas leaned heavily into the dominant discourse of the time and used diffusion to explain the past. Thurston Shaw (1989, pp. 6–7) saw these notions embedded in Rudyard Kipling's (1931, pp. 320–326) 'a white man's burden'; the period during which enlightenment brought European nations into a dark Africa in the same manner that they imagined the Egyptians had done before them. Colonial administrators sought out Egyptian finds in the places they worked as a result of their belief that diffusion is what led to the appearance of archaeological finds in sub-Saharan Africa (e.g., Delafosse 1900; Johnston 1913; Talbot 1926; Seligman 1930; Meek 1931; Palmer 1936; Meyerowitz 1960). Cheik Anta Diop (1960) used this same approach in his hyperdiffusionist reimagining of Africa's past (discussed further in Chap. 6).

There are many early accounts of Africa and its past, briefly discussed in Chapter Chap. 1, that pre-date the onset of colonialism. Probably the earliest made by outsiders was from the Phoenicians who originated in what is now Lebanon and eventually established a capital called Carthage in the late fifteenth century BCE on the North African coastline (Scott 2018). There are records that the Pharaoh Necho II (615–595 BCE) commissioned a fleet of Phoenician ships to set sail and observe if Africa could be circumnavigated. The fleet departed from the Red Sea, settled each year in a new location to plant crops and resupply themselves before moving on, and eventually returned through the Pillars of Hercules, which today is the Strait of Gibraltar between Morocco and Spain (Branigan 1994). Although Phoenician technology was capable of undertaking such a journey, convincing evidence is absent (Issawi 1952, p. 117) and such a tale may appeal more to popular and colonial imaginaries than reality (noted early on by Webb 1906, 1907). However, they did sail down to probably the Equator along the West African coastline and noted, among various things, an erupting volcano, probably Mt. Kakulima in Guinea, and what might have been gorillas or chimpanzees but which they thought were a wild human tribe (Branigan 1994). The latter view was reported by Ptolemy and only dispelled when the Portuguese sailed to the region in the fifteenth century CE.

From the outset of European settlement in Africa, there were attempts, however modest, to record aspects of the continent's past. These early observations were often incidental, shaped by encounters with resident communities who shared their knowledge and material worlds. At the Cape, Dutch settlers noted local customs and traditions as early as the seventeenth century CE (Gabel 1985, p. 242), and reports of rock art also surfaced intermittently. One of the first recorded instances came in 1721 CE, when the Bishop of Mozambique described painted rock shelters to the Royal Academy of History in Lisbon. Yet these fleeting moments of recognition rarely translated into systematic inquiry. Colonel Robert Gordon and his draughtsman Johannes Schumacher, for instance, copied rock paintings in 1777 CE with the assistance of San guides, but their renderings were never published (Gabel 1985). It was not until 1869 CE that George William Stow began recording San art in a more sustained way, though his drawings only reached publication in 1930 (Duffey 2002, 2012). Notably, these African records preceded the recognition of similar European art (Posnansky 1982, p. 345). Other fragments of Africa's past entered European collections through missionary activity, but such examples were rare (Anquandah 1981, 1985; Randsborg 2001). Until the mid-nineteenth century CE, records remained sporadic and unsystematic. It was only after about 1850 CE that more regular commentary and sustained efforts to investigate the African past began to appear. Even then, they were geographically uneven. Southern Africa emerged as an early locus for more consistent engagement, where archaeological observations gradually accumulated into broader regional syntheses.

4.1.1 Southern Africa

Archaeology in southern Africa during the second half of the nineteenth century CE was shaped by uneven practices, Eurocentric ideologies, and the search for both lost treasure and 'white' history. Of all the finds made during this period, which included early investigations of stone tools as well as rock art, none captured European imagination, or became so fiercely contested, as Great Zimbabwe. The site emerged as a focal point for debates about race, civilisation, and Africa's place in global history.

Early antiquarians such as Andrew Anderson (1888) and Edward Dunn (1880) reflected the growing interest in the African past. In 1866, Anderson (1888) travelled north to the Limpopo River region, where he recorded engravings and collected artefacts across South Africa, Botswana, and Zimbabwe, and also visited Namibia. His contributions, though largely forgotten, were substantial (Eastwood and Blundell 1999, p. 19; Mitchell 2001). The collection he sold to the British Museum included 178 stone tools, 29 ostrich eggshell beads, and more from over 50 locations – still the largest single acquisition of southern African material in the museum's holdings (Mitchell 2001, p. 39). Dunn's (1880) work in the 1870s, while similarly extensive, suffered from the absence of provenance and analytical rigour. His work is not as widely recognised as others of his era, such as William Atherstone, Thomas Baines or Thomas and Henry Bowker (Parsons 2013), but he collected a large assemblage of what are important finds, which have subsequently been studied, including painted stones, stone tools (Mitchell 2013), and ceramics (Bollong et al. 1997). Finds were, however, being made across South Africa, such as by John Rickard (1881), an antiquarian and collector studying in East London, Port Elizabeth (Gqeberha), and Riet and Modder River areas (Shepherd 2002), and later Henry Feilden (1905) would collect the first stone tool specimens from Victoria Falls. These accounts demonstrate key trends from the period: the accumulation of material without systematic context, and developing curiosity about the deeper human past.

It was Karl Mauch (1874), a German explorer, who placed southern African archaeology on a global stage. In 1871, guided by local knowledge, Mauch (1874) arrived at Great Zimbabwe (Fig. 4.2). The hilltop site and stone-walled complex was already known to communities in the region, and possibly occupied by Jan Renders in 1868 (Manyanga and Chirikure 2019), and they led Mauch to the site. There he wondered (cf. Burke 1969, p. 139):

> Some more people were questioned about this pot and they, too, told curious stories about it. There was one among these people who came forth with still more important news, namely of the presence of quite large ruins which could never have been made by blacks. Could these be the ruins of the Banyai for which I've been looking?

Mauch (1874) portrayed his visit as a discovery and immediately projected biblical myths onto the ruins. Convinced he had located the palace of the Queen of Sheba and the biblical Ophir, he compared lintel fragments to the cedar wood in his pencil to justify his claims (Burke 1969, p. 190; Matenga 1998, p. 22). These fantasies resonated with European desires for a noble past in Africa that was not African in origin (Fontein 2006). They also appealed to Cecil John Rhodes and his British South Africa Company, who were both enamoured by the site and capitalised on these narratives (Manyanga and Chirikure 2019). After invading Zimbabwe with the Pioneer Column in 1890 CE, Rhodes promoted the idea that Great Zimbabwe was the product of a Caucasian civilisation, thereby justifying settler claims to the land (Fontein 2006; Chirikure 2020). The Rhodesia Ancient Ruins Company, active between 1895 and 1900, formalised looting as policy. One of the famous soapstone birds had already been stolen by Willi Posselt, and at least 50 sites were pillaged in the search for gold (Ransford 1968). These actions caused immense archaeological destruction and were driven by the fantasy of discovering treasure rather than historical understanding.

The excavations that followed at Great Zimbabwe – from Theodore Bent and Richard Hall to David Randal-MacIver and Gertrude Caton-Thompson – revealed the extent to which archaeology was shaped by the ideological currents of the time, and how evidence itself became contested terrain. The first professional investigations at Great Zimbabwe were carried out by Bent (1896) in the 1890s. Initially, he was sceptical of Mauch's (1874) biblical interpretation, and admitted regularly to finding evidence that largely supported a local origin. In fact, he was disappointed in these results and actively sought out evidence in rejection of them. Bent (1896) soon abandoned impartiality and sought evidence for an Arabian or Phoenician origin,

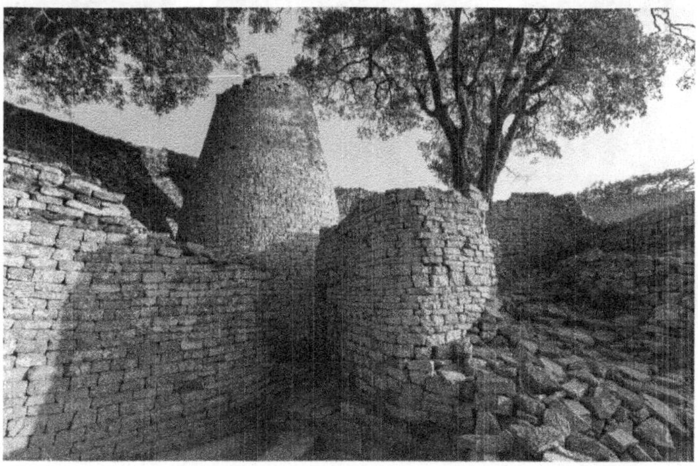

Fig. 4.2 The stone cairn in the valley complex, generally considered to be a female area (photograph: Andrew Moore). *Source* https://commons.wikimedia.org/wiki/File:Conical_Tower_-_Great_Enclosure_III_(33,736,918,448).jpg

which he eventually saw evidence for in the soapstone birds (Fig. 4.3), along with other items such as bowls and monoliths. He ultimately concluded that this came from the Arabian Peninsula and would posit the idea that Phoenicians were involved, tentatively at first. After Bent, Hall (1905) was appointed curator in 1902. His clearance of deposit under the guise of preservation far exceeded the damage done by looters (Garlake 1973, p. 72; Gabel 1985) and his work was unacceptable and accompanied by plundering (Manyanga and Chirikure 2019, p. 76). Hall (1905) insisted that the walls were built by Sabaeans and later he concluded Phoenicians, reinforcing diffusionist and racialised models of history. Though dismissed in 1905, his interpretations had already gained widespread popularity and were being circulated through the media. A turning point came in 1906 with the arrival of Randal-MacIver (1906), supported by the British Association for the Advancement of Science. His excavations identified material culture similar to that of the local Shona, including ceramics and metals, found from the base of the walls through to the upper layers. He proposed a fourteenth century CE date based on imported beads. Despite the data, his findings were resisted, particularly by settlers who saw them as a threat to the colonial narrative (Fontein 2006). Caton-Thompson (1931) later recovered evidence in support of Randal-MacIver's conclusions through her own excavations.

The controversy surrounding Great Zimbabwe exemplifies how archaeology became entangled with colonial power. While some archaeologists challenged Eurocentric myths, others upheld them, and settler resistance often overruled evidence. During the Rhodesian era after 1965, efforts to assert a local origin were censored. Peter Garlake (1973, 1982), who advocated for a Shona-built Zimbabwe, was deported. Locals who adopted these views were also censored (Ndoro 1997). The

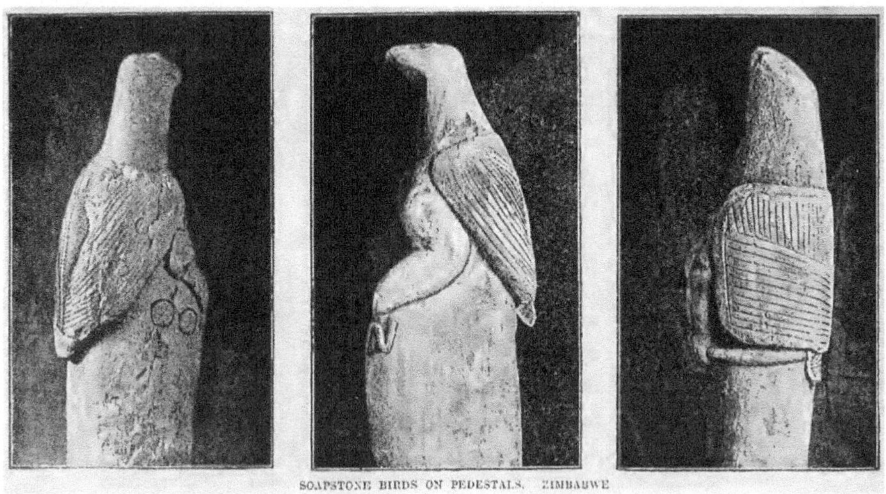

Fig. 4.3 Three soapstone birds from found at Great Zimbabwe, photographed c. 1981. *Source* https://commons.wikimedia.org/wiki/File:Soapstone_birds_on_pedestals.jpg

power placed in Great Zimbabwe was palpable in the late-nineteenth and early twentieth centuries CE, and its role in nation-building was seen as crucial to early statehood success.

Across southern Africa, archaeological investigations during this period were often marked by similar entanglements of racial ideology, speculative interpretation, and emerging scientific interest. One of the earliest debates arose from accumulations of shell middens along the Cape coast. From the 1870s, scholars such as Baines, William Molyneux, and George Leith began excavating sites in the Cape, KwaZulu-Natal, and Mossel Bay, gradually recognising these deposits as the product of human activity (Barham and Mitchell 2008, p. 8). Daniel Kannemeyer's (1890) ethnographic work with San communities in the eastern Drakensberg stands out as an early example of an ethnoarchaeological study. Working with San members offered early interpretive frameworks for understanding stone tools and lifeways in the region. Meanwhile, in 1913, JP Botha unearthed what came to be called 'Boskop Man', a fossilised skullcap that generated intense speculation about racial typologies. Although the skull would later enter broader palaeoanthropological debate, early interpretations focused on fitting indigenous populations into evolutionary hierarchies (Dubow 1995; Derricourt 2009, p. 265). The use of craniometry and physical anthropology to construct racialised narratives of the African past reflected broader trends of scientific racism (Kuljian 2016).

In Zimbabwe, near Bulawayo, the first reported finds were made in 1900, and by 1913 Neville Jones (1926, 1929) had discovered the Hope Fountain site. In 1917–1918, Jones (1926, 1929) excavated Bambata Cave, which at the time represented the most methodical and stratified excavation yet undertaken in the region (Walker 1995). Other finds were also made, such as Henry Balfour's at Victoria Falls, which included the first handaxe in 1903 (Gabel 1985, p. 247), or the work of Louis Péringuey (1911) on collections from around the southern African region. While still lacking in systematic methods, most of these investigations marked an important step toward recognising the deep human history embedded in southern African landscapes. More formalised approaches would come with John Hewitt in the 1920s, whose stratigraphic work on middens and shelters established a more analytical foundation (Deacon and Deacon 1999, p. 5).

4.1.2 East Africa

As with other African regions, archaeology in East Africa focussed on the earlier, expansive human sequence (Kusimba 2024). As a result, the contemporary past, which included urbanism and widescale, global trade, was not fully examined until independence (Horton 1996, p. 1–7; Kusimba 1999; LaViolette and Fleisher 2005). However, despite this general neglect, important kingdoms and centres were well known by the time of European colonisation, not only because of Muslim and Portuguese trade with associated cities, but also because of earlier accounts from the beginning of the first millennium CE (Pwiti 2005, p. 381).

The Aksum Empire in the highlands where modern-day Eritrea and Ethiopia meet was long known but remained largely unexamined by archaeologists until the twentieth century CE. Its capital, Aksum, was referenced by Roman and Byzantine writers from the early first millennium CE, and appears on all major Portuguese maps from the sixteenth century. Despite this visibility, sustained scholarly attention lagged. It was only in the twentieth century, the site was drawn into European consciousness through plunder: during Robert Napier's 1868 military expedition to Ethiopia, known as the Maqdala Expedition, several stelae and other cultural items were taken to Europe (Fig. 4.4) (Burka and Eshetie 2022). Records suggest this looting was premeditated, with correspondence between the British Museum's Department of Greek and Roman Antiquities and the Royal Geographical Society confirming a coordinated plan (Gunning and Challis 2023). It was only after the defeat of the Italian occupation in 1896 by Ethiopian forces that archaeological work at Aksum began in earnest. In the early twentieth century, Emperor Menelik II reached an agreement with Kaiser Wilhelm II, allowing a German team to conduct fieldwork at the site. Headed by Enno Littmann, who left the Princeton expedition in Abyssinia to take up the role, the team worked at Aksum between January 1905 and April 1906, yielding several important discoveries (Littmann et al. 1913; Trüper 2013). Their study coincided with the earliest scientific archaeological investigations at Great Zimbabwe, marking a broader shift in sub-Saharan African archaeology. A French mission followed in the 1920s, but the site was again looted during the Italian fascist occupation of Ethiopia (1935–1941), as Mussolini's forces ransacked cultural heritage across the country, including in Addis Ababa (Pankhurst 1999; Zewde 2002).

Another contested site of significance is Meroe and the Kush Kingdom, which flourished from the early first millennium BCE until its decline around the fourth

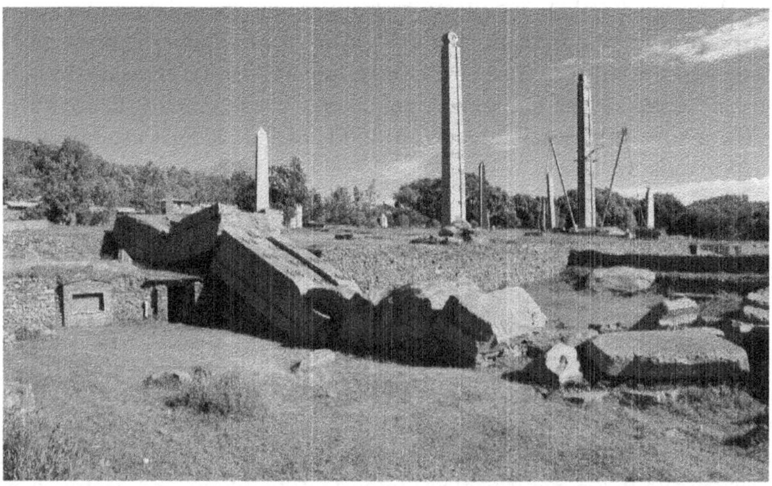

Fig. 4.4 The Aksum stellae with a collapsed stele in the foreground (photograph: Sailko). *Source* https://commons.wikimedia.org/wiki/File:Aksum,_stele_1_(stele_grande)_02.jpg

century CE (Edwards 1998). Like Aksum, Meroe was never lost. Herodotus (2003 translated by Aubrey de Sélincourt) mentioned the kingdom, though his brief and imprecise account, which described Meroe as an Egyptian province beyond the Fourth Cataract, likely reflected his lack of direct experience of the region (Török 2014, p. 4). In the eighteenth century, Scottish explorer James Bruce (cf. Gabel 1985) travelled through Nubia but did not reach Meroe, and thus made no record of its pyramids. The first European descriptions and illustrations came from Frédéric Cailliaud (1822, 2014 the 2014 reference was translated by Andrew Bednarski) during his expeditions between 1817 and 1822 (Fig. 4.5). Around the same time, Linant de Bellefonds documented the site, though his illustrations were only published much later (Gabel 1985). Cailliaud (1822, 2014), an influential early figure in Egyptology, explored much of the Nile Valley, Sudan, and Ethiopia, producing drawings of many now-famous archaeological sites (Mainterot 2011). In the twentieth century, Anthony Arkell (1955) argued in his book *A History of Sudan* that Meroe had been the cradle of the African Iron Age, influencing technologies and cultural practices such as iron-working, architecture, and divine kingship. Although Arkell's ideas retained popularity into the 1960s, they were later recognised as romanticised and unsubstantiated (Trigger 1969). An important early scientific study of Meroe was also conducted by the 1842 Prussian Expedition led by Richard Lepsius (1853), which combined historical and antiquarian research and produced over 800 plates documenting the region's monuments.

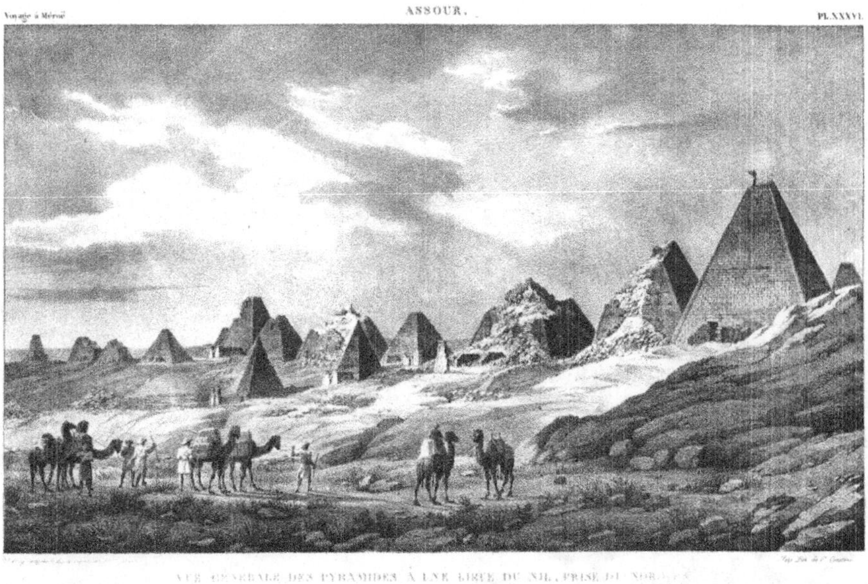

Fig. 4.5 The Royal Necropolis of Meroe, Frédéric Cailliaud, 1821. *Source* https://commons.wikimedia.org/wiki/File:Nubian_pyramids_of_Meroe_in_1821.jpg

Excavations at Meroe were only to begin in the early twentieth century CE. John Garstang and his team (1911) excavated Meroe from 1910 to 1914. They worked in the town area, the Sun and Lion Temples, and in the cemeteries (Fig. 4.6). The famous Meroe pyramids (Fig. 4.7) were excavated later between 1920 and 1923. These were part of the Boston Museum of Fine Arts programme of research conducted by George Reisner (published in the 1950s in five volumes; cf. Trigger 1969). Meroe was not the only Kush site that was excavated. Leonard Woolley and Randall-MacIver (1910) in 1907 to 1908 also excavated sites in Egyptian Nubia, Karanog, that were part of the empire. Urban centres found in the Nile Valley were typically overlooked as archaeologists and historians focussed largely on Egyptian history. Urban places in Egypt were considered more advanced than the upper reaches of the Nile, who were moreover thought to have been colonised by Pharaonic Egypt (Adam and Taha 2022). For example, Archibald Sayce (cf. Pope 2014, p. 5) concluded that the first kings of Meroe were the same masters over Egypt and Ethiopia, and later Reisner (1921) thought it was the Libyan pharaohs that ruled Kush based on similar inscriptions on grave goods. Early perceptions considered the development of complex kingdoms resulting from outsider influence, and Kush was no different.

However, some of the early explorers were less interested in the history of Meroe and more interested in its wealth. An Italian doctor, Giuseppe Ferlini, found gold in Queen Amanishakheto's pyramid in 1834, which he removed and brought back to Europe. It also came to light that he likely fabricated evidence to obfuscate his find spot and intentionally mislead treasure hunters (Markowitz and Lacovara 1996).

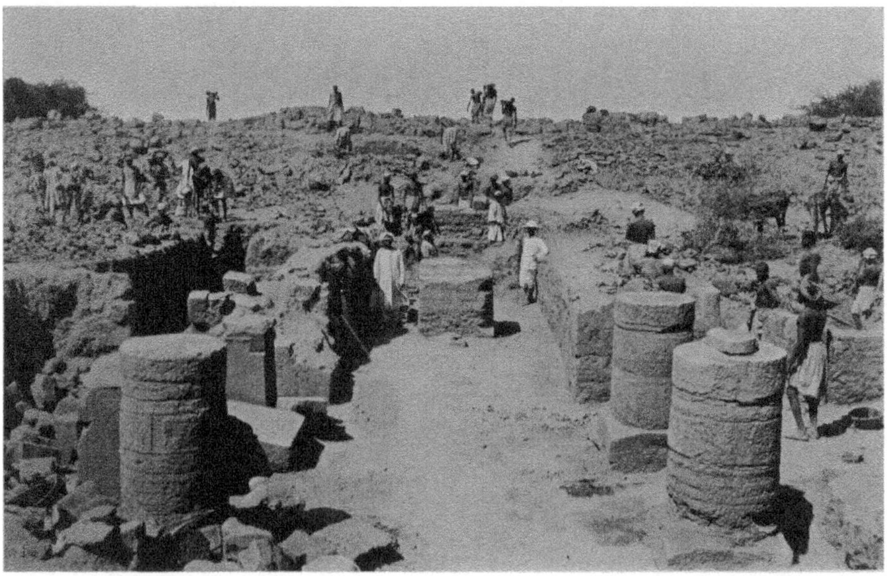

Fig. 4.6 The Temple of Amun after John Garstang's excavations in 1911 CE. *Source* https://commons.wikimedia.org/wiki/File:Meroë,_the_City_of_the_Ethiopians_-_being_an_account_of_a_first_season%27s_excavations_on_the_site,_1909-1910_(1911)_(14,578,447,997).jpg

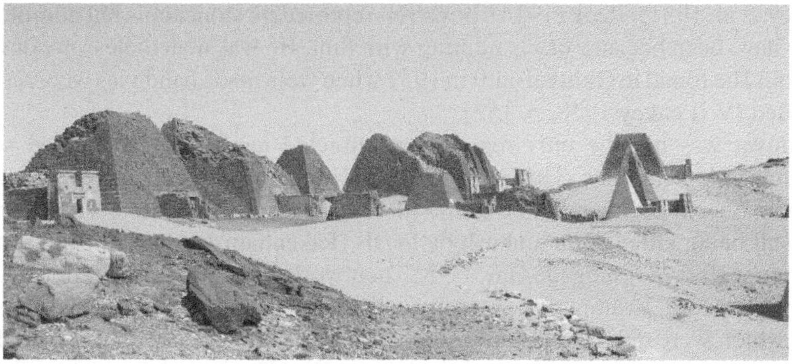

Fig. 4.7 The pyramids of Meroe in their present condition in the Nubian desert (photograph: Fabrizio Demartis). *Source* https://commons.wikimedia.org/wiki/File:Sudan_Meroe_Pyramids_30sep2005_4.jpg

According to Lepsius (1853), Ferlini's find was by chance and the gold was from unexpected locations. However, he mentions Osman Bey, who had soldiers stationed nearby, and his looting of the pyramids led to some being destroyed in his search for treasures. Bey was convinced to stop his destructive ways by Lepsius (1853), but others had already plundered the site, including the governor-general of Sudan, Ahmed Pasha Abu Widan, along with European visitors. By the early twentieth century CE, when archaeology was emerging, the site had been stripped of some of its cultural remains, but fortunately the work of several scholars assisted in recording the site in detail before further damage and loss was incurred.

While East Africa's archaeology is often associated with its large urban centres, empires, and complex civilisations, particularly those that captured the imagination of Western scholars during nineteenth century CE colonisation, these were by no means the only discoveries being made at the time. A wider range of finds, often less monumental but no less significant, also began to emerge across the region. The first stone tools were likely those collected by John Gregory (1901) in 1893, a geologist after whom the Eastern Rift Valley was named (Gregory Rift). He also included a chapter on prehistory in his book *The Rift Valley and Geology of East Africa* (Gregory 1921). In 1895, Félix Jousseaume (cf. Gabel 1984) wrote up a collection of tools from the then British Somaliland that were found by MacConkey several years prior. From 1897, Heywood Seton-Karr (1896) collected stone implements from many sites and areas and sent specimens to 50 different museums. His collections unfortunately contain little provenance data but include rough drawings of some of the artefacts. His work was partly written up but largely left unpublished. By 1913, Hans Reck (1914), a geologist from Berlin, was working in Olduvai Gorge but focussed largely on fossils – he found an articulate modern human skeleton that he mistakenly thought belonged to the middle Pleistocene. Reck's (1914) work was highly influential, in particular because he was the one who proposed to Louis Leakey that beds should be used, which ultimately resulted in the identification of five such beds in the gorge

(Leakey et al. 1931). Reck (1914), however, reported no stone tools but admitted that it may have been because of his training with flint. He was nonetheless unconvinced any would be found in Olduvai until in 1931 when well-made handaxes were retrieved from Bed IV (Leakey 1978, p. 152).

Olduvai was not the only region that attracted geologists who noted significant archaeological finds. The Omo Valley in Ethiopia was another, with geologists Maurizio Sacchi (Sclater 1899), of the ill-fated Bottego expedition which included nearly all being killed in an ambush by locals (Pakenham 1991), and Émile Brümpt (Guillemot 1997) defining the Omo beds. Their work led to the identification of a local Stone Age record. Brümpt, for example, collected specimens from at least 40 sites in 1901, which were described by Breuil and Harper Kelley in 1936 (cf. Gabel 1985). Directly across the river, although unexplored and unrecognised as an archaeological site due to its inaccessibility, was Koobi Fora. It would only be identified in 1967 (Leakey 1976). Other collections were made throughout this period in various areas, including formerly French Somaliland, but they were largely small collections with little provenance data (Gabel 1985). Collectively, these early investigations, from monumental sites like Meroe to scattered surface collections of stone tools, reflect a period of uneven and often opportunistic enquiry, shaped more by geological exploration and colonial curiosity than by systematic archaeological frameworks. Yet, they laid important groundwork for the more rigorous and locally grounded research that would follow later in the century.

4.1.3 North Africa

North Africa occupies a distinctive position in the history of archaeology on the continent. Unlike many other regions of Africa, it has long been familiar to Europe and the Mediterranean world. Proximity across narrow seas fostered enduring contact, trade, and cultural exchange, shaping perceptions of North Africa from antiquity onwards. Yet, familiarity did not prevent distortion. Rather, North Africa became a palimpsest of overlapping identities and claims: imagined in myths such as Atlantis, absorbed into the histories of Rome and Carthage, and later reframed through colonial ideologies that sought to legitimise European conquest. While much of sub-Saharan Africa was presented in European thought as a "dark continent", unknown and uncivilised, North Africa was both familiar and reimagined, seen as a gateway between worlds but interpreted through Eurocentric lenses.

Among the more fanciful interpretations was the Atlantis theory proposed by German ethnologist Leo Frobenius (1911). Frobenius (1911), who travelled repeatedly through North Africa between 1910 and 1935 (Ita 1974), believed Plato's account of Atlantis was based on an actual civilisation located near modern Nigeria and Senegal. He argued that this lost society had influenced African and Mediterranean civilisations, including Egypt and Greece, proposing that the flow of knowledge and technology originated in Africa rather than Europe. While this might seem like a progressive revaluation of Africa's global role, Frobenius (1911) still framed

Atlantis as an ancient 'white' civilisation, positioning African heritage within a Eurocentric narrative and failing to credit indigenous development. His theories, which lacked archaeological or historical evidence (Haberland 2007), reflected his own conflicted positionality: critical of how Africa was misrepresented, yet still beholden to colonial ideas that Africa required external impulses to explain its past achievements.

The familiarity of North Africa to Europeans rested on deep historical links (Fage 1978, p. 34). For millennia, trade across the Mediterranean connected European and African empires, kingdoms, and communities, facilitating exchanges of goods, ideas, and values (Lange 2004, p. 1). This connectivity made North Africa unique on the continent (González-Ruibal 2020, p. 660). Early European travellers, such as Thomas d'Arcos, who visited Tunis in 1681 CE, provided some of the earliest written accounts of North Africa's archaeology, describing sites like Thugga (Dougga) and Thignica (Ain Tounga) (Chaouali 2017, p. 193). Others soon followed, including the English cleric Thomas Shaw (1757), who produced further reports of the region's antiquities (Chaouali 2017, p. 193). However, it was Egypt and the legacies of the Phoenician and Punic eras that came to dominate archaeological attention and imagination.

The Phoenicians, originating in what is now Lebanon, began expanding westwards from around the ninth century BCE. Over time, their influence spread along the North African coast, eventually reaching into the continent's western reaches (Branigan 1994; Pappa 2009). Among their most significant settlements was Carthage, in present-day Tunisia. While its founding date remains obscured by legend, the ninth century BCE is the commonly accepted estimate (Bunnens 2019). Carthage's rise set it on a collision course with Rome, culminating in the protracted Punic Wars between 264 and 146 BCE (de Lisle 2019). Early records suggest that Carthage and Rome initially maintained a cautious coexistence, but as their spheres of influence expanded, particularly over the strategically vital island of Sicily, conflict became inevitable (Hoyos 1998). Roman sources, predictably, depicted themselves as valiant defenders of civilisation, casting the Carthaginians as treacherous adversaries. The Third Punic War ended in catastrophe for Carthage: the city, once the wealthiest in the world (Maróti 1983), was utterly destroyed, its cultural heritage obliterated, and its surviving population of 55,000 sold into slavery (Kiernan 2004). This violent erasure of Carthaginian civilisation marked a profound loss of heritage, knowledge, and technology, the consequences of which still echo today (Scott 2018). Yet, despite its tragic end, Phoenician history continues to resonate across Africa and Europe, with enduring myths such as the story that Phoenician sailors circumnavigated the African continent in the late fifth century BCE (Branigan 1994).

Egypt's archaeological significance, meanwhile, is inextricably linked with Western imperialism. The two developed hand in hand (Reid 1985). European fascination with Egypt soared following the discovery of the Rosetta Stone in 1799 CE, which allowed Jean-François Champollion to decipher hieroglyphs by 1822. Champollion's breakthrough launched Egyptology as a discipline, fuelling a race between European powers to amass Egyptian antiquities. Rival consuls in Cairo, the Englishman Henry Salt and the Frenchman Bernardino Drovetti, competed fiercely in the 1820s to acquire artefacts for their nations. France tightened its grip on Egyptian heritage by installing a French director of antiquities in 1858, a position it monopolised for the next 94 years (Reid 1985, p. 234). Egypt's archaeology became a projection of European imperial interests, deeply entangled with colonial ambitions (Meskell 2000, p. 147).

Elsewhere in North Africa, the French conquest of Algeria in the 1830s accelerated antiquarian interest in the region. This was not a neutral pursuit of knowledge; it was closely linked to colonial objectives. Stressing narratives of African "barbarism" helped justify France's self-appointed "civilising mission." French scholars and officials highlighted Roman history in the Maghreb, portraying Roman civilisation as a noble ancestor to European powers and using it to legitimise modern colonial occupation (Lorcin 2007). Roman roads, fortresses, and infrastructure were not just archaeological interests, they became tools of colonial propaganda, suggesting historical continuity between ancient Rome and modern Europe. Berber communities were likewise absorbed into this narrative, sometimes portrayed as heirs to Roman civilisation and thus more readily assimilable than Muslim groups. The prominence of Roman heritage in Algeria reflected a broader pattern of intellectual colonialism (Fenwick 2012), one that extended into other territories such as the French protectorates of Tunisia (1881) and Morocco (1912), the Spanish protectorate of northern Morocco (1912), and Italian-occupied Libya (1911).

While North Africa's archaeology was comparatively better known than other parts of the continent—thanks largely to Egyptology and Mediterranean historical connections—it was still filtered through Eurocentric perceptions. Like East, West, and southern Africa, it received increasing archaeological attention over time, but always in ways that mirrored the priorities and prejudices of the colonial powers that dominated its excavation and interpretation.

4.1.4 West Africa

West Africa was less well known in antiquity. Compared to eastern Africa, the region was barely mentioned by Greek and Roman writers. While trans-Saharan connections did exist, and contact with Europe via the western coastline developed over time, these routes were neither as direct nor as enduring as those along Africa's northern and eastern fringes. Muslim travellers and traders later provided valuable first-hand accounts of West Africa, though these narratives are uneven in quality and scope (Dueppen 2016, p. 248). European interest intensified with the expansion of maritime trade along the West African coast, but it was not until several centuries later that explorers began venturing into the interior and documenting what they encountered. One of the first to do so was Mungo Park (1799), a Scottish physician who arrived in Africa in June 1795 (Viana 2011). He was appointed by the African Association, a company that explored the continent with the aim of finding resources to exploit, and tasked with travelling the entire length of the Niger River (see also Thomson 1890). He traversed more than 320 km, beginning in the Gambia River, and then into the West African interior (Fig. 4.8). Only a few months into his journey, he was captured

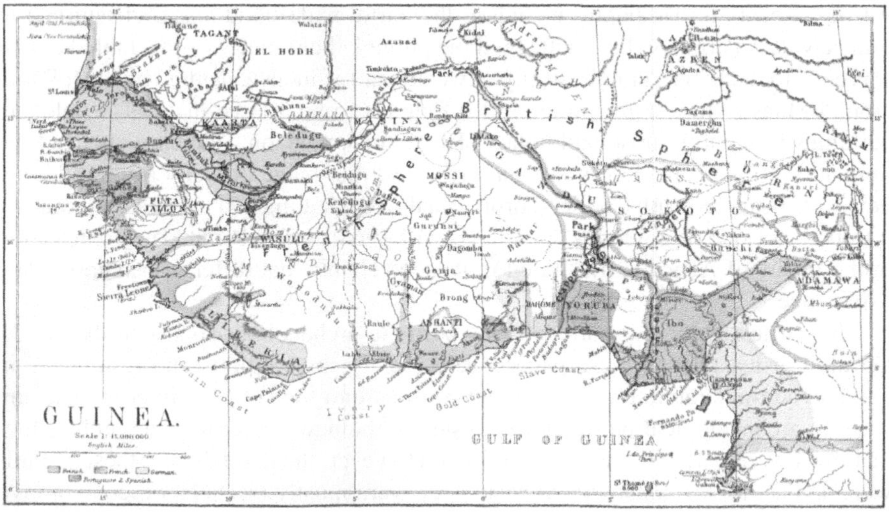

Fig. 4.8 Mungo Park's expedition from the Gambia to the Niger river and into the west African interior. *Source* https://commons.wikimedia.org/wiki/File:Route_de_M._Mungo_Park_depuis_Pisanta..._jusqu%27à_Silla..._-_par_le_major_J._Rennell_-_btv1b8469592g.jpg

by Moors, imprisoned and tortured, before escaping and reaching the Niger River banks in July 1796. On his second voyage, beginning in August 1805, he departed with a large group that included 35 soldiers, but would ultimately lose most of his party to various ailments. It is suspected that he drowned near Yauri, Nigeria, at the Bussa Rapids (Cliff 2022, p. 8). His is one of the earliest accounts of travels in this part of Africa, but his focus was on animals, women, and landscapes, with little on historical sites or places. When he began his journey, Park would not have realised the influence his romantic accounts would have on contemporary travel writers over two centuries later (Cliff 2022).

Park was followed by other explorers. These include Gaspard Mollien (1820), who in 1818 survived the Medusa shipwreck and, on finding himself in Senegal, opted to pursue his childhood dream of exploring Africa (Miles 2008), Alexander Laing (1822) in Sierra Leone, René Caillié (1830) who explored many countries in West Africa including Senegal, Mauritania and Morocco, and the Lander brothers (1832) in Nigeria, from 1804 to 1839. Of these travellers, perhaps the one with the most interesting account of local archaeology, or perhaps most infamous, is Caillié (1830). He had heard that the Geographic Society in Paris would award the first European to travel to Timbuktu and back 10,000 francs. With this goal in mind, he spent a year living with the Braknas tribe, learnt Arabic, and studied Islamic rituals. He was of the opinion that a European would only return safely if he successfully posed as a Muslim. Timbuktu had reached its fame in Europe from the stories of Mansa Musa, who in 1324 CE visited Cairo on his way to Mecca and spent vast amounts of gold (Bell 1972). Caillié (1830) successfully arrived in Timbuktu while travelling in disguise and with a Muslim caravan. In his account he commented on various aspects of Timbuktu, including the earth-made buildings, and returned to France with a narrative that challenged the publicly held image of this fabled city. It was envisioned to be a grandiose city of wealth and affluence, painted by the folklore around Mansa Musa, but Caillié (1830) found it to be a large mass of people and buildings in a barely hospitable place. His commentary on Timbuktu changed the romanticisation of the desert city and presented the image of a city of mud. Laing, however, disagreed with Caillié's surprise at the city, stating that it was as he expected it to be—not one of gold, but of earth (Bovill 1964; Smith 1985). The contestation in the image of Africa is illustrated in these accounts that differ in perception and experience.

The earliest authored works of West African archaeology appear in the 1870s. Up until at least 1900, these papers were largely short reports and resulted from colonial administrators undertaking expeditions into the colony's interior. The aim was not archaeological but intended to survey the new territories, and archaeological finds were part of what was identified. However, those producing these records were archaeological amateurs, at best. They were mostly teachers, officers, or civil administrators, among others, and not necessarily proficient in archaeological reconnaissance (Holl 1990, p. 298). They also largely played a role in French colonialism in West Africa. Émile Hamy (cf. Holl 1990) conducted a number of early studies and was involved in various faculties of the discipline, such as editing journals and volumes, but was posted in West Africa as a medical officer. Maurice Delafosse (1900, 1912) was governor-general of French colonies in the region and he used archaeological knowledge to explain the peopling of West Africa. His publications demonstrate vividly the colonial attitude towards the western colonies (cf. Holl 1990, p. 299). For example, he was dismissive of Muslim intellectual heritage, considered the number of Muslim literary sources to be negligible and of a low quality, and overall undeserving of being considered literature at all (Delafosse 1912, pp. 377–380; cf. Sanni 2012).

Despite not being archaeologists, French officials and army officers were better equipped to identify finds than most others. From the mid-late nineteenth century CE, France was undergoing rapid change in archaeology. New organisations and conferences were appearing, such as the International Congress of Archaeology and Prehistoric Anthropology in 1866, or the journal *L'Anthropologie* in 1872 and *L'Homme Préhistorique* 12 years later (Holl 1990, 298). Many coming from France to Africa arrived with some form of training, they expected all societies to pass through stages of culture as a result of French evolutionary doctrine, and had been excavating Upper Palaeolithic caves in France (Boule 1900; de Morgan et al. 1910). They were the first to carry out excavations outside of Egypt in French Guinea at Grotte de Kakimbon in the mid-1890s and included stratigraphic illustrations (Hamy 1900, 1901). They also excavated the kingdom of Ghana after the conquest of Arab North-West Africa (Bonnel de Mézières 1923), although these finds cannot be traced (Mauny 1970). As a result, the Francophone interest in West Africa laid a strong archaeological foundation for the unfolding of professional archaeology to come in the decades that would follow.

While at first interest in West African was on Stone Age assemblages, often poorly provenanced and interpreted through comparisons with French sequences (see McIntosh and McIntosh 1983), it was the region's art and crafted implements that would ultimately attract greater scholarly attention (Gabel 1985). Certainly one of the most famous example is those of Benin's bronzes. Benin was a prominent kingdom in modern-day Nigeria rising to power in the thirteenth century CE. After 1450, the kingdom interacted with the Portuguese and engaged in regular trade. This would be the beginning of relations with Europe that would persist until the late nineteenth century when it would ultimately lead to the kingdom's demise. The territory of the Kingdom of Benin was incorporated into the British Empire's colonial sphere in 1885, following the conclusion of the Berlin Conference. Over the coming years, British administrators and military activities would overthrow local chiefs and kings and usurp trade authority in the region. In 1897, as a result of continued trade aggravations, the British Punitive Expedition involved an invasion of Benin City, Benin's capital. What precipitated the attack was an ambush of a British trading envoy, although this was used as an excuse to attack the city (Marlowe 2021). The invasion ransacked Benin, plundered its riches and heritage, and led to the collapse of the Benin Kingdom (Aremu and Ediagbonya 2018). The objects best known from this invasion are the Benin Bronzes, which, along with many other crafted items, adorned the city's pillars and shrines, and depicted a great variety of scenes, people, activities, cultural items, and histories. Today, the looted plunder can be found in some 161 museums with comparatively little remaining in Nigeria (Hicks 2020). The value of these works of art was clear to colonial looters, and the necessity to colonise the past along with the present, as the French attempted in Egypt, was enacted in the British approach to the Benin Kingdom.

One of the earliest scholars to attempt to present African heritage in the sub-Saharan region as evidence of sophisticated societies was Frobenius (1913a). His collections are prolific, and he wrote a large number of outputs that included oral histories (although his methods of collections were not ideal). These largely present Ur-histories of Africa involving moon-goddesses and mysticism (Marchand 1997, p. 154). He had interesting polarities. On the one hand, he never questioned the legitimacy of European powers in Africa (Ita 1972, p. 674) and he considered the birth of civilisation and the advancement of technological advancement as linked to Europeans through a much earlier, white connection. However, on the other, he was staunchly against Eurocentric historiography and rejected the 'materialist' appeal that the west held (Marchand 1997, p. 153). He was also acutely aware of the ironies presented by the west, including the focus of his contemporary historians on grand and not daily histories, and the Hegelian historiography – the view that history followed dictates of reason. Frobenius revolted against the west and its framework and depicted Africa, its people, and past with revery (ibid). In so doing, he became an important figure in the later emergence of anti-colonial, Africanist movements, such as Léopold Senghor's *Negritude* (Echeruo 1993; Dubow 2019, p. 33).

Frobenius 1913b travelled through West Africa in 1907 to 1909 and shortly after again from 1910 to 1912. He saw West Africa as composed of two groups: Hamitic (state-forming) and Ethiopian (non-state-forming) people. He created these groups not on racial grounds but cultural; the Hamites had been rendered lazy through the use of slave labour whereas the Ethiopians were hard-working and vigorous (Frobenius 1913a). However, his renderings of these groups reflected his perceptions of the French and Anglo-Saxons (Hamitic-like), and his own people, the Germans (Ethiopian-like), which he emphasised even more after 1918 (Ita 1972, p. 675). These cultural nuances aside, Frobenius was the first European to investigate Ife, for example, and employed a mining engineer to excavate the site. Together they applied a more romantic than scientific approach. He and an assistant excavated (burrowed in his words) at Olokun and found terracotta and a brass head, which they paid six pounds for and a bottle of whiskey (Gabel 1985). Nonetheless, he sought evidence of complex societies in Africa, managed to find support for his ideas, and became contemptuous towards those that were unconvinced of Africa's archaeological importance. Alas, he argued, for example, that Ife was evidence of a Greek colony, c. 1200–800 BCE (the Dark Ages of Greek history) (Posnansky 1982, p. 347; cf. Gabel 1985, 250). The notion that foreign or outsider influence led to African state formation would be redeployed many times by colonial and African writers well after Frobenius (1911) first proposed it (cf. Oliver and Fage 1963; Chap. 4 and 5; Fage 1969, pp. 8–10; and see Kalous 1970). He was unable to truly detach from the colonial perspectives that dominated at the time.

4.1.5 Central Africa

The archaeology of Central Africa, away from the coast at the very least, received less research than many other regions. Issues around accessibility, political instability, and safety all contributed to this lacuna of work. However, some early studies were carried out and led to important findings.

In the Democratic Republic of Congo, the first stone tools to be recorded were very possibly those identified by Georg Schweinfurth (1873) in the Ituri region. He visited the area in the 1870s in search of the 'pygmies', a term now recognised as derogatory, and he met people who called themselves the 'Akka'. He took various measurements to confirm that these were the 'pygmies' that he was searching for and introduced them to the world at large. However, he also collected stone tools and passed these around to other scholars for consideration. Schweinfurth fled the region during the fall of Khartoum and died in North Africa (Ichikawa 2004, p. 104). Another early assemblage was identified by Edward Hore (1892) in 1882. Hore (1892, 1971) was a ship captain who accompanied the Scottish Mission in 1876 to aid in establishing a station at Livingstonia. As part of this, neighbouring regions were being explored by Hore and others, such as the Bishop Steere, including the Lakes Nyassa (Malawi) and Tanganyika, the latter at which he found bored stones. At a similar time, an engineer on Henry Stanley's expedition referred to as Captain Zboinsi (Keith 1919, p. 71), reported stone tools he found eroding from a hill at Manyanga, Lower Congo, in 1885 (Cornelissen 2024). These were recorded during the time when Stanley was aiding Leopold II with the establishment of the Congo

Free State (Gabel 1985, pp. 247–248). By 1899, such collections were common enough that Xavier Stainier (1899) wrote a comprehensive study on Congo's Stone Age prehistory, but this was mostly based on Lower Congo sites with some from the central region; he wrote primarily about the Lupemban and Tshitolian Industries (Clark 1971, p. 68) Another written description was presented in 1901, by Victor Jacques (1901), who described stone tools but did not attempt to define any cultural continuity. Very little work was conducted in the central region until the 1920s and that which was presented relied on small assemblages from surface contexts (Clark 1971, p. 68).

4.2 The Nature of Archaeology and its Influence in Africa

How Africa's past was conceived played a considerable role in how colonial administrations justified their endeavours. From the Egyptian Expedition carried out by Napolean, the past was part of a national agenda. Linked to this, most people carrying out archaeological, historical, or heritage work, were agents of colonialism, such as administrators, explorers, geographers, missionaries, and private companies. They were not necessarily skilled or trained individuals in the field of archaeology. French colonial administrators were better educated in archaeology and history but not highly proficient workers in that regard. Not only did the past allow for the legitimisation of the colonial exercise, but it was a source of wealth. Plundering heritage in Ethiopia, Egypt, Nigeria and Zimbabwe provided sources of revenue for looters as well as companies. Expeditions into 'untouched' African regions setup to explore uncharted territories with the hope of identifying resources that could be exploited also introduced heritage and cultural resources to prying eyes. The commercialisation of the past off the mythology of golden cities and empires led to the formation of companies with the explicit intention of extracting what was of value from heritage sites. Beliefs during the late nineteenth century CE were firmly organised around one key theme; in most cases, white settlers from elsewhere brought to Africa civilisation and technological advancement. Quite often it was this aspect of history that interested stakeholders sought, or appropriated, in their explanations of monumental sites.

The intellectual colonialism that emerged during this period rippled into the next phase of archaeological work. Specifically, the notion that African advancement was co-ordinated through invasions of incoming foreigners. Such a mythology ensconced colonialism in the African terrain. The Roman history in North Africa, Phoenicians in the southern reaches, or a 'white' Atlantis in the area of Nigeria and Senegal couched white occupation of Africa as a kind of birthright, and moreover elevated colonists through a historical stratification to a lofty station in social engineering on the continent.

References

Adam, A., and S. Taha. 2022. Archaeology in Sudan: A Sudanese perspective. In *Oxford research encyclopedia of anthropology*, ed. M. S. Aldenderfer. Oxford: Oxford University Press. https://oxfordre.com/anthropology/display/10.1093/acrefore/9780190854584.001.0001/acrefore-9780190854584-e-565?d=%2F10.1093%2Facrefore%2F9780190854584.001.0001%2Facrefore-9780190854584-e-565&p=emailAGTrCyc.KDHHs&utm_source=chatgpt.com

Anderson, A. A. 1888. *Twenty-five years in a Wagon: Sport and travel in South Africa*. London: Chapman and Hall.

Ankermann, B. 1905. Kulturkreise und Kulturschichten in Afrika. *Zeitschrift für Ethnologie* 37:54–84.

Anquandah, J. 1981. *Rediscovering Ghana's past*. London: Longman.

Anquandah, J. 1985. *Ethnoarchaeological clues to Ghana's great past and—Greater future?* London: Department of Archaeology, University of Ghana.

Aremu, J. O., and M. Ediagbonya. 2018. Trade and religion in British-Benin relations, 1553-1897. *Global Journal of Social Sciences Studies* 4 (2): 78–90.

Arkell, A. 1955. *A history of the Sudan from the earliest times to 1821*. London: University of London.

Barham, L., and P. J. Mitchell. 2008. *The first Africans: African archaeology from the earliest toolmakers to most recent foragers*. Cambridge: Cambridge University Press.

Barnhart, J. 2016. Status competition and territorial aggression: Evidence from the scramble for Africa. *Security Studies* 25:385–419.

Bell, N. M. 1972. The age of Mansa Musa of Mali: Problems in succession and chronology. *International Journal of African Historical Studies* 5 (2): 221–234.

Bent, T. 1896. *The ruined cities of Mashonaland*. London: Longman's Green.

Bollong, C., C. G. Sampson, and A. B. Smith. 1997. Khoikhoi and Bushman pottery in the Cape-Colony: Ethnohistory and later Stone Age ceramics of the South African interior. *Journal of Anthropological Archaeology* 16:269–299.

Bonnel de Mézières, A. 1923. Recherches sur l'emplacement de Ghana et sur le site de Tekrour. *Mémoires présentés par divers savants étrangers à l'Académie* 13 (1): 227–273.

Boule, M. 1900. Étude paléontologique et archéologique sur la station paléolithique du lac Karâr (Algérie). *L'Anthropologie* 11:1–21.

Bovill, E. W. 1964. *Missions to the Niger. vol. I: The journal of Friedrich Hornemann's travels from Cairo to Murzuk in the years 1797–98; The letters of Major Alexander Gordon Laing 1824–26*. Cambridge: Cambridge University Press.

Bowen, T. J. 1857. *Central Africa: Adventures and missionary labors in several countries in the interior of Africa, from 1849 to 1856*. Charleston: Southern Baptist Publication Society.

Branigan, C. 1994. The Circumnavigation of Africa. *Classics Ireland* 1:42–46.

Breuil, H. 1948. The white lady of the Brandberg, South-West Africa, her companion and her guards. *South African Archaeological Bulletin* 3:2–11.

Bulhan, H. A. 2015. Stages of colonialism in Africa: From occupation of land to occupation of being. *Journal of Social and Political Archaeology* 3:239–256.

Bunnens, G. 2019. Phoenicia in the later Iron Age: Tenth century BCE to the Assyrian and Babylonian periods. In *The Oxford handbook to the Phoenician and Punic mediterranean*, ed. C. López-Ruiz and B. K. Doak, 57–74. Oxford: Oxford University Press.

Burka, T., and T. Eshetie. 2022. Heritage management practice in Ethiopia: Is it different? In *Cultural heritage management in Africa: The heritage of the colonized*, ed. G. O. Abungu and W. Ndoro, 159–172. London: Routledge.

Burke, E. E. 1969. *The journals of Carl Mauch 1869–1872*. Salisbury: National Archives of Rhodesia.

Cailliaud, F. 1822. *Travels in the Oasis of Thebes, and in the deserts situated east and west of the Thebaid: In the years 1815, 16, 17, and 18*. London: Richard Phillips & Company.

Cailliaud, F. 2014. *The Lost manuscript of Frédéric Cailliaud: Arts and crafts of the ancient Egyptians, Nubians, and Ethiopians*. Cairo: American University in Cairo Press.

Caillié, R. 1830. *Travels through central Africa to Timbuctoo, and across the great desert, to Morocco, performed in the years 1824–1828*. London: C. W. McAlpin.

Caton-Thompson, C. 1931. *The Zimbabwe culture: Ruins & reactions*. Oxford: Clarendon Press.

Chamberlain, M. E. 1974. *The scramble for Africa*. Harlow: Longman.

Chaouali, M. 2017. Pre-Islamic archaeology in Tunisia: The stakes of a colonial science. *Memoirs of the American Academy in Rome* 62:193–208.

Chirikure, S. 2020. *Great Zimbabwe: Reclaiming a 'confiscated' past*. London: Routledge.

Clark, D. 1971. Problems of archaeological nomenclature and definition in the Congo basin. *The South African Archaeological Bulletin* 26:67–78.

Cliff, N. A. 2022. Lions, landscape and legacy: 'Exploring' Mungo Park's travels in the interior districts of Africa. PhD thesis, Manchester Metropolitan University, Manchester.

Cornelissen, E. 2024. The Stone Age of the Congo Basin. In *Oxford research encyclopedia of African history*, ed. T. Spear. Oxford: Oxford University Press. https://doi.org/10.1093/acrefore/9780190277734.013.1225

De Leon, D. 1886. The conference at Berlin on the West-African question. *Political Science Quarterly* 1:103–139.

de Lisle, C. 2019. The Punic wars. In *The Oxford handbook of the Phoenician and Punic Mediterranean*, ed. C. López-Ruiz and B. K. Doak, 169–182. Oxford: Oxford University Press.

de Morgan, J., L. Capitan, and P. Boudy. 1910. Etude sur les stations prehistoriques du Sud Tunisien. *Revidé l'école d'Anthropologie* 20:267–286.

Deacon, H. J., and J. Deacon. 1999. *Human beginnings in South Africa: Uncovering the secrets of the Stone Age*. Cape Town: David Philip Publishers.

Delafosse, M. 1900. Sur des traces probables de civilisations Égyptiennes et d'hommes de race blanche à la Côte d'Ivoire. *L'A* 11:431–451.

Delafosse, M. 1912. *Haut-Sénégal-Niger*. Paris: Larose.

Derricourt, R. 2009. The enigma of Raymond Dart. *The International Journal of African Historical Studies* 42 (2): 257–282.

Diop, C. A. 1960. *L'Afrique Noire Précoloniale: Étude comparée des systèmes politiques et sociaux de l'Europe et de l'Afrique eoire, de l'antiquité à la formation des états modernes*. Paris: Présence Africaine.

Du Bois, W. E. B. 1896. *The suppression of the African slave—Trade to the United States of America, 1638–1870*. Cambridge: Harvard University Press.

Dubow, S. 1995. *Scientific racism in modern South Africa*. Cambridge: Cambridge University Press.

Dubow, S. 2019. Henri Breuil and the imagination of prehistory: 'Mixing up rubble, trouble and stratigication'. *South African Archaeology Society Goodwin Series* 12:31–43.

Dueppen, S. A. 2016. The archaeology of West Africa, ca. 800 BCE to 1500 CE. *History Compass* 14 (6): 247–263.

Duffey, A. 2002. Pierneef and San rock art. *De Arte* 66:20–41.

Duffey, A. 2012. Reenen van Reenen's (1884-1935) attempt to change the Afrikaner's views of San rock art. *South African Journal of Cultural History* 26 (1): 1–13.

Dunn, E. J. 1880. On the stone implements of South Africa. *Transactions of the South African Philosophical Society* 2:6–22.

Eastwood, E. B., and G. Blundell. 1999. Rediscovering the rock art of the Limpopo-Shashi confluence area, Southern Africa. *Southern African Field Archaeology* 8:17–27.

Echeruo, M. J. 1993. Negritude and history: Senghor's argument with Frobenius. *Research in African Literatures 24*:1–13.

Edwards, D. N. 1998. Meroe and the Sudanic kingdoms. *Journal of African History* 39 (2): 175–193.

Fage, J. D. 1969. *A history of West Africa*. Cambridge: Cambridge University Press.

Fage, J. D. 1978. *A history of Africa*. London: Hutchinson.

Feilden, H. W. 1905. The Stone Age of the Zambezi valley and its relation in time. *Nature* 73:73–77.

Fenwick, C. 2012. North Africa. In *The Oxford companion to archaeology*, ed. N. A. Silberman. Oxford: Oxford University Press. https://discovery.ucl.ac.uk/id/eprint/1495996/1/Corisande%20Fenwick%20ArchaeologyandAuthenticityinAlgeria.pdf

Folorunso, C. A. 2003. Views of ancient Egypt from a West African perspective. In *Ancient Egypt in Africa*, ed. D. O'Connor and D. A. M. Reid, 77–92. London: UCL Press.

Fontein, J. 2006. *The silence of great Zimbabwe: Contested landscapes and the power of heritage*. London: Routledge.

Frobenius, L. 1911. *Auf dem Wege nach Atlantis*. Berlin: Vita.

Frobenius, L. 1913a. *The voice of Africa: Being an account of the travels of the German inner African exploration expedition in the years 1910–1912*. London: Hutchinson & Company.

Frobenius, L. 1913b. *Und Afrika Sprach: Wissenschaftlich erweiterte ausgabe des berichts über den verlauf der dritten reise-periode der Deutschen inner-Afrikanischen*. Hamburg: Hamburgisches Museum für Völkerkunde.

Gabel, C. 1984. Notes on the history of archaeology in sub-Saharan Africa. *Working Papers in African Studies Series* 86:1–24.

Gabel, C. 1985. Archaeology in sub-Saharan Africa. *International Journal of African Historical Studies* 18 (2): 241–264.

Garlake, P. S. 1973. *Great Zimbabwe*. London: Thames & Hudson.

Garlake, P. S. 1982. Prehistory and ideology in Zimbabwe. *Africa* 52:1–19.

Garstang, J., A. H. Sayce, and F. L. Griffith. 1911. *Meroe, the city of the Ethiopians*. Oxford: Oxford University Press.

González-Ruibal, A. 2020. Colonies, missions, violence and trade: The historical archaeology of northeast Africa. In *Routledge handbook of global historical archaeology*, ed. C. E. Orset, A. Zarankin, P. Funari, S. Lawrence, and J. Symonds, 660–680. Abingdon: Routledge.

Gregory, J. W. 1901. *The foundation of British East Africa*. London: Horace Marshall and Sons.

Gregory, J. W. 1921. *The rift valleys and geology of east Africa: An account of the origin and history of the rift valleys of east Africa and their relation to the contemporary Earth-movements which transformed the geography of the world*. London: Seeley.

Guillemot, C. 1997. Recherches paléoanthropologiques dans la basse vallée de l'Omo. *Bull Maison Études Éthiop* 11:69–78.

Gunning, L. P., and D. Challis. 2023. Planned plunder, the British museum, and the 1868 Maqdala expedition. *The Historical Journal* 66 (3): 550–572.

Haberland, E. 2007. *Leo Frobenius on African history, art and culture*. Princeton: Markus Weiner Publishers.

Hall, R. N. 1905. *Great Zimbabwe, Mashonaland, Rhodesia. An account of two years examination work in 1902–4 on behalf of the government of Rhodesia*. London: Metheun.

Hamy, E.T. 1900. Notes sur des haches polies. *Bulletin du Musée d'Histoire Naturelle* 6 : 94–96.

Hamy, E. T. 1901. La grotte de Kakimbon pros Konakry. *L'Anthropologie* 12:380–395.

Hegel, G. F. W. 1894. *Lectures on the philosophy of world history*. London: George Bell.

Herodotus. 2003. *The histories*. Oxford: Penguin Classics.

Hicks, D. 2020. *The Brutish museums: The Benin bronzes, colonial violence and cultural restitution*. London: Pluto Press.

Holl, A. F. C. 1990. West African archaeology: Colonialism and nationalism. In *A History of African Archaeology*, ed. P. Robertshaw, 296–308. Oxford: James Currey Ltd.

Hore, E. C. 1892. *Tanganyika: Eleven years in Central Africa*. London: E. Stanford.

Hore, E. C. 1971. *Missionary to Tanganyika 1877–1888*. London: Frank Cass.

Horton, M. 1996. *Shanga: The archaeology of a Muslim trading community on the coast of East Africa*. Nairobi: British Institute in Eastern Africa.

Hoyos, B. D. 1998. *Unplanned wars: The origins of the first and second punic wars*. Berlin: Walter de Gruyter.

Ichikawa, M. 2004. The Japanese tradition in central African hunter-gatherer studies, with comparative observations on the French and American traditions. In *Hunter-gatherers in history, archaeology and anthropology*, ed. A. Barnard, 103–114. Oxford: Routledge.

Issawi, C. 1952. Arab geography and the circumnavigation of Africa. *Osiris* 10:117–128.
Ita, J. M. 1972. Frobenius in west African history. *Journal of African History* 13:673–688.
Ita, J. M. 1974. Frobenius, Lhote, and Saharan studies: A review article. *African Studies Review* 17 (1): 286–306.
Jacobs, J. M. 1996. *Edge of empire: Postcolonialism and the city*. London: Routledge.
Jacques, V. 1901. *Instruments de pierre du Congo: collection Haas*. Brussels: Hayez.
Johnston, H. 1913. A survey of the ethnography of Africa. *Journal of the Royal Anthropological Institute* 43:375–421.
Jones, N. 1926. *The Stone Age of Rhodesia*. Oxford: Oxford University Press.
Jones, N. 1929. A hitherto undescribed early stone age industry near hope fountain. *Rhodesia. South African Journal of Science* 26 (12): 631–647.
Kalous, M. 1970. Leo Frobenius' Atlantic theory: A reconsideration. *Paideuma* 16:27–51.
Kannemeyer, D. R. 1890. Stone implements: With a description of Bushman stone implements and relics, their names, uses, mode of manufacture and occurrence. *Cape Illustrated Magazine* 1:120–130.
Keith, A. B. 1919. *The Berlin Congo and the Berlin Act*. Oxford: Clarendon Press.
Kiernan, B. 2004. The first genocide: Carthage, 146 BC. *Diogenes* 51 (3): 27–39.
Kipling, R. 1931. *Verse*. London: Hodder and Stoughton.
Kohn, M., and K. Reddy. 2024. Colonialism. In *Standford Encyclopedia of Philosophy*, ed. E. N. Zalta and U. Nodelman. Stanford: Stanford University Press. https://plato.stanford.edu/entries/colonialism/?f%5B0%5D=topic:1&countryid=391&f%5B0%5D=region%3A46
Kuklick, H. 1991. Contested monuments. In *Colonial situations: Essays on the contextualisation of ethnographic knowledge*, ed. G. W. Stocker, 135–169. London: University of Wisconsin Press.
Kuljian, C., 2016. *Darwin's hunch: Science, race and the search for human origins*. Johannesburg: Jacana.
Kusimba, C. M. 1999. *The rise and fall of Swahili states*. Walnut Creek: AltaMira Press.
Kusimba, C. M. 2024. Current themes in the Archaeology of east Africa. *Annual Review of Anthropology* 53 (1): 353–370.
Laing, A. G. 1822. *Travels in the Timannee, Kooranko, and Soolima Countries, in West Africa*. London: John Murray.
Lander, R., and J. Lander. 1832. *Journal of an expedition to explore the course and termination of the Niger*. London: Murray.
Lange, D. 2004. *Ancient kingdoms of west Africa: African-centred and Canaanite-Israelite perspectives*. Dettlebach: JH Röll Verlag.
LaViolette, A., and J. Fleisher. 2005. The archaeology of Sub-Saharan urbanism: Cities and their countrysides. In *African archaeology: A critical introduction*, ed. A. B. Stahl, 327–352. Oxford: Blackwell Publishing.
Leakey, L. S. B., A. T. Hopwood, and H. Reck. 1931. Age of the Oldoway bone beds. *Tanganyika territory. Nature* 128:724.
Leakey, M. D. 1978. Olduvai Gorge 1911–75: A history of the investigations. *Geological Society, London, Special Publications* 6 (1): 151–155.
Leakey, R. E. 1976. New hominid fossils from the Koobi Fora formation in Northern Kenya. *Nature* 261 (5561): 574–576.
Lepsius, R. 1853. *Discoveries in Egypt, Ethiopia and the Peninsula of Sinai, in the Years 1842–1845: During the mission sent out by his majesty, Frederick William IV of Prussia*. London: Richard Bentley.
Littmann, E., D. Krencker, and T. von Lüpke. 1913. *Deutsche Aksum-Expedition: Herausgegeben von der Generalverwaltung der Königlichen Museen zu Berlin*. Berlin: Reimer.
Lorcin, P. 2007. Rome and France in Africa: Recovering colonial Algeria's Latin past. *French Historical Studies* 25:295–329.
Mainterot, P. 2011. *Aux Origines de l'égyptologie. Voyages et collections de Frédéric Cailliaud, 1787–1869*. Rennes: Presses Universitaires de Rennes.

Manyanga, M., and S. Chirikure. 2019. The Mapungubwe–Great Zimbabwe relationship in history: Implications for the evolution of studies of socio-political complexity in southern Africa. *South African Archaeological Society Goodwin Series* 12:72–84.

Marchand, S. 1997. Leo Frobenius and the revolt against the west. *Journal of Contemporary History* 32:153–170.

Markowitz, Y., and P. Lacovara. 1996. The Ferlini treasure in archeological perspective. *Journal of the American Research Center in Egypt* 33:1–9.

Marlowe, E. 2021. Review of Dan Hicks, the Brutish museums: The Benin Bronzes, colonial violence and cultural restitution. *International Journal of Cultural Property* 28 (4): 575–586.

Maróti, E. 1983. On the causes of Carthage's destruction. *Oikumene* 4:223–231.

Matenga, E. 1998. *The Soapstone birds of great Zimbabwe: Symbols of a nation*. Harare: African Publishing Group.

Mauch, K. 1874. *Reisen im Inneren von Südafrika: 1865–1872: Mit einer originalkarte*. Gotha: Justus Perthes.

Mauny, R. 1970. *Les Si&les Obscurs de l'Afrique Noire*. Paris: Fayard.

McIntosh, S. K., and R. J. McIntosh. 1983. Current directions in West African prehistory. *Annual Review of Anthropology* 12:215–258.

Meek, C. K. 1931. *A Sudanese kingdom*. London: Kegan Paul, Trench, Tubner.

Meskell, L. 2000. The practice and politics of archaeology in Egypt. *Annals of the New York Academy of Sciences* 925 (1): 146–169.

Meyerowitz, E. L. 1960. *The divine kingship in Ghana and ancient Egypt*. London: Faber and Faber.

Miles, J. 2008. *The wreck of the Medusa: The most famous sea disaster of the nineteenth century*. London: Grove Press.

Mitchell, P. J. 2001. Andrew Anderson and the nineteenth century origins of southern African archaeology. *Southern African Humanities* 13:37–60.

Mitchell, P. J. 2013. Stone Age sub-Saharan Africa. In *World archaeology at the Pitt rivers museum: A characterization*, ed. D. Hicks and A. Stevenson, 16–34. Oxford: Archaeopress.

Mollien, G. T. 1820. *Travels in the interior of Africa, to the sources of the Senegal and Gambia performed by command of the French Government in 1818*. London: Henry Colburn & Company.

Mommsen, W. J. 1995. *Imperial Germany 1867–1918: Politics, culture, and society in an authoritarian state*. London: Arnold.

Ndoro, W. 1997. Great Zimbabwe. *Scientific American* 277:94–99.

Oliver, R., and J. D. Fage. 1963. *A short history of Africa*. New York: New York University Press.

Pakenham, T. 1991. *The scramble for Africa: The white Man's conquest of the dark continent from 1876 to 1912*. New York: Random House.

Palmer, H. R. 1936. *The Bornu Sahara and Sudan*. London: Juhn Murray.

Pankhurst, R. 1999. Ethiopia, the Aksum obelisk, and the return of Africa's cultural heritage. *African Affairs* 98 (391): 229–239.

Pappa, E. 2009. Reflections on the earliest Phoenician presence in north-west Africa. *Talanta* 41:53–72.

Park, M. 1799. *Travels in the Interior of Africa, in the Years 1795, 1796, and 1797*. London: JW Myers.

Parsons, I. 2013. Artefacts that travel: The changing contexts and meanings of archaeological objects collected by Edward J. Dunn. *Southern African Humanities* 25:53–63.

Péringuey, L. 1911. *Annals of the South African museum. vol VIII. The Stone Ages of South Africa as represented in the collection of the South African museum*. London: West Newman.

Perry, W. J. 1923. *Children of the Sun*. London: Metheun.

Pope, J. W. 2014. *The double kingdom under Taharqo: studies in the history of Kush and Egypt, c. 690–664 BC*. Leiden: Brill.

Posnansky, M. 1982. African archaeology comes of age. *World Archaeology* 13:345–358.

Pwiti, G. 2005. Southern Africa and the east African coast. In *African archaeology: A critical introduction*, ed. A. B. Stahl, 378–391. Oxford: Blackwell Publishing.

Pwiti, G., and W. Ndoro. 1999. The legacy of colonialism: Perceptions of the cultural heritage in southern Africa, with special reference to Zimbabwe. *African Archaeological Review* 16:143–153.

Randal-MacIver, D. 1906. *Medieval Rhodesia*. London: MacMillan & Co.

Randsborg, K. 2001. Archaeological globalization: The first practitioners. *Acta Archaeologica* 72 (2): 1–53.

Ranger, T. 1993. The Invention of tradition revisited: The case of colonial Africa. In *Legitimacy and the state in twentieth-century Africa*, ed. T. Ranger and O. Vaughan, 62–111. London: Palgrave Macmillan UK.

Ransford, O. 1968. *Bulawayo: Rhodesia's historic battleground*. Cape Town: A. A. Balkema.

Rash, F., and G. Horan. 2021. Cutting up the world pie and what happened next. In *The discource of British and German colonialism*, pp. 3–25 ed. F. Rash and G. Horan. London: Routledge.

Rashid, N. 2014. British colonialism in east-Africa during nineteenth century. *Journal of Humanities and Social Science* 19:8–11.

Reck, H. 1914. Erste vorläufige Mitteilung über den Fund eines fossilen Menschenskelets aus Zentralafrika. *Sitzungsberichte der Gesellschaft Naturforschender Freunde zu Berlin* 3:81–95.

Reid, D. A. 1985. Indigenous Egyptology: The decolonization of a profession? *Journal of American Oriental Society* 105:233–246.

Reisner, G. A. 1921. The royal family of Ethiopia. *Museum of Fine Arts Bulletin* 19:21–38.

Rickard, J. C. 1881. Notes on four series of Paleolithic implements from South Africa. *Cambridge Antiquary Society* 7:57–66.

Robinson, R. E., and J. Gallagher. 1966. *Africa and the Victorians: The official mind of imperialism*. London: MacMillan & Co.

Rodney, W. 1972. *How Europe underdeveloped Africa*. Washington: Howard University Press.

Sanderson, G. N. 1975. The European partition of Africa: Coincidence or conjuncture? In *European Imperialism and the Partition of Africa*, ed. E. F. Penrose, 1–54. London: Frank Cass.

Sanni, A. O. 2012. Reviewed work: The hidden treasures of Timbuktu: Historic city of Islamic Africa, by John O. Hunwick, Alida Jay Boye. *British Journal of Middle Eastern Studies* 39:144–146.

Schweinfurth, G. 1873. *The heart of Africa*. London: Sampson Low, Marston Low, and Searle.

Sclater, P. L. 1899. Results of the second Bottegò expedition into eastern Africa. *Science* 10 (261): 951–955.

Scott, J. C. 2018. The Phoenicians and the formation of the western world. *Comparative Civilizations Review* 78:25–40.

Seligman, C. G. 1930. *Races of Africa*. London: Thornton Butterworth.

Seton-Karr, H. W. 1896. Discovery of evidences of the Palaeolithic Stone Age in Somaliland (Tropical Africa). *Journal of the Anthropological Institute of Great Britain and Ireland* 25:271–275.

Shaw, T., 1757. *Travels, Or Observations Relating to Several Parts of Barbary and the Levant*. London: A. Millar in the Strand, and W. Sandby in Fleet-Street.

Shaw, T. 1989. African archaeology: Looking back and looking forward. *African Archaeological Review* 7 (1): 3–31.

Shepherd, N. 2002. Disciplining archaeology; the invention of South African prehistory, 1923-1953. *Kronos: Journal of Cape History* 28 (1): 127–145.

Smith, G. E. 1915. *The migration of early culture*. Manchester: University of Manchester.

Smith, G. E. 1933. *The diffusion of culture*. London: Watts.

Smith, R. L. 1985. The image of Timbuktu in Europe before Caillié. *Proceedings of the Meeting of the French Colonial Historical Society* 8:12–22.

Solomon, A. 2014. Africa. In *The history of archaeology: An introduction*, ed. P. Bahn, 119–136. London: Routledge.

Stainier, X. 1899. *L'âge de la Pierre au Congo*. Brussels: Imprimerie Charles van de Weghe.

Talbot, P. A. 1926. *The peoples of Southern Nigeria*. London: Oxford University Press.

Thomson, J. 1890. *Mungo park and the Niger*. G. Phillip and son.

Török, L. 2014. *Herodotus in Nubia.* Leiden: Brill.
Trigger, B. G. 1969. The myth of Meroe and the African Iron Age. *African Historical Studies* 2 (1): 23–50.
Trüper, H. 2013. Wild archives: Unsteady records of the past in the travels of Enno Littmann. *History of Human Sciences* 26:128–148.
Uzoigwe, G. N. 1985. Reflections on the Berlin west Africa conference, 1884-1885. *Journal of the Historical Society of Nigeria* 12:9–22.
Viana, L. 2011. The tropics and the rise of the British Empire: Mungo Park's perspective on Africa in the late eighteenth century. *História, Ciências, Saúde-Manguinhos* 18:33–50.
Walker, N. J. 1995. *Late Pleistocene and Holocene hunter-gatherers of the Matopos: An archaeological study of change and continuity in Zimbabwe.* Uppsala: Societas Archaeologica Upsaliensis.
Webb, E. 1906. On the pretended Phoenician circumnavigation of Africa. *Geographical Journal* 28 (3): 297–298.
Webb, E. J. 1907. The alleged Phoenician circumnavigation of Africa: Considered in relation to the theory of a South African Ophir. *English Historical Review* 22 (85): 1–14.
Williams, E. 1966. *Capitalism and slavery.* New York: Capricorn Books.
Woolley, L., and D. Randall-MacIver. 1910. *Karanog, the Romano-Nubian Cemetery.* Philadelphia: University of Pennsylvania.
Ypi, L. 2013. What's wrong with colonialism. *Philosophy & Public Affairs* 41 (2): 158–191.
Zewde, B. 2002. *A history of modern Ethiopia, 1855–1991.* Athens: Ohio University Press.

Chapter 5
The Emergence of Archaeology in Africa

Abstract Moving into the early—mid twentieth century CE, this chapter charts the consolidation of archaeology on the continent before independence. It follows the establishment of surveys, departments, and journals; the growth of field methods; and the discipline's crossroads with history, linguistics, and the natural sciences. Regional differences show uneven institutionalisation linked to colonial administration, resource geographies, international funding, and colony relations. Case studies illustrate how typologies, chronologies, and migration models were advanced and later revised through new datasets and critiques. The chapter emphasises both advancements and limitations existing within archaeological practices and thinking, notably between existing amateur approaches and the rise of professional archaeology. It ends by situating "pre-independence archaeology" as a period that generated key archives and advanced methods but also inculcated problems that later generations would contest: ownership, voice, and interpretive frames.

> [S]cientists in Europe and elsewhere are only willing to accept the statements of visitors with a brief knowledge of the country, rather than to augment these with the detailed work of those who know South Africa and local conditions, and have a knowledge of hundreds of sites over a period of years. (Goodwin 1946, P. 38–39)

From the late nineteenth century CE, into the first two decades of the twentieth century, South African archaeological finds were placed into European sequences. Louis Péringuey (1911), during this period, published regular works that compared finds to Aurignacian or Magdalenian Industries and described Neolithic elements in local assemblages. Often, the antiquity of these finds was considered recent when compared to their European counterparts. Some local terms emerged, such as 'Stellenbosch' and 'Orange River' types. In spite of these, the schema that supported the local occurrence of stone tools was based on European approaches and terminology. Not all agreed with this framework. Alfred Haddon (1906, p. 492) in his address to the British Association for the Advancement of Science in 1905 suggested that "until the stratigraphical evidence has been more satisfactorily studied it would be rash to speak of a South African palaeolithic period as being necessarily synchronous with that of Europe". Not only was there an issue with context but also analysis. Pieces were described as similar to those found in Europe, but assemblages were not being

T. Forssman, *Archaeology in Africa: Why the Past Matters*, Archaeology of Africa,
https://doi.org/10.1007/978-3-032-13365-6_5

systematically typed, morphological attributes were not strictly recorded, and the seriation of assemblages had not been attempted.

Within this context, a major development to take place was the appointment of the first professionally trained archaeologist in South Africa. John Goodwin, a South African born archaeologist trained at the University of Cambridge under Haddon and Miles Burkitt, was recruited to the University of Cape Town by Alfred Radcliffe-Brown in 1923. From Goodwin's arrival, Péringuey persuaded him to sort and compare the stone tool collections at the university and South African Museum. Goodwin set about this work and began forming ideas around South Africa's prehistory and its Stone Age sequence (Schlanger 2003). His earliest work to deal with this was titled *South African stone implement industries* (Goodwin 1926, p. 784), which was originally published in twelve articles under the title *Sermons in Stones*. In his final work he reported that "several of the keenest students of stone implements in South Africa" agreed that "sufficient evidence is now available for a clear distinction" between different industries. They agreed to adopt new terminology for the Earlier and Later Stone Age, but recognised that no geological basis to approximate dates existed. Whereas initially Goodwin (1926) had only written of an Earlier and Later Stone Age, the work of scholars such as Neville Jones (1926) in Zimbabwe led to the emergence of the Middle Stone Age, first used in 1927 (Goodwin 1958; Shepherd 2002b, p. 135). Before Goodwin could fully outline his schema of the Stone Age, Burkitt (1928) published his work titled *South Africa's Past in Stone and Paint* after a three month visit to the country in 1927. Goodwin would resent this for years to come, as he had already planned his book (Malan 1970, p. 91), and expressed his dismay at being excluded from Burkitt's production (Schlanger 2003). He would go on to make the statement used to open this chapter.

Goodwin's 1926 paper at the Pretoria conference led to further discussions with an engineer and keen amateur archaeologist: Clarence van Riet Lowe (Shepherd 2002b). Van Riet Lowe's interest in the past had been stimulated by a trip to Egypt while serving as a soldier in World War I. Back in South Africa, he found stone implements while building bridges and requested assistance from Alfred Radcliffe-Brown in interpreting them, who passed his letter on to Goodwin. This began a lengthy collaboration (Malan 1970). The first milestone of their work together was the most definitive publication at the time on the South African Stone Age, and probably the first archaeological book written within the country. It was titled *The Stone Age Cultures of South Africa* (Goodwin and Van Riet Lowe 1929) and presented the outline that Goodwin and others had been discussing for at least three years. Later, van Riet Lowe would share many discussions with Jan Smuts that would eventually lead to the formation of the Bureau of Archaeology that was to conduct research, promote archaeology, and network scholars. It was established in 1935 and led by van Riet Lowe (Malan 1970, p. 91). The 1929 book and the work that led to its publication neatly characterised African archaeology in the early twentieth century CE as the field came of age: amateur versus professional archaeologists (Stevenson 2012).

Goodwin and van Riet Lowe's (1929) work keenly illustrates the challenge of bringing together amateur and professional archaeologists at the time. Until then, amateur archaeology had dominated research. It was driven by non-specialists, those interested in the past, and people mostly working for, or with, colonial administrations. On the other hand, the dawn of professional archaeology glimmered. In *The Stone Age Cultures of South Africa,* Goodwin and van Riet Lowe (1929) grappled with assemblages collected from the surface with little systematisation and mostly from a short distance to South Africa's Cape, the authors struggled to confidently determine chronology, their relative dating attempts were unsatisfactory, and their means of determining mixing between assemblages absent. Above all, none of their assemblages came from sealed, stratified contexts; although they did compare their finds to stratigraphic sequences from two cave sites (Summers 1972). The only measure they used to determine the value of a collection was its number of artefacts (Goodwin 1958). They were victim in many respects to the vocational work that characterised the retrieval of the many assemblages or collections that they investigated across the country.

Amateur archaeologists that had for many years worked on African sequences were confronted with the professionalisation of the field. The disciplinary crossroad, however, was marshalled by colonial interests. These presented archaeologists with several challenges in the form of access to funds, government and organisational support, institutional and global interests, and commercial prospects. As in the past, the many challenges plagued archaeological studies, and they continued to do so as the discipline went through the complicated process of disentangling amateur and professionalism in archaeology locally. Moreover, the continent was still in the throes of colonialism and opposition arose towards this, intensifying during the inter-war years. Part of this was recognising local history and the significant cultural sequences, developments, and advances that took place on the continent. However, these issues, and many others, ebbed and flowed between national landscapes, language boundaries, and larger regions, with some being more prevalent than others during different periods or under varying contexts.

5.1 Disciplinary Crossroad for African Archaeology

Early archaeological practices were often influenced by colonial ontologies, most especially how these were applied to Africa. Many of the initial practitioners were associated with colonial missions and often had vested interest in their success (De Barros 1990, p. 158; Holl 1990, pp. 207–208; Robertshaw 1990b, p. 4; Shepherd 2002a, p. 193; Giblin 2013a, p. 254), although not always explicitly or directly. In Uganda, for example, Edward Wayland (1934) conducted among the first archaeological investigations while examining the nation's geology history for the colonial administration. Similarly, a geological prospector's wife in Rwanda, Boudiné Boutakoff (1937), when accompanying her husband became interested in local archaeology and published the first report on the finds made in the country (Giblin 2013b, p. 505). Like earlier attempts at understanding archaeology in Africa, these examples, and many other studies (for examples see Gabel 1985; Shaw 1989;

Musonda 1990), were carried out by amateurs and professionals in other fields. Before the mid-twentieth century, this began to change. More rigorous excavation techniques, standardisation in typologies and terminology, and regional and inter-regional perspectives emerged (Gabel 1985, p. 251). The focus of the discipline was still largely on classification and chronology, the latter largely based on relative techniques. However, the early practices of archaeology in Africa still fell within a "colonial paradigm" (Shaw et al. 1993, p. 22); an exotic gaze dominated explanatory frameworks, largely looking north or even east (Kirkman 1954; Clarke 1962; Chittick 1974, 1984).

When professional archaeology appeared, it was focussed on the search for migrations and diffusions. Such a perspective suited perceptions of Africa where a unilinear cultural evolution was suspected and political ends were sought (see Renfrew 1989, pp. 3–4). Such a model made it possible to explain the appearance of 'unexpected' finds in what was considered by some to be a cultural backwater (Holl 1990, p. 300). The Sahara Desert, for example, offered a further explanatory lens. Except for some, the vast desert was seen as largely impenetrable. It was thought to have blockaded cultural goods moving north from 'primitive' southern cultures, whereas 'advanced' northern societies were suitably capable of moving themselves and their goods through the region (cf. Deacon 1990, p. 255). From this perspective the view that eastern and southern pastoral groups descended from northern, 'civilised' people was justified (Robertshaw 1990b, p. 84). Similarly, the empires of West Africa were imagined to be descendent from Muslim or Jewish migrants who were throught to have travelled south (De Barros 1990, pp. 162–164; Holl 1990, p. 300), as opposed to Frobenius's (1911) Atlantis theory (see below). Scholars at the time perpetuated this view with great agility used to avoid simpler explanations. Charles Seligman (1930), for example, professed that all sub-Saharan accomplishments were the direct result of pre-historic Hamitic migrations. In this Hamitic hypothesis, groups from Egypt and the Middle East were thought to have diffused into Africa bringing with them the various advances in the recent past. Such views led to mischaracterisations of indigenous people in contemporary Africa (Giblin 2013a, p. 255 citing Robertshaw 1990b, 1990a):

> Maasai pastoralists became wandering Jews, Saharan and Sahelian settlements became Negro, Hamite, or Berber based on lithics or rock art, Maghrebi lithic traditions were given European antecedents, and Egyptian influence was identified in West African stone ruins and lithic industries, while ancient Greeks became the colonizers of Ife, southern African rock art, Asian or European, and metallurgy in sub-Saharan Africa Arabian, and Swahili coastal states and monuments in the east African interior the products of a northeastern Azanian civilization.

The 'Hamitic' origins were placed variously in Pharaonic Egypt (Seligman 1930) or possibly in an earlier Nilotic history from which the former emerged (Frankfort 1948). They were thought to have produced stone and earthen monuments in East Africa (Huntingford 1933, 2017) as well as state formations in West Africa and Zimbabwe (e.g., Irstam 1944), and they possibly had Stone Age histories as well (Cole 1954). Many groups around Africa were beneficiaries of the Hamitic spread from the Nile Valley region that filtered into other parts of the continent. The diffusion of crafts, knowledges and skills were used to explain a vast array of developments and innovations. For example, iron smelting was thought to come from a single source, linked to Meroe (Shinnie 1967), and that megalithic constructions as far south as Zimbabwe were linked to Cushites (Murdock 1959); this while Oliver and Fage (1963) countered prevailing diffusion models by emphasising historical connections between the Nile Valley and the Kingdoms of Nubia and Kush. Similarly, towns in Africa were linked to Muslim connections and not local innovations. Muslims, it was thought, brought with them new developments, socio-political complexity, and technological advances. However, although the Hamitic hypothesis has been discredited by academics, it still persists in political discourse in East Africa (Taylor 1999).

Partly driving the proliferation of the diffusion-migration approach was amateur archaeology (Trigger 1990, p. 312). In addition, this was imbued with prejudicial and narrow perspectives of Africa's past. The use of skull measurements to enforce racial superiority is one such example founded in so called biological sciences (Renfrew 1989, p. 4). However, cultural sequences were strongly impacted by such prejudices as well, such as early views of Great Zimbabwe, but so was the interpretation of, among other things, rock art.

A famous example is from Namibia. Henri Breuil (1948) visited a site in the Brandberg Massif and provided interpretations of what was called the white lady (in fact a male) (Fig. 5.1), in which he compared the human images and their actions to Cretan ceremonial practices. He interpreted the white pigment as an indication of race. Following on from this, he visited parts of what is now Zimbabwe and concluded that there are many other similar examples, further supporting his contentions and arguing for a vast array of northerners heading south but eventually 'disappearing' over centuries of "cross-breeding" (Breuil 1954, p. 41). His views, underpinned by the notions that local communities were incapable of such advanced artistic innovation, were well supported by some scholars, but notably not Goodwin and van Riet (Dubow 2019). These exotic views did not venture far from earlier projections of Africa's past and its connection with the 'white world' (e.g., Frobenius 1913; Seligman 1930). These ideologies persisted for most of the first half of the century. In as late as the 1960s, Grafton Smith and William Perry (cf. Daniel 1962) argued that all of Africa outside of the Nile Valley has benefited from either diffusion or migration to the extent that local innovation and invention was entirely absent, and later Charles Binns (1974) would argue that the Zulu in South Africa's KwaZulu-Natal were associated with the lost tribe of Israel.

What the exotic model did, by extension, was exclude sub-Saharan Africa from the northern regions as well as from global histories. Sub-Saharan groups were considered stranded between a desert and the oceans with no ability to escape these confines. While this perspective might not seem all that significant initially, it is vitally important that such a view was scaffolded into general perceptions of the continent from the late nineteenth century CE onwards. Generating and purporting the notion that Africa's lack of advancement, cultural achievements, and historic reverence cast the continent into a socio-cultural and evolutionary doldrum that suited colonialism. Africa lacked the ability to elevate itself. Its primitive state was seen as victim to

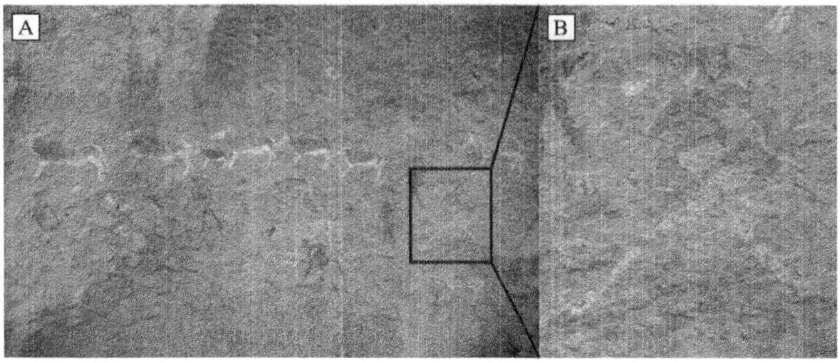

Fig. 5.1 (A) The white lady of the Brandberg scene with a procession of humans and antelope, and (B) An enlarged image of the white lady (photograph: Tim Forssman)

internalised preconditions. Therefore, external factors were needed to 'help' Africa escape its quagmire. Constructing the continent's past in this way reinforced the idea that positive change could only be advanced by outside, civilised forces (De Barros 1990, p. 160; Robertshaw 1990c, p. 84). Diffusionist ideologies were central to colonial administrators' legitimisation of their involvement on the continent (Giblin 2013a, p. 255).

These frameworks rooted in Eurocentric ideologies, pseudo-scientific racial typologies, and an obsession with external origins shaped early archaeological interpretations across the continent. Yet, as archaeology began to take root regionally, local case studies began to both reflect and challenge these entrenched paradigms. The relationship between amateur and professional and foreign and local frameworks took hold in many parts of Africa where excavations contested interpretations, and tensions appeared between colonial narratives and emerging archaeological practices.

5.1.1 Southern Africa

In southern Africa, South Africa's context was incomparable to its neighbours. Except for Botswana and Lesotho, which were British protectorates, all other countries were occupied by various European nations: South Africa and Zimbabwe by Britain, Namibia (then South-West Africa) by Germany, Mozambique by Portugal, and Madagascar by France. At the turn of the twentieth century CE, South Africa became a brutal battleground between white settler societies and Britain. What is presently called the South African War, but which was previously known as the Boer War, began on 11 October 1899 and would last until the signing of the Treaty of Vereeniging on 31 May 1902 (Judd and Surridge 2002). By this time, about 28,000 white people, mostly children, and between 14,000 and 20,000 black people perished in concentration camps (Warwick 1983; Kessler 1999; Mongalo and Du Pisani 1999). Additionally, about 7000 Boer troops and 22,000 soldiers fighting for the British died

(Morgan 2002). It was a highly attritional war fought between a small number of local soldiers, around 88,000 in total, and nearly half a million from Britain and various colonies, and led to mass destruction of infrastructure, property, and livestock across the terrain of war. The conflict enraged after a period of strife, uneasiness, and tension between European 'outsiders' (*uitlanders*) living in the republics and Boer administration. The war had considerable impact on the character of colonialism within the country.

Two related issues are worth mentioning that pertain to the relationship between locals and colonial administrators. First, after the war the Boers generally split into two factions: those who accepted defeat and saw it most appropriate to move forward as a British colony, and the *'bittereinders'* or bitter-enders, who wanted to continue their fight for independence. Most administrators fell into the former group, and they were intent on demonstrating their allegiance with Britain. In 1907, they gifted the world's largest diamond, the Cullinan (3106 carats), to King Edward VII "as a symbolic token to heal the rift between Britain and South Africa following the Boer War" (Mechkarini et al. 2023, p. 825). The diamond was split into nine, with many smaller diamonds, and the largest was placed in the British crown jewels, notably the Star of Africa in the crown itself (Smith 2003, p. 531). The second issue is the treatment of local black communities during and after the war. Initially, the South African War was considered a 'white man's' war that involved only Europeans and their local descendant groups (Marks 2001). However, Boer generals claimed that the British were deploying vast numbers of black troops in combat. Recent estimates place this at 100,000 to 120,000 black troops, of which 30,000 were armed. The Boers, despite their protestations, also used black troops and deployed about 14,000 individuals (20% of the Boer forces) (Warwick 1983; Nasson 2003). Despite their involvement in the war, when it concluded, they were excluded from reparative endeavours, political roles, or economic assistance (Warwick 1983). In fact, it has been argued that growing fear that the 'black threat' would overcome the by-then-Afrikaner rule in the 1940s contributed to the appearance of South Africa's *apartheid* regime under the National Party (Wessels 2016). These two very different relations between groups in South Africa and colonial administrators illustrates the stratified nature of colonial influence across a nation's society. It also forms the backdrop that heritage fields were set against, and which imbricated with those fields in various ways.

South Africa's National Party (1948–1994) government perpetuated several beliefs used to legitimise their occupation of the region and dominion over it. They described the land as empty until the arrival of *voortrekkers*; European-descent groups that migrated from the Cape to establish their own territories in the interior. In their construction of the past, black 'hoards' arrived in the southern region of Africa in the seventeenth century CE at the same time that the Dutch established a refreshment station in the Cape (Gerstner 1991). European groups' movement to occupy territories initially along the coastal region but eventually in land was perceived to be at the same time as arriving African communities. These views conveniently justified widespread land occupations associated with white expansionism. The nineteenth century CE *Groot Trek* (Great Trek) is perhaps one of the most foundational occurrences in recent South African history. It involved numbers of dissenting Boer settlers, unhappy with losing the colony to the British, vacating the Cape in search of their own territories leading to the widespread settlement of the interior region (Fig. 5.2). The trek reformed the way Boers related to God, one another, the land, and others living in the region. The many conflicts between themselves and local communities fashioned their relationships going forward and would influence their politics in the second half of the twentieth century AD (Templin 1999).

Archaeology in South Africa developed earlier than in most sub-Saharan regions, owing in part to the presence of a growing colonial settler population and the establishment of universities (Shaw 1989, p. 7). By the mid-twentieth century, it had become a prominent and internationally recognised field, with a small cohort of foreign scholars engaging with the region's archaeological record. The discipline even showed promise as a site for challenging Eurocentric frameworks and rethinking Africa's past. This momentum was supported by figures like Smuts, who, despite his own ideological complexities, allowed a degree of academic freedom and remained largely indifferent to rising anti-colonial sentiment and African nationalism in the sciences. His support provided space for archaeologists to pursue research from a relatively non-partisan perspective. However, following Smuts' death in 1950 and the rise of the National Party, this fragile autonomy quickly eroded. The new government, steeped in extreme settler nationalism (see Esterhuysen 2006), reversed much

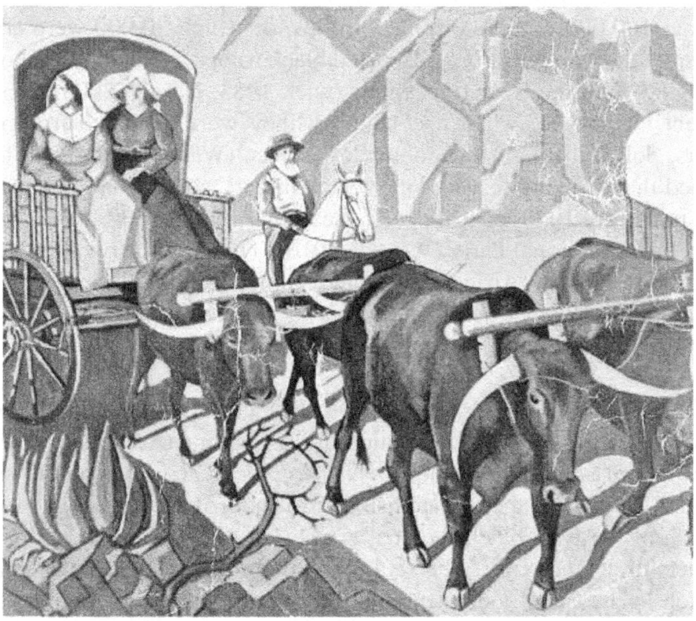

Fig. 5.2 A painting by Jacobus Pierneef from 1938 commemorating the centenary celebration of the Groot Trek (Great Trek). *Source* https://commons.wikimedia.org/wiki/File:JH_Pierneef_-_Die_Groot_Trek_1938.jpg

of the earlier progress. Goodwin lamented the withdrawal of support, especially the cancellation of Smuts' invitation to host the Pan-African Congress (Shepherd 2003, p. 833). Under the National Party, archaeology was sidelined in favour of nationalist historical narratives that centred on Afrikaner identity. State-sanctioned celebrations such as the re-enactments of the Groot Trek, the Battle of Blood River, and the arrival of Jan and Maria van Riebeeck became dominant commemorative events (Rassool and Witz 1993; Templin 1999). The past was no longer something to be uncovered in the soil but something to be mythologised on the surface. The discipline of archaeology stagnated. Goodwin, increasingly isolated, shifted his focus to Nigeria and trained only one doctoral student (Revil Mason), creating just three jobs for his students (Berry Malan, Mason, and Peter Beaumont) before his death in 1959 (van Riet Lowe had died earlier, in 1956) (Shepherd 2003). By 1961, Ray Inskeep (1961, pp. 225–227), addressing the Annual Meeting of the South African Museums, acknowledged that while South African archaeology had once been at the forefront of research on the continent, it now lagged.

The 'discovery' of Mapungubwe on the southern banks of the Limpopo River overlapped with these two political phases in South African archaeology. The history of research at the site illustrates the clash of prevailing views at the time and the contestation between amateur and professional archaeology. The site was first reported in 1933 by the van Graan family. They came upon it while hunting in the region and approached a local resident, Mowena (or Mokoena), asking for water, noticing what they thought was an unusual ceramic vessel at his hut. He explained that it had come from a nearby, ancient settlement to which he could not lead them because it was sacred. However, eventually a young relative offered to show the family the site when they presented remuneration, and he led them to the now famous hill – although he stopped short saying he was frightened and would not go any further. The van Graan group ascended the hill and scoured its flat top finding a trove of archaeological remains, including ceramics, gold, and dry-packed stone walling. They excavated sections of the site themselves until they realised the significance of their finds. One of the family members was a student at the University of Pretoria at the time and on returning to campus he informed Leo Fouché of their 'discovery'. His reports prompted a visit to the site and ultimately its excavation (Carruthers 2006; Tiley-Nel 2022).

In April of 1933, Fouché (1937) began excavations at Mapungubwe (Fig. 5.3). He and his team excavated a limited area on the hill itself as well as in the area of the court below. The excavations were conducted by a large team, including van Riet Lowe, John Schofield, Alexander Galloway, Guy Gardner and Jones, who led the field programme (Fouché 1937). Many finds were made, including gold and Chinese celadon, suggesting an age around 1200 CE. However, most of the team members, including Fouché, were not trained archaeologists, and the work that they carried out was not conducted at a level that would have been acceptable even at the time. Soon after their study was complete, P. W. Van Tonder (see Fouché 1937), a field assistant at first (Tiley-Nel 2011), and then he and Gardner (1963), who in fact was an archaeologist, began their excavations. Between 1934 and 1940 they excavated and removed a huge amount of deposit from the hilltop area; Schofield (1937) had conducted limited excavations here in 1934 with additional excavations in the court area and focussed his research primarily on ceramics. The various programmes of research included amateur approaches followed by professional investigations, but both were marred with romantic and political hues, pilfering Africa's past for contemporary, nationalist agendas (see the overview by Meyer 2000).

Mapungubwe's occupants were disputed, much like those of Great Zimbabwe. One of the earlier interpretations was that Boskop Man was responsible for Mapungubwe. Galloway (1959) thought the human remains, his part of the study, were 'Bantu-Hottentot' and not 'Bantu-Negroid'. This was a convenient interpretation at the time because it was accepted at that stage that Boskop Man had become extinct. As only a relic of the past, there were no descendants to lay claim to the site or history, which suited the political scenario in South Africa at the time (Dubow 1995). Gardner (1963) later suggested it was a Khoekhoe group, indigenous herders, that had been responsible for Mapungubwe. This led to the notion that the Iron Age spread ahead of black communities through Khoekoe people. These contentions, additionally, drew into question differences between the Iron Age and Stone Age, and ultimately contributed to a still-held separationist approach when dealing with these overlapping phases and their associated identities (Forssman 2023). Such interpretations, like those before it, adopted a clear nationalist slant (Dubow 1995). Both arguments denied contemporary, Bantu-language speaking groups a connection with those who established and occupied Mapungubwe (Schoeman and Pikirayi 2011). Archaeological finds, however, challenged the notions that Mapungubwe was not connected to African communities in South Africa, and more emphatically that the land was not empty (Marks 1980). Research through to the 1960s was largely problematic, or in contestation with political views, before a lengthy period of disinterest in the site persisted until the late 1990s.

Just across the Limpopo in Zimbabwe, archaeological research had taken root with a focus on both the Stone Age and state societies like Great Zimbabwe. Key figures such as Cran Cooke, Geoffrey Bond, Roger Summers, and Keith Robinson contributed to refining the region's cultural sequence through work at sites like Khami, Inyanga, and Great Zimbabwe (Robinson 1959; Cooke 1960; Summers et al. 1961). However, despite this progress, archaeology across southern Africa remained highly regional. Outside of South Africa and Zimbabwe, much of the subcontinent received limited scholarly attention. Botswana, for example, was largely overlooked despite its rich archaeological record, including important late Holocene sites comparable to those of its neighbours (Mitchell 2024). In Mozambique, over 90 Stone Age sites were identified between the 1930s and 1950s, but little of this work was followed up; even by 2000, it remained underrepresented in continental syntheses (Rodrigues 1998, 2004; McBrearty and Brooks 2000, p. 478). Caimane, excavated in 1984, was the only site to yield a full sequence from the Earlier Stone Age through to the Iron Age (Morais 1984). Though research was carried out, it remained far less intensive and coordinated than in neighbouring countries.

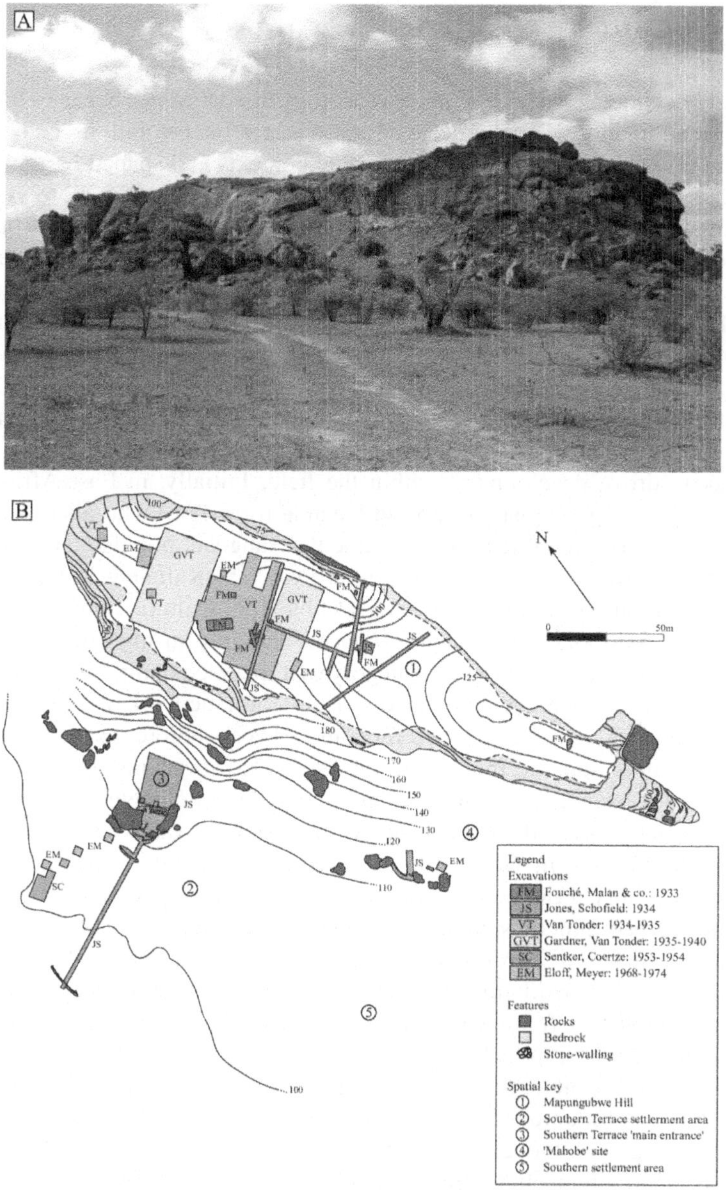

Fig. 5.3 (A) Photograph of Mapungubwe Hill looking northwards (photograph: JJ van Zyl). *Source* https://en.m.wikipedia.org/wiki/File%3AMapungubweHill.jpg?utm_source=chatgpt.com, and (B) A reproduced map showing the history of excavations at Mapungubwe Hill from 1933 to 1974 (the photograph was taken from approximately the 100 m contour) (map produced by Tim Forssman)

5.1.2 *East Africa*

In the early twentieth century CE, the archaeology of East Africa began to take shape through a combination of geological explorations, personal ambitions, and emerging scientific curiosity. Though rooted in colonial contexts and shaped by the interests of external scholars, this period also marked the beginnings of a more systematic and professional approach to uncovering the region's past. Early frameworks were experimental, often speculative, and later overturned, yet they laid the groundwork for what would follow. Central to this story are the individuals and teams whose work defined East African archaeology between the wars, as well as the evolving methodologies that gradually moved the field from isolated discovery towards collaborative scientific inquiry.

The archaeology of East Africa become known to a wider scientific community through geological surveys carried out in the region. As with other areas, a handful of characters drove development within the field. Initially, in East Africa it was Wayland (1934), a geologist working in Uganda from 1919 who also focussed on local prehistory. His work led him to define the Sangoan, but also the Kafuan and Magosian Industries, which have since fallen away. The Kafuan was thought to be a pre-Oldowan Industry, known then as the Pebble Tool Culture, but was abandoned as a result of the tools likely being produced naturally in high-fracture environments. Magosian was found to be a category that included a mixture of Middle and Later Stone Age assemblages. Wayland's (1934) climatic work and its correlations with industries in Uganda dominated for some 30 years before they were discarded in favour of more suitable models in the 1950s. However, his approach laid the groundwork for later research into the interplay between climate, environment and human societies. Wayland's work resulted in a book by van Riet Lowe (1952) in the series *The Pleistocene Geology and Prehistory of Uganda*, which presented the country's prehistory. Prior to this, the only book of its kind was Terence O'Brien (1939) presenting a general summary of Ugandan prehistory in 1939. Early archaeological approaches were therefore launched by non-specialists but with a background in earth sciences. The work nonetheless laid the formative steps towards professionalism, but established frameworks that would later be overturned, such as early typologies and climatic models.

The most significant contributors to Africa's past from this period, and arguably one who did more for unravelling humanity's story in Africa (Tobias 2003), however, were the Leakeys. Although a Cambridge-trained English archaeologist, Louis Leakey considered himself "more of a Kikuyu than an Englishman in many ways" (Leakey 1937; cf. Tobias 2003, p. 41); he was initiated into Kikuyu life (Posnansky 2012, p. 34). He was raised in Kikuyu territory by missionary parents and was accustomed to Kikuyu ways, such that he later consulted with the Kenyan government during the Mau Rebellion between 1952 and 1960, which involved Kikuyu people (Leakey 1952, 1954). In 1923, after injuring himself in a rugby match, he was advised to take a year's leave and ended up, the following year, working with William Cutler, a member of the British Museum East African Expedition, on a fossil collection

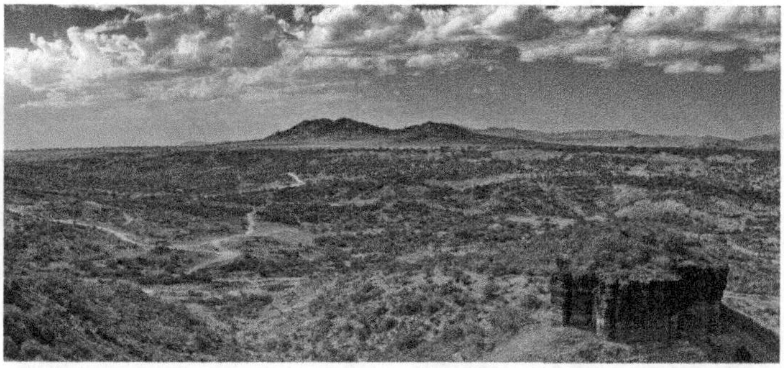

Fig. 5.4 A view of Olduvai Gorge in northern Tanzania (photograph: Noel Feans). *Source* https://commons.wikimedia.org/wiki/File:Olduvai_Gorge_or_Oldupai_Gorge.jpg

study in Tanganyika Territory. He obtained a first in Archaeology and Anthropology in 1926 and then led the East African Archaeological Research Expeditions from that year until 1935. His work during this time, which included excavations at what are now renowned sites such as Olduvai Gorge (Fig. 5.4) and Gamble's Cave, along with many others, laid the foundation for later archaeological and palaeontological studies (Tobias 1973, 2003, p. 42). It also led to the production of his first outline of the Stone Age, in the same year that Goodwin and van Riet Lowe (1929) completed their study (Leakey 1929), which subsequently was converted into his book, *The Stone Age Culture of Kenya Colony* (Leakey 1931). He classified a handaxe culture, afterwards called the African Acheulean, as well as flake and blade-and-burin cultures, and the Mesolithic and Neolithic Industries.

What L. Leakey is perhaps most credited for is his work with Mary Leakey in Olduvai (Fig. 5.5). Wilhelm Kattwinkel, a German entomologist, was the first European scholar to note the occurrence of stone implements and fossils in Olduvai during his work there in 1911. It was Hans Reck (1914a 1914b) who first collected fossils in the gorge prior to the First World War, but the war stalled work after Reck had piqued interest in the region back home in Germany. On their next research visit to Olduvai, the 1931–1932 East African Expedition, Reck and L. Leakey, with others, resulted in L. Leakey finding the first handaxe in situ with his Kikuyu team-members. By 1951, hundreds had been found and eleven stages of handaxe evolution were defined (Leakey 1951). After the first visit, Reck "formally handed over the scientific rights to work in the Gorge to Dr. [L.] Leakey" (Gabel 1985, p. 258). L. Leakey and Wayland returned the following year, and in 1935 the Leakeys, with a larger team, spent several months working in the gorge, but this turned out to be the last extended visit as a result of financial issues and the onset of the Second World War, delaying the publication of their findings (Leakey 1951).

L. Leakey was undoubtedly one of the most influential characters in African archaeology and palaeontology. He was "the dominant pioneer adventurer-explorer of humanity's distant past" (Posnansky 2012, p. 34). When he wrote *Adam's Ancestors* (Leakey 1934), Africa's past was vastly unknown and its possibilities gradually

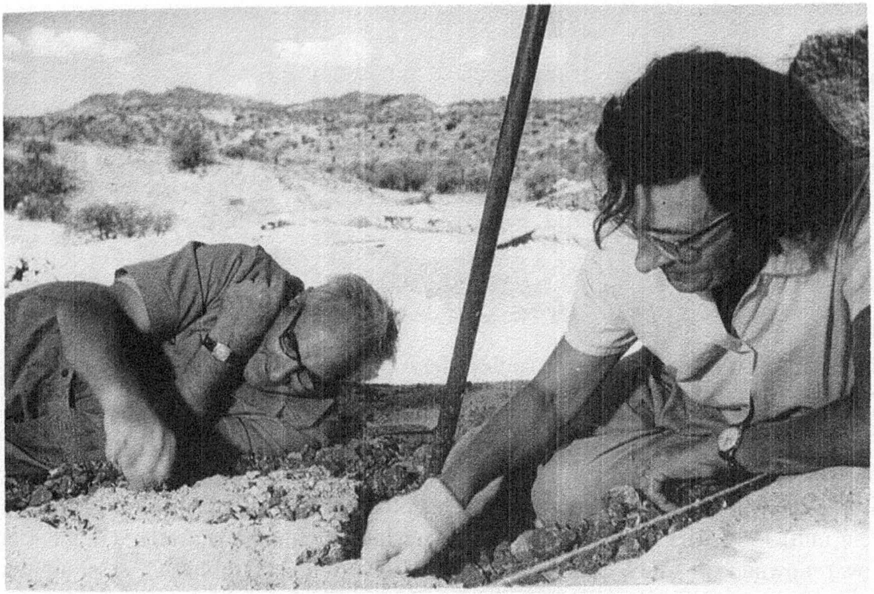

Fig. 5.5 Louis and Mary Leakey excavating in Olduvai Gorge, Tanzania, c. 1952–1953. *Source* https://commons.wikimedia.org/wiki/File:Mary_Douglas_Nicol_Leakey_(1913-1996)_and_her_husband_Louis_Seymour_Bazett_Leakey_(1903–1972).jpg

coming to the fore. From early on, L. Leakey recognised the incredible role Africa played in the human story. Phillip Tobias (1973, p. 6) described him as single-minded, with restless energy, and a visionary who "sparkled with an effervescent enthusiasm". By his death in 1972, he had authored some 20 books and near-on 170 articles, and supported a swathe of students in various ways. He was also involved in Jane Goodall's, Diane Fossey's and Jill Donisthorpe's influential work. His organisation of the third Pan-African Prehistory Congress in Nigeria represented a significant moment in the history of the discipline, and his role as chair in the following years succeeded in fostering a continental identity for the discipline. L. Leakey also courted controversy, specifically with unsubstantiated claims he made about finding early man, but these are partly a consequence of the times he worked in, archaeological science, and his enjoyment of the limelight (Posnansky 2012). But these incidents are few in what was an incredibly important career and ultimately chapter in learning about human history in Africa.

M. Leakey, a distant relative of John Frere who pioneered work on Europe's stone tool industry, first ventured to Africa in 1933. She and her mother travelled to Cape Town, South Africa, to meet Goodwin and visit South African and Zimbabwean sites. There she assisted Goodwin excavate Oakhurst Shelter and later studied under Jones in Bulawayo. From here she went to Kenya in 1935 and joined L. Leakey at Olduvai, whom she had first met in 1933 at the Royal Anthropological Institute. The two would marry the following year and marking what J. Desmond Clark (2001,

p. 598) called "the beginning of the most important partnership in the search for and discovery of the fossils, biological, and cultural evidence of the human ancestral record". M. Leakey directed research at Olduvai, and later Laetoli, and through her work advanced understanding of the gorge's prehistorical record, and held the project together after L. Leakey passed in 1972 (Clark 2001, p. 596). Clark (2001, p. 612) described her as tireless, rigorous, and excellent in her endeavours. She also possessed a foresight unlike many others; at a time when bone fragments were being discarded, she retained them and refitted long bones which showed the significance of marrow extraction. She was also keenly liked by members of her teams for her patience, compassion, and kindness.

M. Leakey's (1959) best-known fossil find was in 1959 when she discovered 'Dear Boy', *Zinjanthropus boisei* but now *Paranthropus boisei*, the first major hominin fossil find in Olduvai from a site called FLK Zinj. The human cranium remains were recovered from Bed I and thought to date to 1.75 million years ago. The co-occurrence of stone tools led M. Leakey (1959) to suggest that the hominin had possibly produced tools, but these were later associated with *Homo habilis*. The first of this species was also discovered by M. Leakey's son, Jonathan, near to FLK Zinj during her excavations in 1960 and is now the type specimen OH7 (Leakey et al. 1964). Subsequent to these discoveries, more than 400 hominin fossils were found in the gorge (Gaur 2015, p. 673). Another important finding that M. Leakey was involved in was the discovery of fossils at Laetoli, which led to the identification of a tuff dating to about 3.5 million years ago that included tracks from insects and mammals, as well as a 25 meter hominin trail, probably *Australopithecus afarensis* (Hay and Leakey 1982). This important track shows with certainty the bipedalism of australopithecines (Clark 2001, p. 610).

The Leakeys began an archaeological dynasty, which has been followed by their family. As the accounts by Tobias (1973, 2003) and Clark (2001) state several times, they were incredible servants to the field of prehistory, and laid the foundations for future studies from infrastructure to local interest, while revolutionising approaches to archaeology as well as understandings of the past. As in southern Africa and other parts of the continent, they were the characters that drove the discipline forward, professionalising palaeosciences as they did so, and introduced it to a wider audience.

5.1.3 North Africa

Archaeology in the Maghreb was heavily influenced by what was happening in France at the time (Sheppard 1990, p. 173). Much of the work was carried out by amateur or avocational archaeologists—doctors, military personnel, and teachers—who had been sent to North Africa to serve in the colonies or in territories in the process of colonisation, such as Algeria. By the 1920s, several archaeological societies had been established, and publications in the French journal *L'Anthropologie* had become regular. These contributions largely sought to fit the North African Palaeolithic sequence into frameworks developed in France. However, these attempts led to misinterpretations and rival claims, neatly captured in one disagreement known as the Aurignacian Debate.

In 1909, Jacques de Morgan, an established archaeologist of the Near East and Egypt, began research in eastern Algeria and Tunisia. He published findings on stone tools from southern Tunisia, identifying an earlier assemblage of blades, burins, and thick scrapers, and a later assemblage comprising small scrapers, ostrich eggshell, and polished bone tools (de Morgan et al. 1910, p. 273). He noted that parts of this assemblage resembled the French Aurignacian Industry described by Breuil (1905, 1912). de Morgan et al. (1910, p. 117) termed this the Capsian, and explained the similarities from a 'palaeoethnological' perspective, then a contemporary term aligned with evolutionary thinking, proposing independent development, a view shared by Émile Gobert (1910), a local doctor with archaeological interests. Both argued that similar environmental conditions in France and North Africa led to comparable assemblages (Sheppard 1990, p. 176). However, these views were immediately challenged.

French amateur archaeologists rejected the notion that independent development was more likely than contact and diffusion. De Morgan's co-author, Louis Capitan, disagreed with him, believing that these similarities indicated exchanges of people or ideas across the Mediterranean (de Morgan et al. 1910, p. 226). Breuil (1912, p. 183) elaborated further, comparing the Capsian to the Middle Aurignacian, and proposed that it had spread from North Africa into Europe via Spain, influencing the French Aurignacian. Historical societies in the Maghreb enthusiastically embraced these diffusionist models, perhaps motivated by the prospect that African traditions might predate and even influence those of Europe (Sheppard 1990, p. 177). Excavations by Albert Debruge (1923) at Mechta El Arbi near Constantine in eastern Algeria (1914, 1923) recovered an assemblage lacking burins and geometric microliths, as well as a bone industry that he attributed to an intrusive Neolithic occupation. Earlier finds at the site included skulls thought to be Neanderthaloid (Mercier and Debruge 1912), but subsequent analyses rejected this, concluding that the skulls were likely of a later age (Mercier 1915; Pond et al. 1928). This undermined the argument for diffusion from North Africa to France, since these finds post-dated comparable European assemblages.

Further complicating matters were notable geographic differences across North Africa. Sites in eastern Algeria, for example, yielded geometric microliths – small, crescent-shaped stone tools – recorded by Debruge (1923), while these were absent at western sites. Maurice Reygasse (1920, p. 515) interpreted this pattern as evidence of an Aurignacian tradition in the east, proposing three cultural phases based on technological characteristics (e.g., early blade, microlithic, and later debitage industries). However, Gobert (1910) questioned whether the absence of microliths in some areas reflected genuine cultural variation or was simply a result of inadequate excavation methods, such as the failure to sieve sediments properly. These debates were clearly complicated by the prevailing determination to align the North African archaeological sequence with French typologies, reinforcing assumptions of diffusion and cultural influence across the Mediterranean.

A central problem in these debates, as across much of Africa at the time, was the absence of reliable chronology. For example, the Logan Museum's expedition in

Algeria during the 1920s conducted extensive surveys, covering 2800 km by vehicle and a further 500 km by camel, recording numerous sites (Pond et al. 1928). These were followed by systematic surface collections and analyses. However, there was no methodical approach to establishing the age of the assemblages or their stratigraphic contexts. It remained unclear whether the sites represented palimpsests or discrete occupational episodes, and it was often assumed that the artefact scatters were time-constrained accumulations (Sheppard 1990). At some sites excavations were conducted in three-metre-wide trenches, and sediments were screened through angled sieves, following Debruge's (1923) methods. The upper 15 cm were treated as a single surface unit, while the remainder of the trenches were excavated in arbitrary layers corresponding to the thickness of the mound, using 3 × 2 m squares. Alonzo Pond and the museum's director, George Collie, carried out these excavations with remarkable methodological care for the time, employing approaches that would not be seen again in North Africa for another two decades (Sheppard 1990, p. 1980).

Building on the Logan Museum's work, Raymond Vaufrey (1933, 1955) excavated small areas at multiple sites, often in collaboration with Gobert, and focused on formal, retouched tools to characterise industries. His work established the standard outline of the Capsian sequence for the next 30 years. Vaufrey (1933) developed a relative chronology and argued against the Aurignacian hypothesis on typological and geological grounds. Notably, he identified Capsian tools within wadi alluvium deposits, indicating a younger age than previously thought; a view that Breuil (1937) later endorsed, agreeing that this disproved the supposed link to the Aurignacian. Vaughfrey (1933) also mapped the geographic distribution of the Capsian and its three phases, developing a spatial framework that remains reasonably accurate (Camps 1974, p. 117).

The Aurignacian Debate in the Maghreb illustrates how early archaeological efforts, shaped by colonial ambitions and disciplinary immaturity, struggled to move beyond fitting African sequences into European frameworks. Yet, as methodologies improved and data accumulated, simplistic models of diffusion or evolution began to give way to more nuanced understandings. The gradual professionalisation of the field, marked by advances in excavation techniques and growing attention to chronology, allowed North African industries like the Capsian to be recognised on their own terms. This case study thus reflects a broader shift: from speculative, agenda-driven interpretations towards a more rigorous, evidence-based approach that laid the groundwork for a genuinely African archaeology.

5.1.4 West Africa

West African archaeology from the early twentieth century CE until the 1940s was exploratory, descriptive and fragmentary, rather than systematic. There were excavations but the majority of work relied on surface collections and surveys. Prior to the 1920s, West African archaeology was rooted in British and French colonialism, each with its own character. British colonies were separate and distinct, whereas the

French colonies were intended to be assimilated into the host territory (Kense 1990). As a result, French amateur and professional archaeology emphasised comparison and integration. Finds made often by administrators or teachers (see McIntosh and McIntosh 1995, p. 15), for example, were largely sent back to scholars in France, who may never have visited Africa, where they were studied and placed in French sequences. Interest was largely in prehistory as the continent was not thought to have an important contemporary past, and even its prehistory was considered backward and stagnant (Fage 1980). These views trickled down from the pejorative notions held of local communities, who were often connected to the Stone Age past, and any advances that were noted were ascribed to external influences (De Barros 1990). In British West Africa, research into the local archaeology was mostly carried out by geologists and amateurs at first, and largely in isolation (Kense 1990). The consequence of much of this was an emphasis on climatic variation and geomorphological processes (Kense 1990). Most work was concentrated in areas with improved visibility and not the forested savannah or tropical regions (Mauny 1953).

West African archaeology began to change from the 1930s, with the establishment of *Institut Francais d'Afrique Noire* in 1936 (Thiaw 2013, p. 356). The institute centralised scientific work in French West-African colonies, but was still troubled with stray finds, small assemblages, single site studies, and troublesome chronologies. Its first director was Theodore Monod (1936), a naturalist, engaged in archaeological and historical research. In 1937 he was joined by Raymond Mauny, whom he coached and who was to make a notable contribution. While Mauny (1961, p. 13) served in the Second World War he used his off-time to visit libraries in the places he visited across North Africa and develop his knowledge of African archaeological sequences. On his return, in 1947, he was appointed as the head of the archaeology and prehistory section of the institute. However, until the late 1950s, his work as well as others at the institute, proposed diffusionist thinking since at the time Senegal was considered the backwaters of the Muslim world. There was little consideration for local innovation or development and the general thinking was that items such as luxuries were imported (McIntosh 2001). Studies did not attempt to understand regional patterns (McIntosh and McIntosh 1981) and collections were primarily unsystematic (De Barros 1990). A notable advantage during this time was provided by aerial photographs taken by the French military that led to the identification of a number of sites in urban areas (Gard and Mauny 1961). Because of the threats that development posed, collections at these sites was often undertaken, but were largely unsystematic (Thiaw 2013).

Increasingly after the war, systematic archaeological studies began appearing. Isolated excavations included Bernard Fagg's (1972) work at Rop Shelter, Nigeria, published in 1940 and 1944, and cave studies by Robert Delcroix and Vaufrey (1939) in French Guinea. In Ghana, Thurston Shaw (1944) excavated Bumpra (Bosumpra) Cave in 1940, the country's first excavated microlithic site. Ceramic traditions associated with stone tools were also reported by Robert Wild (1934) in Ashanti and Jean-Baptiste Jauze (1944a, 1944b) in Cameroon. From the 1940s onwards, West African archaeology began to take on a more systematic character. Oliver Davies's

(1967) definition of the Kintampo Industry in 1950, with clear links to domesticated animals, marked a step towards more integrated cultural reconstructions. Major discoveries such as the enigmatic Nok terracottas, first published by B. Fagg (1945) in 1945, and further finds of Ife heads just before the war, deepened understanding of early West African artistry. Shaw's (1970) excavations at Igbo-Ukwu uncovered rich ritual deposits, comparable to Ife in complexity, suggesting a sophisticated society possibly contemporary with, or even preceding, the well-known southern Nigerian civilisations. By the late 1940s, archaeology in West Africa had come of Age and its practice advanced rapidly after that, as Chapter 6 discusses. However, for the early twentieth century CE, archaeology in West Africa was not as advanced as other regions, largely due to the perception at the time that the region was peripheral.

5.1.5 Central Africa

In central Africa, north of the Zambezi River saw little archaeological work. That which was carried out, was widely scattered geographically, but did include foundational studies. Jean Colette (1929) began his work in what was then Belgian Congo. His excavations began in 1925 with the help of six prisoners who would be rewarded if they left their finds in situ (Couttenier 2012). Between 1925 and 1927, he excavated Kalina Point (now Gombe Point), Kinshasa. The site yielded stratified deposits and a substantial cultural sequence (Colette 1929). The context enabled Colette to examine shifts over time at the site and establish cultural change (Bequaert 1938), although he had no way of determining absolute chronology. His study nonetheless provided early insights into local tool technology (Clark 1971; Gabel 1985, p. 256). He analysed 18,652 knapped flakes and sent 779 back to Tervuren (Couttenier 2012). At first, he explained these using diffusion-migration approaches, reflecting current trends in the field of archaeology for the time. However, later he distanced himself from such ideas and proposed independent, innovation, which was an approach very much ahead of its time (Colette 1935). Colette was a leader in Central African archaeology and contributed significantly to our understanding of the past from this region. The meticulous approach he took to excavation and studying sites was advanced for its day and laid the foundation for archaeological endeavours.

Although not being confined to a single region, the most prolific archaeologist of this period in Central Africa was Clark. In 1937 he accepted a position as secretary at the Rhodes-Livingstone Institute and curator of the David Livingstone Memorial Museum in what then was Northern Rhodesia (now Zambia). Initially, he had little interest in local archaeology, but this would change (Clark 1989). He served in these posts from 1938, and later as director of the museum until 1961. In his years there he oversaw substantial constructions and renovations to the museum, expanded the staff, developed exhibitions and a library, and grew the archaeological and ethnographic collections. The Second World War broke out and during his service he spent time in Ethiopia, Kenya, Madagascar, and Somalia, and took the opportunity to conduct extensive, on-foot archaeological surveys. The results from work in the Horn of

Africa during this period, along with pre-war studies he had conducted in the Zambezi Valley beforehand, formed the basis of his doctoral work (cf. Gabel 1985, pp. 255–256; Toth and Schick 2003). He eventually excavated significant archaeological sites, such as Kalambo Falls, Mumbwa Caves, and Twin Rivers, among others.

Clark's work was revolutionary in African archaeology, least of all because he was examining a region scarcely touched by others. He implemented a new approach to excavations first proposed by M. Leakey (cf. Toth and Schick 2003, p. 680). Clark became interested in largescale horizontal excavations to identify behaviour patterns. With such an approach, at Kalambo he recovered a cultural sequence that included Acheulean, Sangoan, Middle and Later Stone Age, and Iron Age traces from a stratified context allowing him to study cultural change (Clark 1954, 1974). The exceptional preservation also allowed him to consider human-environment interactions over the span of Kalambo's occupation (Clark 1964). Clark was yet another pioneering character in African archaeology that shaped the discipline and introduced it to a far wider audience than otherwise (Toth and Schick 2003). His greatest impact, however, was in the period that followed the Second World War.

Much of the work carried out in Central Africa was, however, done by non-specialists or amateurs who mostly described finds. For example, Oswald Menghin (1925) and later O'Brien (1936) studied stone tools from Central Africa; Menghin described what he called the "Tumbakultur", while O'Brien referred to similar assemblages in Uganda as the "Tumbian". These industries were eventually subsumed under the term "Sangoan", based on Wayland's (1924, 1934) work at Sango Bay on Lake Victoria, where heavy-duty picks and robust tools were characteristic. Comparable assemblages have since been found across much of southern and Central Africa (Taylor 2022), indicating a wide distribution of heavy-duty Earlier-to-Middle Stone Age transition technology. In 1934, Francis Cabu collected artefacts from Kasai and Katanga and brought them to Johannesburg, where they were examined by van Riet Lowe and Breuil (Van Riet Lowe 1944). These finds were subsequently classified as the Lupemban and Tshitolian Industries, which represent important technological stages following the Tumbian/Sangoan traditions (Gabel 1985). Outside of the Congo, archaeological work in Angola was minimal but noteworthy: Jean Janmart, working for the *Companhia de Diamantes de Angola*, undertook systematic geological and archaeological surveys in the Lunda region, producing several early monographs on the area (De Matos et al. 2021). In Central Africa, the first stone tools were discovered in 1930 by Alfred Lacroix and Félix Éboué, with Breuil publishing his analysIs of Lacroix's finds in 1933 (Gabel 1985, p. 253). A Senegalese-style megalithic culture was also identified in the Central African Republic, and though only lightly investigated at the time, it has since been subject to more sustained research (Holl 2022). These studies, while laying an important foundation, were not always systematic, largely conducted as by-products of other work or by non-specialists, and did not lead to larger, robust syntheses of local archaeology.

5.2 Pre-Independence Archaeology in Africa

Archaeology in the first half of the twentieth century CE experienced significant growth, marked by the rise of professional practice and its gradual spread across the continent. From the 1930s onwards, and especially after the Second World War, the field benefited from expanding infrastructure and growing research capacity. Post-1945, archaeological practice shifted from reliance on accidental discoveries towards more systematic surveys, supported by improved recovery techniques, the integration of scientific methods, increasing attention to environmental and ecological contexts, and ongoing efforts to build regional syntheses (Gabel 1985, p. 260).

This more deliberate approach marked a clear departure from earlier practices, though the pace of change was uneven across the continent. South Africa, which had previously led the continent in archaeological development, experienced a marked decline following the election of the National Party, which prioritised research into the Afrikaner past while in many instances neglecting broader histories. Elsewhere, however, momentum gathered as classification work continued up to and beyond the advent of radiocarbon dating in the 1950s, which at last enabled absolute chronologies. Yet, the radiocarbon revolution in Africa progressed slowly (Loftus et al. 2019), largely because early laboratories were located overseas, primarily in the United States. As late as 1959, fewer than 50 radiocarbon dates had been obtained for sub-Saharan Africa, but this number expanded fifteen- to twenty-fold over the following 12 years (Gabel 1985, p. 260).

The rapid growth in dating capacity not only allowed African sequences to be better integrated with global archaeological frameworks but also opened the door to challenging long-held Eurocentric narratives about Africa's past. The increasingly systematic nature of archaeological research, combined with scientific advances and widening geographic coverage, made it progressively more difficult to maintain outdated colonial assumptions about the continent's deep history. However, this was not yet to crumble as diffusionist ideas persisted as did the notion that marginal regions in Africa existed and foreign influences are to be credited for their upliftment.

As archaeological methods became more refined and scientific data accumulated, the discipline edged towards an uncomfortable realisation: unlike many other fields, archaeology was uniquely positioned to contest colonial views of land, people, culture, and Africa's precolonial history. Rather than reinforcing colonial expansion and legitimisation, archaeology risked exposing the inaccuracies at their core. At the same time, when narratives were carefully managed, archaeology could be used to reinforce political agendas (Shepherd 2002a, p. 197). Yet, archaeologists themselves were rarely overtly nationalistic or advocates of colonialism (Robertshaw 1990b,1990a, p. 78). Nonetheless, archaeology remained, shaped by the political climate and the position each region held within the global system (Trigger 1984, p. 255).

The period was also marked by ongoing tension between amateurs and emerging professionals, which kept the field divided. Some clung to exotic theories rooted in nineteenth-century visions of Africa's past, while others increasingly argued for local origins and indigenous development. The division was not simply between amateurs and professionals, since many reputable scholars also supported diffusionist theories. Frictions emerged too between foreign and local practitioners. Malan (1957), for instance, criticised the impression Breuil's publications left, wrongly suggesting that no local archaeologists disagreed with his conclusions. A central issue in these debates was the reliability of evidence. Goodwin, for example, took aim at Breuil's excavation methods, accusing him of mixing contexts and undermining the credibility of his results (Dubow 2019, p. 36).

Until the 1950s, archaeology across Africa remained largely the domain of settler societies (Shepherd 2002b, p. 40). While African archaeologists were beginning to receive training, all professional practitioners at this time were European or of European descent. As a result, the frameworks and narratives applied to Africa's past reflected European values and perspectives, even as they sought to describe African histories. African voices were not yet shaping the character of the discipline, and its intellectual foundations remained distinctly European. Though today archaeology is enriched by a greater diversity of perspectives, its roots in the colonial era remain evident.

References

Bequaert, M. 1938. *Les fouilles de Jean Colette à Kalina*. Tervuren: Musée Royal de l'Afrique Centrale.

Binns, C.T. 1974. *The warrior people: Zulu origins, customs and witchcraft*. Cape Town: Howard Timmins.

Boutakoff, B. 1937. Premières exploration méthodiques des gisements de l'âge de la pierre au Ruanda-Urundi. Abris sous roche, ateliers et stations en plein air. *Institute Colonial Belge, Bulletin des Séances* 8:179–201.

Breuil, H. 1905. Essai de stratigraphie des dépôts de l'âge du renne. *Comptes rendues congrès préhistoriques français* 1:74–80.

Breuil, H. 1912. Les subdivisions du paléolithique supérieur et leur signification. In *Congrès international d'anthropologie et d'archéologie préhistoriques-compte-rendu de la XIVème session, Genève*, vol. tome 1:165–238. Geneva: Imprimerie Albert Kündig.

Breuil, H. 1937. *Les subdivisions de paléolithique supérior et leur signification*. Paris: Lagny.

Breuil, H. 1948. The white lady of the Brandberg, South-West Africa, her companion and her guards. *South African Archaeological Bulletin* 3:2–11.

Breuil, H. 1954. Rock paintings of South Africa. *Anthropological Quarterly* 27 (2): 31–42.

Burkitt, M. 1928. *South Africa's past in stone and paint*. Cambridge: Cambridge University Press.

Camps, G. 1974. *Les civilisations préhistoriques de l'afrique du nord et du sahara*. Paris: Doin Editeurs.

Carruthers, J. 2006. Mapungubwe: An historical and contemporary analysis of a World Heritage cultural landscape. *Koedoe* 49 (1): 1–13.

Chittick, H. N. 1974. *Kilwa: An Islamic trading city on the East African coast*. Nairobi: British Institute in Eastern Africa.

Chittick, H. N. 1984. *Manda: Excavations at an Island Port on the Kenya coast*. Nairobi: British Institute in Eastern Africa.

Clark, J. D. 1954. An early Upper Pleistocene site at the Kalambo Falls on the northern Rhodesia/Tanganyika border. *South African Archaeological Bulletin* 9 (34): 51–56.

Clark, J. D. 1964. The influence of environment in inducing culture change at the Kalambo Falls prehistoric site. *South African Archaeological Bulletin* 19 (76): 93–101.

Clark, J. D. 1971. Problems of archaeological nomenclature and definition in the Congo basin. *South African Archaeological Bulletin* 26:67–78.

Clark, J. D. 1974. *Kalambo Falls prehistoric site, Vol. II: The later prehistoric cultures*. Cambridge: Cambridge University Press.

Clark, J. D. 1989. J. Desmond Clark. In *The Pastmasters: Eleven modern pioneers of archaeology*, ed. G. Daniel and C. Chippindale, 137–152. New York: Thames & Hudson.

Clark, J. D. 2001. Mary Douglas Leakey: 1913–1996. *Proceedings of the British Academy* 111:595–614.

Clarke, J. D. 1962. Africa south of the Sahara. In *Courses towards urban life*, ed. J. Braidwood and G. Willey, 1–33. New York: Wenner-Gren Foundation.

Cole, S. 1954. *The prehistory of East Africa*. Harmondsworth: Penguin.

Colette, J. 1929. Le préhistorique dans le Bas-Congo. *Bulletin de la Société d'Anthropologie de Bruxelles* 44:42–47.

Colette, J. 1935. Complexes et convergences en préhistoire. *Bulletin de la Société d'Anthropologie et de Préhistoire* 50:49–192.

Cooke, C. K. 1960. Report on archaeological sites Bubye/Limpopo valleys of southern Rhodesia. *South African Archaeological Bulletin* 15 (59): 95–109.

Couttenier, M. 2012. Sociétés scientifiques, musées, universités. *Les nouvelles de l'archéologie* 128:23–27.

Daniel, G. 1962. *The idea of prehistory*. London: C.A. Watts.

Davies, O. 1967. *West Africa before the Europeans: Archaeology & prehistory*. London: Metheun.

De Barros, P. 1990. Changing paradigms, goals and methods in the archaeology of francophone West Africa. In *A history of African archaeology*, ed. P. Robertshaw, 155–172. Oxford: James Currey Ltd.

De Matos, D., A. C. Martins, J. C. Senna-Martinez, I. Pinto, A. G. Coelho, S. S. Ferreira, and L. Oosterbeek. 2021. Review of archaeological research in Angola. *African Archaeological Review* 38 (2): 319–344.

de Morgan, J., L. Capitan, and P. Boudy. 1910. Etude sur les stations prehistoriques du Sud Tunisien. *Revidé l'école d'Anthropologie* 20: 105–136, 206–221, 267–287, 336–347.

Deacon, J. 1990. Weaving the fabric of Stone Age research in southern Africa. In *A history of African archaeologyy*, ed. P. Robertshaw, 39–58. London: James Currey Ltd.

Debruge, A. 1923. Essai de chronologies sur 'les escargotières'. *Recl. des Notes et Mémoires de la Société Archéologique de Constantine* 44:61.

Delcroix, R., and R. Vaufrey. 1939. *Le Toumbien de Guinée Française. L'Anthropologie* 49:265–312.

Dubow, S. 1995. *Scientific racism in modern South Africa*. Cambridge: Cambridge University Press.

Dubow, S. 2019. Henri Breuil and the imagination of prehistory: 'Mixing up rubble, trouble and stratigication'. *South African Archaeology Society Goodwin Series* 12:31–43.

Esterhuysen, A. B. 2006. Let the ancestors speak: An archaeological excavation and re-evaluation of events prior and pertaining to the 1854 siege of Mugombane, Limpopo Province, South Africa. PhD thesis, University of the Witwatersrand, Johannesburg.

Fage, J. D. 1980. Evolution de l'histographie de l'Afrique. In *Histoire general de l'Afrique I: Méthodologie et préhistoire Africaine*, ed. J. Ki-Zerbo, 45–53. New York: UNESCO.

Fagg, B. 1945. A preliminary note on a new series of pottery figures from Northern Nigeria. *Africa* 15 (1): 21–22.

Fagg, B. 1972. Rop rock shelter excavations 1944. *West African Journal of Archaeology* 2:1–12.

Forssman, T. 2023. Africa, South: Forager and farmer interactions in the late Holocene. In *Encyclopedia of archaeology*, ed. T. Rehren and E. Nikita, 159–168. London: Academic.

Fouché, L. 1937. *Mapungubwe, ancient Bantu civilization on the Limpopo: Reports on excavations at Mapungubwe (Northern Transvaal) from February 1933 to June 1935*. Cambridge: Cambridge University Press.

Frankfort, H. 1948. *Kingship and the Gods*. Chicago: University of Chicago Press.

Frobenius, L. 1911. *Auf dem Wege nach Atlantis*. Berlin: Vita.
Frobenius, L. 1913. *The voice of Africa: Being an account of the travels of the German inner African exploration expedition in the years 1910–1912*. London: Hutchinson & Company.
Gabel, C. 1985. Archaeology in sub-Saharan Africa. *International Journal of African Historical Studies* 18 (2): 241–264.
Galloway, A. 1959. The skeletal remains of Mapungubwe. In *Mapungubwe: Ancient Bantu civilization on the Limpopo: Reports on excavations at Mapungubwe (Northern Transvaal) from February 1933 to June 1935*, ed. L. Fouché, 127–174. Cambridge: Cambridge University Press.
Gard, J., and R. Mauny. 1961. Découverte de tumulus dans la région de diourbel (Sénégal). *Notes Africaines* 89:10–11.
Gardner, G. A. 1963. *Mapungubwe*. Pretoria: Van Schaik.
Gaur, R. 2015. Louis Leakey and Mary Leakey: The first family of palaeontology. *Resonance* 20:667–679.
Gerstner, J. N. 1991. *The thousand generation covenant: Dutch reformed covenant theology and group identity in colonial South Africa, 1652–1814*. Leiden: Brill.
Giblin, J. 2013a. Politics, ideology, and indigenous perspectives. In *The Oxford handbook of African archaeology*, ed. P. J. Mitchell and P. J. Lane, 253–265. Oxford: Oxford University Press.
Giblin, J. D. 2013b. A reconsideration of Rwandan archaeological ceramics and their political significance in a post-genocide era. *African Archaeological Review* 30:501–529.
Gobert, É. 1910. Reserches sur le capsien lre série. *Bulletin de la Société Préhistorique Française* 6:595–604.
Goodwin, A. J. H. 1926. South African stone implement industries. *South African Journal of Science* 23 (12): 784–788.
Goodwin, A. J. H., and C. Van Riet Lowe. 1929. *The Stone Age cultures of South Africa*. Cape Town: AMS Press.
Goodwin, J. 1946. *The loom of prehistory*. Cape Town: South African Archaeological Society.
Goodwin, J. 1958. Formative years of our prehistoric terminology. *South African Archaeological Bulletin* 13 (49): 25–33.
Haddon, A. C. 1906. Anthropology at the South African Meeting of the British Association for the Advancement of Science, 1905. *Science* 23 (587): 491–497.
Hay, R. L., and M. D. Leakey. 1982. The fossil footprints of Laetoli. *Scientific American* 246 (2): 50–57.
Holl, A. F. C. 1990. West African archaeology: colonialism and nationalism. In *A History of African Archaeology*, ed. P. Robertshaw, 296–308. Oxford: James Currey Ltd.
Holl, A. F. C. 2022. Burial protocols, megaliths production, and ancestor-hood in ancient Senegambia (ca. 1450 BCE–1500 CE). In *Studying Africa and Africans today*, ed. A. F. C. Holl, 203–224. Bhanjipour: BP International.
Huntingford, G. W. B. 1933. The Azanian civilization of Kenya. *Antiquity* 7:153–165.
Huntingford, G. W. B. 2017. *The Southern Nilo-Hamites: East Central Africa Part VI*. London: Routledge.
Inskeep, R. R. 1961. The present state of archaeology in South Africa. *South African Museums Association Bulletin* 7:225–227.
Irstam, T. 1944. *The king of Ganda*. Stockholm: Ethnographic Museum.
Jauze, J.-B. 1944a. Notes d'archéologie Camerounaise. *Bulletin d'Information et Correspondance de l'IFAN* 23:12–13.
Jauze, J.-B. 1944b. Contribution à l'étude de l'archéologie du Cameroun. *Bulletin de la Société d'Etudes Camerounaises* 8:105–136.
Jones, N. 1926. *The Stone Age of Rhodesia*. Oxford: Oxford University Press.
Judd, D., and K. Surridge. 2002. *The Boer War*. London: John Murray.
Kense, F. J. 1990. Archaeology in anglophone West Africa. In *A history of African archaeology*, ed. P. Robertshaw, 135–154. London: James Currey Ltd.
Kessler, S. V. 1999. The black concentration camps of the Anglo-Boer War 1899-1902: Shifting the paradigm from sole martyrdom to mutual suffering. *Historia* 44 (1): 110–147.

Kirkman, J. S. 1954. *The Arab city of Gedi: Excavations at the great mosque. Architecture and finds.* Oxford: Oxford University Press.
Leakey, L. 1931. *The Stone Age cultures of Kenya colony.* Cambridge: Cambridge University Press.
Leakey, L. S. B. 1929. An outline of the Stone Age in Kenya. *South African Journal of Science* 26:749–757.
Leakey, L. S. B. 1934. *Adam's ancestors: The evolution of man and his culture.* London: Metheun.
Leakey, L. S. B. 1937. *White African: An early autobiography.* London: Hodder and Stoughton.
Leakey, L. S. B. 1951. *Olduvai Gorge: A report on the evolution of the hand-axe culture in beds I-IV.* Cambridge: Cambridge University Press.
Leakey, L. S. B. 1952. *Mau and the Kikuvu.* London: Metheun.
Leakey, L. S. B. 1954. *Defeating Mau Mau.* London: Metheun.
Leakey, L. S. B., P. V. Tobias, and J. R. Napier. 1964. A new species of genus *Homo* form Olduvai Gorge. *Nature* 202:7–9.
Leakey, M. D. 1959. A new skull from Olduvai. *Nature* 184:491–493.
Loftus, E., P. J. Mitchell, and C. B. Ramsey. 2019. An archaeological radiocarbon database for southern Africa. *Antiquity* 93 (370): 870–885.
Malan, B. D. 1957. Review of White Lady of the Brandberg. *Antiquity* 3:51–52.
Malan, B. D. 1970. Remarks and reminiscences on the history of archaeology in South Africa. *South African Archaeological Bulletin* 25 (99/100): 88–92.
Marks, S. 1980. South Africa: The myth of the empty land. *History Today* 30 (1): 7–12.
Marks, S. 2001. White masculinity: Jan Smuts, race and the South African war. *Proceedings of the British Academy* 111:199–224.
Mauny, R. 1953. Les recherches archéologiques en A.O.F., particulierement de 1938 á 1952. *Bulletin de l'Institut Français d'Afrique Noire* 15:684–730.
Mauny, R. 1961. *Tableau Géographique de L'ouest Africain au Moyen Age, D'aprèS des Sources Écrites, la Tradition et L'archéologie.* Dakar: Mémoires de l'Institut Français d'Afrique Noire.
McBrearty, S., and A. S. Brooks. 2000. The revolution that wasn't: A new interpretation of the origin of modern human behaviour. *Journal of Human Evolution* 39 (5): 453–563.
McIntosh, R. J., and S. K. McIntosh. 1981. The Inland Niger Delta before the empire of Mali: Evidence from Jenné-Jeno. *Journal of African History* 22:1–22.
McIntosh, S. K. 2001. Africa, Sudanic Kingdoms. In *Encyclopedia of archaeology, history and discoveries*, ed. T. Murray, 71–78. Santa Barbara: ABC CLIO.
McIntosh, S. K., and R. J. McIntosh. 1995. Background to the 1981 research. In *Excavations at Jenne-Jeno, Hambarketolo and Kaniana: The 1981 season*, ed. S. K. McIntosh, 1–26. Berkley: University of California Press.
Mechkarini, S., D. Siân Rutherford, and B. Sèbe. 2023. Unmasking the colonial past: Memory, narrative, and legacy. *Journal of Imperial and Commonwealth History* 51 (5): 825–841.
Menghin, O. 1925. Die Tumbakultur am unteren Kongo und der westafrikanische Kulturkreis. *Anthropos* 20:516–557.
Mercier, G. 1915. L'Homme de Mechta-Châteaudun (Algérie). *Bulletin de la Société Préhistorique de France* 12 (3): 160–166.
Mercier, G., and A. Debruge. 1912. La station préhistorique de Mechta-Chateaudun. *Recueil des Notes et Mémoires de la Société Archéologique de Constantine* 46:287–307.
Meyer, A. 2000. K2 and Mapungubwe. *South African Archaeological Society Goodwin Series* 8:4–13.
Mitchell, P. J. 2024. *The archaeology of Southern Africa.* Cambridge: Cambridge University Press.
Mongalo, B. E., and K. Du Pisani. 1999. Victims of a white man's war: Blacks in concentration camps during the South African War (1899-1902). *Historia* 44 (1): 148–182.
Monod, T. 1936. Travels in the western Sahara, 1934-35. *Geographical Journal* 87 (6): 534–539.
Morais, J. 1984. Mozambican archaeology: Past and present. *African Archaeological Review* 2:113–128.
Morgan, K. O. 2002. The Boer War and the media (1899–1902). *Twentieth Century British History* 13 (1): 1–16.

Murdock, G. P. 1959. *Africa: Its peoples and their culture history*. New York: McGraw-Hill.
Musonda, F. 1990. African archaeology: Looking forward. *African Archaeological Review* 8:3–22.
Nasson, B. 2003. *Abraham Esau's War: A black South African war in the Cape, 1899–1902*. Cambridge: Cambridge University Press.
O'Brien, T. P. 1936. Notes on the Stone Age cultures of Uganda. *Man* 36:41–44.
O'Brien, T. P. 1939. *The prehistory of the Uganda protectorate*. Cambridge: Cambridge University Press.
Oliver, R., and J. D. Fage. 1963. *A short history of Africa*. New York: New York University Press.
Peringuey, L. 1911. Annals of the South African museum. Volume VIII. In *The Stone Ages of South Africa as represented in the collection of the South African museum*. London: West Newman.
Pond, A. W., A. Romer, and F. Cole. 1928. *A contribution to the study of prehistoric man in Algeria, North Africa*. Beloit: Logan Museum Bulletin.
Posnansky, M. 2012. Adam's ancestors, Louis Leakey, and African archaeology's quest for validation. In *Backdrift: Annual review of the Costen Insitute of Archaeology at UCLA*, ed. G. E. Areshian, 34–43. Costen Institute of Archaeology: Los Angeles.
Rassool, C., and L. Witz. 1993. The 1952 Jan Van Riebeeck Tercentenary festival: Constructing and contesting public national history in South Africa. *Journal of African History* 34:447–468.
Reck, H. 1914a. Erste vorläufige mitteilung über den fund eines fossilen menschenskelets aus Zentralafrika. *Sitzungsberichte der Gesellschaft Naturforschender Freunde zu Berlin* 3:81–95.
Reck, H. 1914b. Zweite vorläufige mitteilung über fossile tier-und menschen-funde aus Oldoway in Zentralafrika. *Sitzungsberichte der Gesellschaft Naturforschender Freunde zu Berlin* 7:305–318.
Renfrew, C. 1989. *Archaeology and language: The puzzle of Indo-European origins*. London: Penguin Books.
Reygasse, M. 1920. Études de palethnologie maghrébine. *Recueil des Notes et Mémoires de la Société Archéologique de Constantine* 52:513–570.
Robertshaw, P. 1990a. A history of African archaeology: An introduction. In *A history of African archaeology*, ed. P. Robertshaw, 3–12. Oxford: James Currey Ltd.
Robertshaw, P. 1990b. The development of archaeology in East Africa. In *A history of African archaeology*, ed. P. Robertshaw, 78–94. Oxford: James Currey Ltd.
Robertshaw, P., 1990c. The development of archaeology in East Africa. In *A History of African archaeology*, ed. P. Robertshaw, 78–94. Oxford: James Currey Ltd.
Robinson, K. 1959. *Khami ruins*. Cambridge: Cambridge University Press.
Rodrigues, M. C. 1998. Os primordios da investigaçao arqueologica em moçambique e o prof. *Santos Júnior. Portvgalia* XIX–XX:265–278.
Rodrigues, M. C. 2004. A arqueologia em moçambique nas "Missoes Científicas" da antiga Junta de Investigaçao do Ultramar de 1936–1972. PhD thesis, Universidade de Coimbra, Coimbra.
Schlanger, N. 2003. The Burkitt affair revisited. Colonial implications and identity politics in early South African prehistoric research. *Archaeological Dialogues* 10 (1): 5–26.
Schoeman, M. H., and I. Pikirayi. 2011. Repatriating more than Mapungubwe human remains: Archaeological material culture, a shared future and an artificially divided past. *Journal of Contemporary African Studies* 29 (4): 389–403.
Schofield, J. 1937. The pottery of the Mapungubwe District. In *Mapungubwe: Ancient Bantu civilization on the Limpopo: Reports on excavations at Mapungubwe (Northern Transvaal) from February 1933 to June 1935*, ed. L. Fouché, 119–124. Cambridge: Cambridge University Press.
Seligman, C. G. 1930. *Races of Africa*. London: Thornton Butterworth.
Shaw, T. 1944. Report on excavations carried out in the cave known as 'Bosumpra' at Abetifi, Kwahu, Gold Coast Colony. *Proceedings of the Prehistoric Society* 10:1–67.
Shaw, T. 1970. *Igbo-Ukwu: An account of archeological discoveries in eastern Nigeria*. Evanston: Northwestern University Press.
Shaw, T. 1989. African archaeology: Looking back and looking forward. *African Archaeological Review* 7 (1): 3–31.
Shaw, T., P. J. J. Sinclair, A. Andah, and A. Okpoko, eds. 1993. *The archaeology of Africa: Food, metals and towns*. London: Routledge.

Shepherd, N. 2002a. Disciplining archaeology; the invention of South African prehistory, 1923-1953. *Kronos: Journal of Cape History* 28 (1): 127–145.

Shepherd, N. 2002b. The politics of archaeology in Africa. *Annual Review of Anthropology* 31:189–209.

Shepherd, N. 2003. State of the discipline: Science, culture and identity in South African archaeology, 1870–2003. *Journal of Southern African Studies* 29 (4): 823–844.

Sheppard, P. J. 1990. Soldiers and bureaucrats: The early history of prehistoric archaeology in the Maghreb. In *A History of African Archaeology*, ed. P. Robertshaw, 173–188. London: James Currey Ltd.

Shinnie, P. 1967. *Meroe, a civilization of the Sudan (ancient people and places)*. London: Thames & Hudson.

Smith, G. 2003. The allure, magic and mystery: A brief history of diamonds. *Journal of the Southern African Institute of Mining and Metallurgy* 103 (9): 529–534.

Stevenson, A. 2012. An amateur's prehistory: A view from James A Swan's South African collections. *South African Archaeological Bulletin* 67:52–58.

Summers, R. 1972. Progress of prehistoric studies in southern Africa. *South African Archaeological Society Goodwin Series* 1:3–5.

Summers, R., K. Robinson, and A. Whitty. 1961. Zimbabwe excavations. *Occasional Papers of the National Museums of Rhodesia* 3:15–332.

Taylor, C. C. 1999. *Sacrifice as terror: The rwandan genocide of 1994*. Oxford: Berg.

Taylor, N. 2022. Sangoan. In *Oxford research encyclopedia of anthropology*, ed. M. S. Aldenderfer. Oxford: Oxford University Press. https://oxfordre.com/anthropology/display/10.1093/acrefore/9780190854584.001.0001/acrefore-9780190854584-e-30

Templin, J. A. 1999. The ideology of a chosen people: Afrikaner nationalism and the Ossewa Trek, 1938. *Nations and Nationalism* 5:397–417.

Thiaw, I. 2013. Colonization and the development of archaeology in Senegal. In *European archaeology abroad: Global settings, comparative perspectives*, ed. S. van der Linde, M. H. van den Dries, N. Schlanger, and C. G. Slappendel, 349–374. Leiden: Sidestone Press.

Tiley-Nel, S. 2011. *'Sermons in stones, poetry in potsherds': The history of the Mapungubwe collection at the University of Pretoria*. Pretoria: University of Pretoria Museums.

Tiley-Nel, S. 2022. *Past imperfect: The contested early history of the Mapungubwe Archive, South Africa*. Oxford: British Archaeological Reports International Series.

Tobias, P. V. 1973. Louis Seymour Bazett Leakey 1903-1972. *South African Archaeological Bulletin* 28 (109/110): 3–7.

Tobias, P. V. 2003. Louis Leakey, self-styled white African: Appreciation and some personal recollections. *Transactions of the Royal Society of South Africa* 58 (1): 41–50.

Toth, N., and K. Schick. 2003. John Desmond Clark (1916–2002). *American Anthropologist* 105 (3): 679–682.

Trigger, B. G. 1984. Alternative archaeologies: Nationalist, colonialist, imperialist. In *Contemporary archaeology in theory: A reader*, ed. R. Preucel and Ia. Hodder, 615–631. Oxford: Blackwell Publishing.

Trigger, B. G. 1990. The history of African archaeology in world perspective. In *A history of African archaeology*, ed. P. Robertshaw, 303–319. Oxford: James Currey Ltd.

Van Riet Lowe, C. 1944. Notes on Dr. Francis Cabu's collection of stone implements from the Belgian Congo. *Transactions of the Royal Society of South Africa* XXX:169–174.

Van Riet Lowe, C. 1952. *The pleistocene geology and prehistory of Uganda: Part II*. Colchester: Benham.

Vaufrey, R. 1933. *Notes sur le capsien. L'Anthropologie* 43:457–483.

Vaufrey, R. 1955. *Préhistoire de l'afrique du nord et maghreb*. Tunis: Publication de l'Institut des hautes études de Tunis.

Warwick, P. 1983. *Africans in the Boer War: Black people and the South African War, 1899–1902*. Cambridge: Cambridge University Press.

Wayland, E. J. 1924. Palaeolithic types of implements in relation to the Pleistocene deposits of Uganda. *Proceedings of the Prehistoric Society of East Anglia* 4 (1): 96–112.

Wayland, E. J. 1934. Rifts, rivers, rains and early man in Uganda. *The Journal of the Royal Anthropological Institute of Great Britain and Ireland* 64:333–352.

Wessels, A. 2016. The Anglo-Boer War (1899 – 1902) and its traumatic consequences. In *Breaking intergenerational cycles of repetition: A global dialogue on historical trauma and memory*, ed. P. Gobodo-Madikizela, 160–173. Opladen: Barbara Budrich Publishers.

Wild, R. P. 1934. Stone Age pottery from the Gold Coast and Ashanti. *Journal of the Royal Anthropological Institute of Great Britain and Ireland* 64:203–216.

Chapter 6
Archaeology Comes of Age During Africa's Independence

Abstract Spanning the independence decades, this chapter traces the changing practice of archaeology as African nations underwent profound transformations. Universities and heritage bodies expanded; African scholars and students increasingly shaped agendas; and collaborations diversified. Methodologically, chronometric dating, settlement archaeology, palaeoenvironmental studies, archaeometallurgy, and historical archaeology grew, while community-based and ethnoarchaeological approaches complicated earlier narratives. Regionally, trajectories varied with political economy and conflict, but across the continent, research questions shifted toward local histories of production, mobility, religion, and urbanism. The chapter also confronts enduring colonial legacies — collections abroad, legal regimes, extractive funding — and the dilemmas of nation-building, where archaeology could be mobilised for identity work as well as critical history. Growing in this period was an expanded capacity to ask better questions of richer archives while negotiating constraints that independence did not magically dissolve.

> [H]istory is not to be equated with any one version of the past. The past is always a created ideology with a purpose, designed to control individuals or motivate societies or inspire classes. Nothing has been so corruptly used as concepts of the past. (Plumb 1969, p. 7)

In the nineteenth century CE, European traders along the Benue River in present-day Nigeria acquired delicate tin straws from local communities along the river banks. The origin of the metal was at first unknown. It was only in the early twentieth century that it was discovered that the tin had been extracted from the rich alluvial deposits of the Jos Plateau. Once identified, this region drew the attention of large-scale mining enterprises, which soon transformed the landscape in search of valuable ores. In 1939, Bernard Fagg was stationed at Jos as an administrative officer. He had received a degree in archaeology from the University of Cambridge and was keen to explore the region as he had read about its archaeology during his studies. He and his wife, Catherine, began cataloguing miscellaneous finds collected from mining activities and stored at the mining headquarters in Jos by the Chief Inspector of Mines. They recorded a wide range of artefacts, including iron objects, ceramics, Later Stone Age tools, and an unusual sculpture of a monkey's head found in 1928. The Faggs' interest in these finds led them to travel the region in search of more, speaking to local men mining alluvium, and excavating a rock shelter near Rop during their leave

T. Forssman, *Archaeology in Africa: Why the Past Matters*, Archaeology of Africa,
https://doi.org/10.1007/978-3-032-13365-6_6

in 1944. That same year, the Director of the Geological Survey contacted B. Fagg to report a find held by the mining engineer. In B. Fagg's words (1956, quoted from A. Fagg 2014, p. 81):

> ... I found out where the engineer lived and went to visit him ... I was quite astonished at what I saw ... It was a head in baked clay or, as it is more often called, terra cotta, very slightly less than life-size ... and had a compelling, almost magnetic, expression in its stylised features. Here was a great work of art. I was at once struck by its similarity in style to a fist-sized terra cotta depicting the head of a monkey, which had been found many years before in the course of mining at Nok....

This find led him to visit the lease holder of the mine and be shown a complete head that he had placed in his garden. Further inspections of the mine led to finding many more fragments as well as potsherds, polished stone axes, worked iron, and tin beads. These finds were reported to the Royal Anthropological Institute in a paper on northern Nigeria, after which colonial authorities appointed B. Fagg as the first Government Archaeologist and Assistant Surveyor of Antiquities (Fagg 2014, p. 82). Excavations carried out by B. Fagg and a geologist, Geoffrey Bond, in an area of the minefield reserved for archaeological work resulted in the first in situ find of a well-preserved terracotta figurine along with fragments of other cultural objects. A tentative age of at least 2000 years was suggested based on Bond's investigation of the deposits. Similar finds had by this time been made at 13 other sites where alluvium had been mined or investigated, and although chronology and context were problematic, B. Fagg (1956) felt that they were all part of the same culture. The Nok Culture was introduced to the world at large in 1947 by the *Illustrated London News* in an article titled *Primitive art of a problematic age: Nigerian heads now at the British Museum* (Fagg 2014, p. 81). The number of known sites and their distribution grew substantially in the 1950s once the finds became well known and recognisable throughout the region.

B. Fagg returned in the mid-1960s to advance his research into the Nok Culture. He used a proton magnetometer to record magnetic anomalies below the surface. From 60 sites that were recorded, 56 were excavated and the findings included nine furnaces, furnace debris and slag and various cultural objects. An additional furnace outside of the magnetometer's survey area was later identified. These ten furnaces became the focus of sustained work, but this was halted between 1966 and 1967 due to political disturbances in Nigeria. However, it was only in 1969 that Angela Fagg, also an archaeologist and the daughter of Bernard, found a habitation site. Excavations revealed a wide range of domestic and craft activities, including evidence of smelting (Shaw 1981, p. 161). The team included a range of specialists, such as geomagnetic investigators and iron-smelting experts, and samples for radiocarbon dating were taken. In the 1970s, thermoluminescence dating was developed and B. Fagg (1977) used the opportunity to date individual figurines. As with the earlier advent of radiocarbon dating, B. Fagg (1977) was keenly interested in using contemporary archaeological science to investigate and understand the past (Franke 2016, pp. 258–259). His study is an early example of an ensemble team of scientists working co-operatively to investigate an archaeological occurrence.

The Nok Culture is enigmatic. At the time of its discovery, it was generally thought that complex society was a recent development in West Africa. It was also unclear to whom the terracottas belonged as they were not known to any contemporary groups. B. Fagg's (1977) investigations, however, challenged the idea that these items were relatively young. His analysis of soils from find spots, the later radiocarbon dating of plant matter embedded in terracottas, and thermoluminescence dating of the original Jemaa head all indicated ages of around 500 BC (Shaw 1981; Jemkur 1986; Franke 2016). Some of these dates represented the early attempts at radiocarbon dating sub-Saharan African archaeology (Fagg 1959; Shaw 1968); earlier samples had been submitted from North Africa (Wendorf 1992). As an aside, radiocarbon dating grew slower in Africa than elsewhere in the world but rapidly increased from the late 1960s (Shaw 1968). The chronology for the Nok Culture predated by some measure all notions of complex society in Nigeria, and appeared unrelated to finds from Benin or Ife and elsewhere in the country. It was not immediately accepted, however, and the artefact associations were also questioned (Shaw 1963). B. Fagg and his colleagues had, nonetheless, found an unknown civilisation through luck and good fortune but also as the result of advances in archaeological science (Atwood 2011).

After B. Fagg's work, research into the Nok Culture was discontinued for many years. Unfortunately, in the interim, the value that these items obtained led to widespread looting. The Nok Culture was worse hit than perhaps any other cultural entity (Breunig and Rupp 2010), outside of probably Egypt. It is estimated that thousands of terracotta Nok sculptures, and likely many other finds as well, were extracted from subsurface, secured contexts by locals with the aim of selling them to foreign markets. Syndicates were even established employing large numbers of locals to search for Nok finds within the territory (Darling 2000). Many of the finds turning up in collections in Europe and the United States had never been recorded or even seen by officials before (Darling 2004, p. 101). The emergence of fakes ultimately stalled the looting as it was too difficult to discern the real from the replica (Breunig and Rupp 2010, p. 48).

The Nok finds emerged at an important intersectional period: the crossroads between colonisation and independence. Discovering the early history of the Nok Culture and its deep, complex societal roots would not have suited colonial exploits or interests. In other parts of the continent, notably Zimbabwe, archaeological finds supported notions of deep time and cultural richness were suppressed in various ways. The Nok Culture would likely have suffered a similar fate, had it not emerged at a time when such finds supported African independence, challenged colonial hegemony over African landscapes, and celebrated African history. Nok, like other finds on the continent, defied colonial sentiments and the claims that Africa lacked a history. Crucially, the emergence from colony to independent state took place as archaeological science was advancing, and vitally this included the ability to establish accurate, absolute chronologies for the first time (Clark 1964). The coalescence of new ideologies and scientific developments made possible far deeper understandings of Africa's past. But, the past was still to truly break free from colonial mindsets, constructions, and renderings, only to be thrust into a new role on the continent – legitimising new African leadership and pride (Emeni and Nukueye 2019, p. 14).

African history was being rewritten in response to new political agendas (Blench 2015, p. 150).

6.1 Archaeological Transformations

Just as the Second World War marked a watershed in the process of independence, so too did it signal a turning point in the sciences. Advances in scientific method and techniques in the post-war period offered a response to growing frustrations with traditional approaches, opening the door to major advances across many disciplines. Archaeology, in particular, was in need of such transformation amid mounting discontent over the direction of the field. Yet despite these developments, the colonial scramble for Africa and its aftermath sustained many longstanding misconceptions about the continent's past, misconceptions rooted in the era of slavery and shaped by colonial agendas. Africans were often excluded from serious historical consideration, relegated instead to anthropology's search for the primitive or the savage. Archaeology had the potential to challenge these views and reshape perceptions of Africa, but its findings did not align with colonial narratives. The past it uncovered was not one colonial administrators were willing to acknowledge. As Frantz Fanon (1967) observed in the wake of colonialism, history was a tool used to advance and legitimise colonial ideologies.

African archaeology transitioned in the 1960s into an early state of maturity (Robbins 1993, p. 21). At its beginning, archaeologists were few in number, led by a handful of individuals who performed a large amount of work, given the lack of resources in Africa, but left significant blank spots (Gabel 1985, p. 251). However, the discipline saw tremendous growth from pre- to post-independence Africa. Merrick Posnansky (1982, p. 345) noted that by 1982 the number of practising professional archaeologists in Africa had swollen from less than 35 in the 1960s to over 100; J. Desmond Cark (1994, p. 16) echoed these sentiments in his autobiography. Although a staggeringly small number by today's standards, this figure nevertheless represented a nearly three-fold increase during a time of massive socio-political transformation. Additionally, a wider diversity of approaches began appearing in Africa, spurred on by post-colonialism (Schmidt 2009; Lane 2011). The growth in the field of archaeology at this important juncture in nation re-claiming and building presented an interesting potential for collaborative ideologies in such a context.

From the Sahel to the Swahili coastline, archaeologists began examining interactions, social change, and complexity with a nuanced perspective that did not hinge on exotic assumptions (McIntosh and McIntosh 1981; Horton 1987). Approaches also branched away from strictly diffusion-migration hypotheses. For example, an early attempt at doing so was Catherine Coquéry-Vidrovitch's (1969) model that considered the interplay between local and global networks in West Africa more intimately. Unlike in diffusionist approaches, she examined the intersectionality of African state formation and the need for control over long-distance trade. She argued that the low agricultural production yield in Mali, despite an abundance of land, could not support the emergence of a socio-politically complex state. To do so, trade relations with far off groups were used to build centralised polities and buoy elite groups. The means to do so was the acquisition of exotic and scarce items. These were redistributed as 'rewards' to followers. Such a model was soon after adopted to explain the Kongo Kingdom and its own appearance (Ekholm 1972), but eventually came to be applied widely across Africa where local groups used available resources to obtain foreign goods (Hall 1987; Loubser 1991; Huffman 1986; Robertshaw 2003). These conclusions sat in opposition with the notion that foreigner groups introduced advances in sub-Saharan Africa.

Arguably the most significant advance that occurred in the history of archaeology, at least for the period predating the written record, which is much of Africa's past, was the advent of absolute dating. In Europe, there had been a longer history of archaeological research, and other techniques and methods were used to determine chronology (see Renfrew and Bahn 2020, Chapter 4). But, this was not the case in Africa where chronology plagued scholars (Shaw 1989, p. 11). When Willard Libby developed radiocarbon dating in 1946, the possibility emerged of developing far more accurate chronologies. In addition, it pushed human pasts deeper into prehistory and traced associated change, development, and advances far more rigorously over time. In Africa, as elsewhere, chronology enabled significant strides in challenging earlier conclusions about the continent's history (Clark 1979). B. Fagg's (1977) dating of Nok terracottas both demonstrated greater antiquity than previously thought and challenged notions of African history in the area. The opportunity to determine the calendar age of a find or site meant that archaeologists could now verify their various relative date ranges with greater scrutiny and dispute the subjective beliefs that at times permeated their formation. Moreover, the impact of stringent chronologies was to have penetrating consequences across a vast region in which history had no depth, and in this way was ahistoric, and where settler authorities had subverted archaeological sequences in favour of colonial justifications. Chronology also made it possible to place African sequences in global frameworks (Giblin 2013, p. 255), from which it was also able to draw further connections (Mitchell 2005a). Despite these advantages, the wider application of radiocarbon dating across Africa was slow. By the late 1960s, two decades after its introduction, only a limited number of dates had been produced (Shaw 1968), and its broader uptake beyond southern and eastern Africa only gathered pace from the 1970s (Musonda 1990, pp. 5–6).

After the Second World War, archaeology continued to focus heavily on categorising findings. A major aim was, and mostly still is, the development of typological systems to group artefact assemblages into distinct cultural and technological phases. However, this emphasis on classification raised persistent challenges across the African continent. Early efforts to categorise the past often relied on European taxonomic models, which were poorly suited to local contexts and rarely incorporated indigenous naming systems. The Third Panafrican Congress in 1955 (Clark 1957) and the Burg Wartenstein Symposium in 1965 (Bishop and Clark 1967, pp. 687–901) attempted to establish a more standardised nomenclature, but a consensus was not found (Shaw 1967). As a result, archaeologists working in different regions faced difficulties both in adopting shared terminology and in developing locally grounded systems. The application of European terms in African contexts frequently led to definitional inconsistencies and explanatory limitations, as these terms often carried assumptions that did not align with local historical realities.

The advent of absolute dating along with new intellectual frameworks, notably processual archaeology, led scholars to recognise the important role that climate played in shaping human societies in the past (Binford 1962). Although archaeologists had considered the impact the environment had on human populations prior to the mid-twentieth century, growing geoarchaeological interest and collaborations with geologists and geographers assisted with building climatic models after the Second World War (Clark 1981). Clark (1960) was an early proponent of emphasising the import role the environment had on evolution in East Africa (e.g., Grove and Warren 1968). The recognition that hominins deployed adaptive strategies with behavioural and evolutionary outcomes shaped archaeological interpretations (Butzer 1964). During the Holocene epoch, researchers observed that periods of increased precipitation led to the "greening" of the Sahara Desert, facilitating movements of hunter-gatherer groups and later pastoral communities across the expanded habitable regions. Early studies focused on how these environmental changes influenced human mobility and subsistence strategies in the Sahara. For instance, they examined the role of climatic fluctuations in shaping the behaviours of Holocene hunter-gatherers (cf. Gallinaro and Biagetti 2016, p. 437). Additionally, analyses of sediment cores from African lakes provided insights into past precipitation levels, shedding light on their impact on settlement patterns (Hance 1970) and the development of trade networks, such as those involving salt (Good 1972). Stone tool technological change was also aligned with broad climatic shifts that led to new opportunities and adaptive requirements. This was a key interpretation in explaining Later Stone Age change over a short, rapid period from one industry to the next in southern Africa; its co-occurrence with environmental change drove the need for human behavioural and technological adjustments (Clark 1970; Deacon 1972). Frameworks such as this and others were, however, later accused of oversimplifying a complex archaeological sequence that was the result of communities with great degrees of agency, stylistic and functional tools, and who responded to localised opportunities (Parkington 1980).

Key challenges awaited archaeologists using environmental models, as they still do today. Clark (1960) noted in the first paragraphs of his seminal work on the topic that chronological frameworks need to be built on firm foundations. He also argued that they should be continent-wide, but this assumed a greater degree of homogeneity that we know today never existed. Clark (1960) also noted the need for satisfactory classification work regarding industry typologies. In reality, issues such as inter-analyst bias, experience, typological cross-referencing, and comparability have hindered attempts to ensure that classification of finds remains consistent between assemblages. This is further exacerbated by geographic distances, chronological periodisation, and language barriers. Finally, Clark (1960) argued for the important role of ethnographic research in determining human responses to environmental change. This is a critical consideration and came at a time when many scholars had not yet placed such importance on indigenous knowledge systems.

The post-Second World War period saw several strides in archaeology in Africa. The emergence of independence in the years that followed altered the character of archaeology. It led to new possibilities of research, support for studies into the last few millennia, African-led initiatives, and growing interest in Africa's past beyond topics of interest from a western perspective. The development of radiocarbon dating had a significant impact, and shifts in theoretical and methodological fields contributed to the further professionalisation of the field. Archaeology was still challenged by colonial legacies, limited funding and resources, and under-developed infrastructure. However, the field was in a position of growth in most regions on the continent, and this would assist in increasing access, resources, personal, training, and research in a spread of fields (Posnansky 1982). This period redefined archaeology in Africa and made it possible to more recognisably highlight the continent's complex history and centrality in the human story (e.g., McIntosh and McIntosh 1983).

6.1.1 Southern Africa

After the Second World War, archaeology in South Africa was increasingly constrained by the political climate of apartheid. The government prioritised Afrikaner nationalist narratives and withdrew support for research into deeper African pasts and for participation in international scholarly exchanges (Shepherd 2003). Most archaeologists steered clear of conflict with state ideology, instead directing their focus toward remote prehistories and the technical aspects of material analysis, which kept the discipline largely apolitical and marginalised (Inskeep 1961; Hall 1990, pp. 73, 75). On the few occasions when archaeological findings did challenge state-endorsed narratives, they were dismissed by the government, which remained committed to its own ideologically driven version of history (Lucas 2006, p. 56). By the 1980s, South African archaeology faced growing isolation abroad. Although local archaeologists were not necessarily complicit in apartheid, the World Archaeological Congress in 1985 revoked their invitation in protest at the regime's racist laws (Mitchell 2005b). The decision, made to prevent wider boycotts, backfired: over 400 delegates protested against what they saw as a political intervention that stifled academic exchange (Tobias 1985). Ironically, this marginalisation of archaeology, both domestically and internationally, created a vacuum that political actors were quick to fill. In the absence of robust, empirically grounded narratives, alternative histories emerged to serve ideological ends (Giblin 2013, p. 257).

Control over the school curriculum further enabled the state to dictate historical knowledge in both black and white education systems. White scholars were legally prohibited from entering black schools, effectively preventing archaeologists from sharing their findings through public or community outreach (Hall 1990,

p. 73). The government was acutely aware of the potential political power of archaeological knowledge, fearing that it could be appropriated by movements such as Black Consciousness to legitimise African historical claims and contest white hegemony. Despite this potential, archaeology was rarely employed to challenge apartheid ideology (Giblin 2013, p. 258). One influential contribution that relied on history, heritage and the past was Credo Mutwa's (1964) *Indaba, My Children*, which sought to reclaim African identity and history in the face of apartheid repression. His work deliberately challenged Eurocentric and state-sanctioned histories, blending oral tradition, myth, folklore, and fiction into a complex narrative that defied easy separation between fact and fiction (Chidester 2002; Steyn 2003). His text became a form of cultural resistance, offering a spiritual and symbolic counter-narrative to the apartheid hallucinations of the past, but was itself victim to its own imaginations.

Towards the end of apartheid, South African archaeologists, who were themselves keen to rewrite African history (Shepherd 2003), did not harness the past in a way that aided meaningfully the politics of the present. Meanwhile, in Zimbabwe, the past became a crucial tool for branding the nation once it became independent. In 1962, Winston Field and Ian Smith orchestrated a takeover of Southern Rhodesia, which they named Rhodesia, and although the British government did not intervene immediately, they did not recognise Rhodesia as an independent nation. Smith (1997) claimed that the earlier Pioneer Column, a group of colonists spearhead by Cecil Rhodes to occupy Zimbabwe, found a land of animals only and no human groups. By his reasoning, it was empty land and there for whoever claimed it first. As such, their occupation and colonisation of Zimbabwe was argued to be legitimate (Beach 1983). It was not long after that liberation struggles began. The first battle took place in 1966 and conflict continued until independence in 1980, after which the country was renamed Zimbabwe. Robert Mugabe described the responsibility he and his party officials held as the 'burden of history' (cf. Ndlovu-Gatsheni 2012, p. 5).

The new government set to reform the nation through their patriotic, 'historic mission'. They renamed it Zimbabwe after its most famous archaeological site, Great Zimbabwe, to root the independent country's image and identity in African culture and history (Garlake 1984; Matenga 1998). Great Zimbabwe was the region's precolonial 'golden age' and modern Zimbabwe was presented as a direct descendent of the ancient state (Thondhlana et al. 2021, pp. 287–288). Iconography was appropriated and deployed in different forms (Fig. 6.1), as it had been by previous regimes (Thondhlana et al. 2021, p. 288), and when the two primary liberation movements joined to become the Zimbabwe African National Union – Patriotic Front (ZANU-PF) they adopted Great Zimbabwe's conical tower in their branding (Ndlovu-Gatsheni and Willems 2009). The tower became a symbol of unity and post-colonial rule (Fontein 2006). The various invocations of Great Zimbabwe in the political idolatry of Zimbabwean leaders reveal the enduring power of the past within national discourse (Kristiansen 1993).

Even in Botswana, which was a British protectorate, the past became an important tool. Soon after Botswana became a self-government in September 1966, the new president, Sir Seretse Khama, stated in an address at what is now the University of Botswana (Phaladi 1998, p. 233):

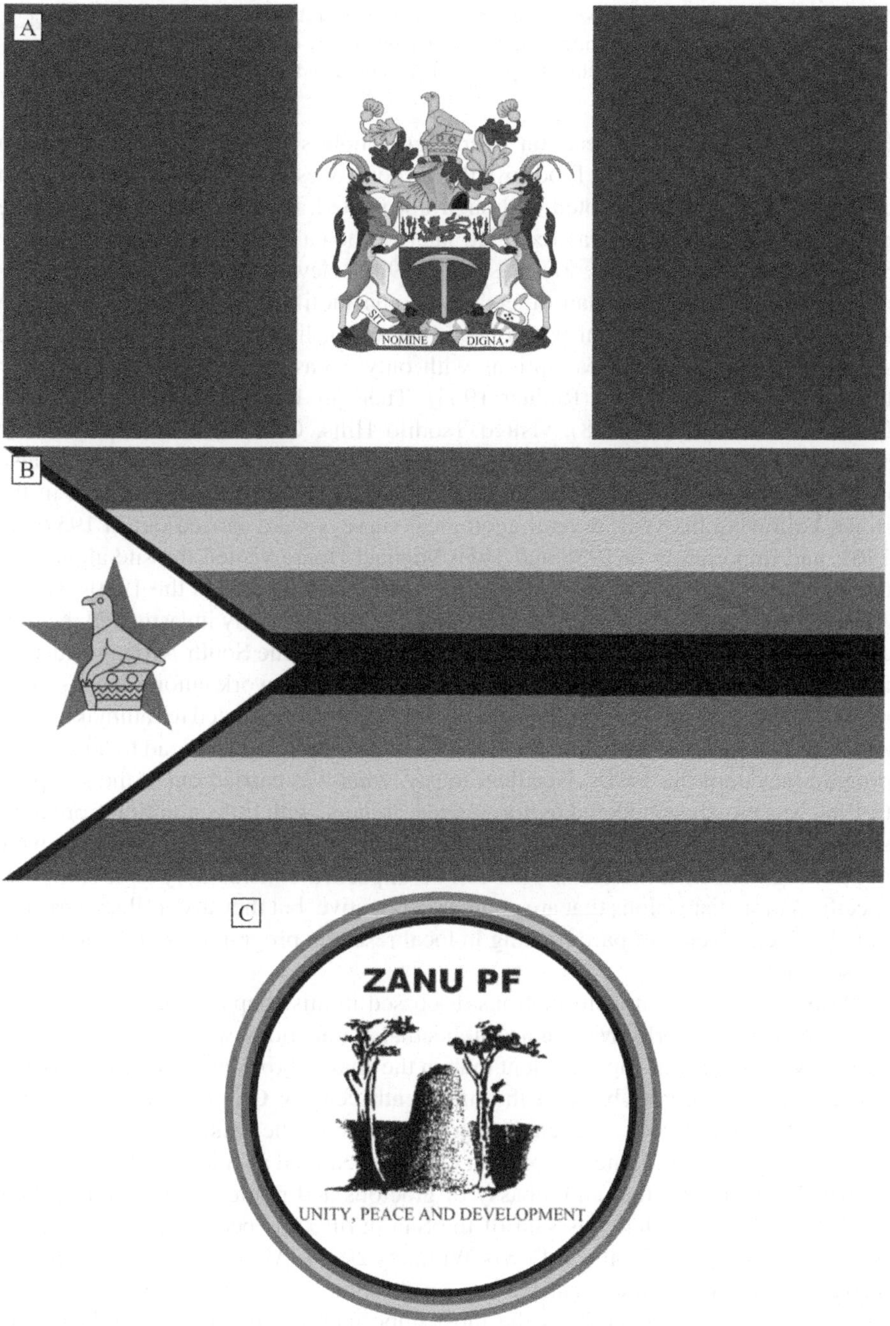

Fig. 6.1 A soapstone bird from Great Zimbabwe is included in both the (**A**) Rhodesian (1968–1979) and (**B**) National flag of Zimbabwe (1980 onwards), whereas the conical tower is used in (**C**) The ZANU-PF logo

> We should write our own history books, to prove that we did have a past, and that it was a past that was just as worth writing and learning about as any other. We must do this for the simple reason that a nation without a past is a lost nation, and a people without a past are a people without a soul.

His speech was in part a reaction to foreign scholars being the authors of much of Botswana's history. The Tsodilo Hills in north-western Botswana serves as an example. They were first noted, although not visited, by Livingstone in a map he produced, but its rock art was recorded later in the early twentieth century CE by Siegfried Passarge (1907, p. 97). Passarge (1907) viewed several paintings, determining some to be older than others, and some motifs of a young age based on an image of what he thought was a horse. However, little sustained interest in the site followed these early descriptions with only occasional visits – partly due to the region's inaccessibility (Rudner 1965). Then, in 1955, the ethno-romanticist, Laurens van der Post (1958), visited Tsodilo Hills. Convinced that spirits were present, he inserted a message into a lime-juice bottle and left it behind. He also identified evidence of habitation around the hills and ancient animal paths in the stone. Following his visit, several geological surveys were carried out in 1957 and 1961, and importantly in 1958 and 1959 Michael Hoare visited the site alone, and then with a larger team, to explore the hills and record the art. In the 1960s, Henri-Alexander (S.M.) Junod (1963) and Ione Rudner (1965) briefly investigated the hills and the latter collected specimens that were brought to the South African Museum in Cape Town for investigation. Megan Biesele's (1974) work among local groups identified myths in which the hills featured, including those related to rainmaking and ancestral connections. The slow trickle of work at Tsodilo did not lead to larger field programmes until the 1990s. Needless to say, what was carried out at the site prior to 1980 was mostly conducted by foreign researchers, with little attention from local scholars, as President Khama noted. At the time, there was concern that Africans were not writing their own histories. This can be unpacked considerably as it enmeshes specific nationalist visions that are counter-productive, but they also reflect a frustration that locals were not participating in local research programmes and knowledge construction.

While many of the transformations discussed in this chapter gained momentum after the Second World War, their intellectual foundations were often laid much earlier. Nowhere is this more evident than in the study of rock art in southern Africa, which traces its origins back to the nineteenth century CE. John Barrow (1801, p. 239) admired San rock art even though he considered the artists to be 'savages'. In another early account, James Alexander (1837) attempted an interpretation of a rock art panel, concluding that an embassy of gracious and polite females were asking for peace. Much of what was said of the San during this period was deprecating, dismissive, and prejudicial (cf. Lewis-Williams 2006). Although little attempt was made to stop the injustices carried out on the San, or halt their destruction, one study stands out and is perhaps the most important and remarkable collection of ethnographic and linguistic information from the region to this day. Wilhelm Bleek and Lucy Lloyd (1911) worked with /Xam-speaking San who had been incarcerated at the Breakwater Prison in the Cape Colony. Their interest was the /Xam language and to record it Bleek developed a phonetic script that accompanied a transliteration. All in all, they produced over 12,000 pages of texts and notes. The answers that the informants gave Bleek when he questioned them provided a deeper insight into the complexity of San society than had been considered by probably any other European by then.

At the same time, Joseph Orpen was a Chief Magistrate in Nomansland, now part of South Africa's Eastern Cape Province. In 1873, he joined the Frontier Armed Mounted Police with the mandate to capture the fugitive Langalibalele, a Hlubi chief who refused to pay tax and relinquish his weapons to the colonial authorities in Natal, South Africa (King 2015). Orpen became interested in the rock art that he occasionally found in the Maloti-Drakensberg Mountains. With the help of Qing, a southern San guide on this expedition into the Maloti Drakensberg Mountains of Lesotho, he was able to gain insights into the meaning of the art. Although he did not think much of the significance of his actions, they would come to shape our understanding of rock art. Orpen (1874) traced several panels and wrote down Qing's statements about them. He sent his journal to the *Cape Monthly Magazine* editor, who passed them onto Bleek in Cape Town. Bleek showed the reproduced drawings to his informants and received an interpretation, which he duly recorded, noting various similarities. Some years later he received additional rock art reproductions from George Stow, who had been visiting rock art sites for several years by that time (Solomon 2006), which would confirm what he had thought: the San had a complex society with a deep and rich cosmology that was reflected in their artwork (Lewis-Williams 2006).

By the mid-twentieth century, these remarkable findings had been forgotten and shifts in archaeology had driven thought away from ethnography. The emphasis on systematising research promoted investigations of stratigraphy and typology, or superpositioning of images and styles in rock art, with an overarching aim to obtain objective understandings of the past. Additionally, Stone Age sequences were of primary interest and attracted most of the research interest. John Goodwin (1953) described rock art research in *Method in Prehistory* as being ripe for amateurs. Rock art studies entered a phase of quantitative assessments and speculative interpretations often invoking the activities of daily San life. Rock art research unfortunately was left behind by archaeology.

While rock art studies were struggling to find their way, Patricia Vinnicombe (1967, p. 141) expressed her concern: "If … the study of rock art is to make a meaningful contribution to the field of archaeology where quantitative techniques and statistical methods are becoming increasingly important, an analytical approach is essential". She attempted to use rock art to identify clan or group regions, ecological zones occupied by specific animals, or the artists' behaviour patterns. What ensued was a period of intense fieldwork and recording to generate data that complimented the excavated record. However, what emerged was growing frustration at the clear limitations a quantitative and objective approach was having, namely its inability to say much at all about the meaning of the rock art itself (Lewis-Williams 2006).

As quantitative approaches continued, further attempts to examine specific patterns, such as superpositioning, led frustratingly to few real answers. As such,

Lewis-Williams (1972, p. 65) concluded in an early quantitative paper that to understand what moved the mind of the artist scholars need to turn to the "albeit fragmentary, mythology" that Bleek and Lloyd (1911) had collected. Evaluating nineteenth and twentieth century CE ethnographies was the next task. From careful examination of them and of the detailed, well-recorded rock art record across southern Africa, it became clear that using San spirituality, cosmology, myth and folklore allowed for richer understandings of the art than could be achieved using quantitative approaches. The works of Vinnicombe (1976), Lewis-Williams (1981), and Thomas Dowson (Lewis-Williams and Dowson 1990), to name some early pioneers, developed what has been called the shamanistic model or ethnographic method (Solomon 2006). While it is not wholeheartedly accepted by all (Skotnes 1994; Jolly 1996; Solomon 1998, 2008; McCall 2007; Bahn 2010), it is the most powerful theoretical turn in rock art studies and has influenced research around the globe (Lewis-Williams 2002; Bahn 2010; Cruz Berrocal 2011) and in other archaeological fields as well (Pearce 2012). Ultimately, rock art research came to reinvent itself as archaeology was doing so, but could only achieve this once it broke away from certain theoretical pillars in the field of archaeology and adopted ethnographic analogical frameworks (Lewis-Williams 1984).

6.1.2 East Africa

Prior to the 1960s, the archaeology of East Africa was deeply bounded within a colonial frame. Sonia Cole's (1954) book *Prehistory of East Africa*, and particularly its revised edition (1964), reflected a late colonial perspective in which local African communities were largely denied a recent past of complexity and achievement. Published shortly before the independence of many East African nations, the book emphasised deep prehistory, especially the Stone Age, as the most significant period in Africa's past. Cole (1964, p. 40) described this period as "by no means the cultural backwater that it became later", reflecting a tendency at the time to celebrate early human evolution while dismissing later African cultures. As such, the book contributed to broader colonial narratives that minimised African historical agency and implicitly supported the logic of white dominance. Other examples of this colonial framing include the work of L. Leakey and his collaborators (Leakey 1935, 1950; Leakey and Leakey 1945; Leakey et al. 1948), who interpreted many prehistoric burials as "Caucasoid" or "Mediterranean" in type, reflecting the racial classifications of the time. L. Leakey also argued that certain artefacts, such as glass beads, indicated Mediterranean or other foreign influences, consistent with a broader diffusionist model in which complex cultural elements were assumed to have arrived from outside Africa. During this period, influential myths such as the Hamitic hypothesis were widespread. For example, myths in which 'Megalithic Cushites' (Murdock 1959) and 'Azanians' (Huntingford 1933) appeared, a term derived from the Graeco-Roman name for East Africa, Azania (Chami 2021). These groups were presented as the originators of monumental architecture and earthworks across Kenya

(Robertshaw 1990, p. 84), yet were framed as entirely distinct from contemporary African populations. This kind of thinking relied on moderate diffusionism to account for cultural complexity and contributed to a broader pattern of denying African people agency in their own past, an approach that began to be challenged more forcefully from the 1960s onward.

Transitioning to independence led to alternative nationalist ideologies or accounts of lineage histories (Finneran 2013, p. 43). As part of the post-colonial drive was the aim to view the African past from an African viewpoint using African sources (Posnansky 1969). The Cwezi Dynasty in Uganda illustrates this perfectly. The Bacwezi capital was thought to be Bigo bya Mugenyi (often referred to as Bigo earthworks or just Bigo). The site was first reported in 1909 by Douglas Baines in a publication intended for colonial officers. His report presented the oral tradition that he had been told of Bacwezi at (Schmidt 2014, p. 448). However, it was deeply flawed, but this went unnoticed and it was accepted as the official version of Bacwezi history (Schmidt 1990, p. 259). As a result, most scholars argued that the Cwezi were rulers of an early fourteenth and fifteenth century CE state (Oliver 1953), with at least one person claiming that they were mythical in nature (Wrigley 1958). The dominant notion was that early or pre-Cwezi herders invaded western Uganda and through superiority or military strength overcame local farmer groups that were organised into clans. In absorbing and consolidating diverse groups, the Cwezi Dynasty emerged and expanded from the Mubende region in Uganda, extending south into Tanzania and east toward the Kenyan border region (Nyakatura 1973).

Oral histories have long linked the Cwezi Dynasty to the later Bito rulers, creating a narrative of political and spiritual continuity (Robertshaw and Taylor 2000). The Bito are believed to have been of Nilotic origin, migrating into western Uganda as pastoralists and integrating with existing farming communities. They are typically credited with founding the Bunyoro-Kitara Kingdom in the fifteenth and sixteenth centuries CE. Bunyoro became a dominant regional power, noted for its extensive trade networks, military strength, and political influence. Under Bito leadership, fragmented polities in the Great Lakes region were consolidated into a more centralised state. The earlier Cwezi, meanwhile, retained spiritual significance in oral traditions; they were believed to have been deified and associated with fertility, agriculture, and rain. The genealogical links between the Cwezi and the Bito served to legitimise Bito rule, presenting it as a divinely sanctioned succession. By the nineteenth century, the Buganda Kingdom had gained favour with European colonisers, leading to the decline of Bito political dominance. At the time of Uganda's independence in 1962, the newly formed government promoted a national narrative that used the Cwezi as symbols of a "glorious and united past" (Robertshaw 1996, p. 8).

Archaeological evidence, however, did not support the claimed link between the Cwezi and the Bito, and thus the national narrative that the past was being cast into. One of the first systematic studies at Bigo was by Peter Shinnie (1960). He mapped and excavated the site, and recovered evidence for extensive earthworks, distinct pottery, iron tools, and faunal remains composed largely of cattle bones. Posnansky (1966, 1969) followed Shinnie in excavating Bigo. He coined the term Bigo Culture and helped further establish the site's chronology, which broadly aligned with the

Cwezi Dynasty. Both Shinnie and Posnansky excavated in an area called Mound I, which is today a shrine. However, neither mentioned it being such at the time of their excavations. It therefore appears that its history as a shrine originates in the post-colonial era when the Bito mythicised link with the Cwezi propagated (Reid 1991, pp. 75–76). Not far from Bigo is Ntusi, where Andrew Reid (1991) and John Sutton (1993) focussed their studies. Both worked at the site after independence once archaeologists had returned to Uganda in 1986 (Robertshaw and Taylor 2000, p. 5). They examined the domestic attributes of the site as well as evidence of trade and settlement organisation. Each argued that the site was a major centre based on the range of finds that they made and the size of the settlement. Finally, Robertshaw and others (e.g., Robertshaw 1994, 1997, 2002, 2010; Robertshaw and Taylor 2000) integrated environmental data, material analyses and oral traditions to argue that a decentralised set of polities existed that were connected via shared cultural and ritual practices. Robertshaw (2002, 2010) argued against the notion that the Cwezi ruled a large territory in a centralised manner, and instead that small-scale polities in competition with one another existed using resources such as cattle, agriculture, and trade.

The emphasis on empires and civilisations in African national narratives may reflect the influence of global, particularly Western, historiographical frameworks that prioritise state formation and monumental complexity (Robertshaw 1996). In response to colonial-era depictions of Africa as a 'dark continent' devoid of significant precolonial change, postcolonial states often sought to counter such portrayals by highlighting imperial achievements. Yet, in regions where centralised empires were absent, histories of decentralised polities, dynamic economies, and diverse spiritual landscapes reveal equally rich and complex trajectories. These narratives, while less easily mobilised for nation-building purposes, underscore the continent's varied and sophisticated pasts. Recognising this diversity requires not only attention to local historical particularities but also openness to broader cultural sequences and comparative patterns across regions.

Ethiopia differs from most African countries. Between 1936 and 1941 it was colonised by the Italians, but other than this short period it remained independent despite numerous attempts at colonising the region (Selden 2013). It has, however, captured the minds of Europeans under various guises: Abyssinia, Aethiopia, Ethiopia, and Prester John's realm (Finneran 2013, p. 43). Ethiopia is also one of the oldest Christian states in the world, with a long relationship with both Asia and Europe. For these reasons, and others, it does not wholly see itself as 'African' (Finneran 2003). The country itself is incredibly diverse, like many African states, and includes over 80 ethnic groups and languages (Adamu 2013, p. 18). The country was not forged through colonialism but territorial expansion of the Abyssinia empire (Van Der Beken 2007, p. 106). The aim was to ensure peace and stability by establishing a nation. To do this, a national identity was needed and this privileged Christian, Semitic speakers at the expense of other groups (Finneran 2013, p. 43). A widely read guidebook on Ethiopian culture dedicated only two pages to the history of the country outside of the Christian highlands (Girma Kidane and Wilding 1977). Very similarly to the use of the past elsewhere on the continent, in Ethiopia it was hewn as a monolithic entity to engender a certain angle orchestrated by political elites, and this became the dominant narrative.

Aksum is a wonderful example of the trajectory East African archaeology followed in the twentieth century. Aksum was a northern town in Ethiopia that reached its opulence between the third and seventh centuries CE (Phillipson 2003, 2012, pp. 69–71). During this period, it was the capital of a centralised kingdom that ruled over a large region and was an important political, religious and trading centre. The full size of its territory varied over time; in some instances, it reached the Sudanese Meroitic territory, and it also controlled parts of southern Arabia. One of the incredible features of Aksum was the early advent of minted coins, in the late third century CE, that contain names of successive kings accompanied by their titles and regalia (Fig. 6.2). Stone inscriptions also provide written insights into the Aksumite civilisation, including military and religious aspects. Additionally, visitors from the Byzantine Empire recounted their experiences at Aksum, which offer a rare glimpse into local society at the time. Aksum society initially followed a modified religious belief from south Arabia, which likely entered the region early in the first millennium BCE, but Christianity was later adopted in the fourth century CE and has remained the dominant religion ever since (Munro-Hay 1991).

Archaeological interest in Aksum began relatively early. The Deutsche Aksum-Expedition carried out the first serious archaeological study in the Horn of Africa in 1906. During this expedition, Aksum was excavated and the buildings, stelae, stone thrones and other features were documented. The next phase of work was in 1939, during the Italian occupation of Ethiopia, and was followed by the Imperial Ethiopian Government launching a largescale study after their expulsions, lasting from the 1950s until the 1970s. From 1972 to 1974, the British Institute in East Africa conducted excavations (Munro-Hay 1989), after which archaeological work ceased, and began again from 1993 until 1997 under David Phillipson (2000, 2012). Initially, archaeological research identified two main periods, separated from one another based on the adoption of Christianity. The early, Pre-Christian Phase, dated to the first to fourth centuries CE, and the succeeding Christian Period continued until the seventh or eighth centuries CE. Dating the site was based on textual records and coinage in the absence of chronologies.

The Christian governments of Ethiopia positioned Aksum as the foundation of national and religious identity, using its legacy to legitimise contemporary rule (Munro-Hay 1991). Leaders of the Solomonic Dynasty, for example, claimed direct descent from Aksumite kings and biblical figures, asserting that Menelik I, regarded as Aksum's founder, was the son of King Solomon and the Queen of Sheba (Adamu 2009). Pre-1991 regimes celebrated Aksum as the birthplace of Ethiopian civilisation and prominently featured it in nationalist discourse. Its historical status as a powerful and enduring Christian kingdom was used to reinforce narratives of resilience and independence, particularly in contrast to the colonial histories of other African nations (Munro-Hay 1991; Phillipson 2012). In this framing, earlier pre-Christian periods were often marginalised or treated merely as precursors to the Christian Aksumite era. During the early to mid-twentieth century CE, when foreign archaeological teams began working at Aksum, their activities were closely monitored by the government to

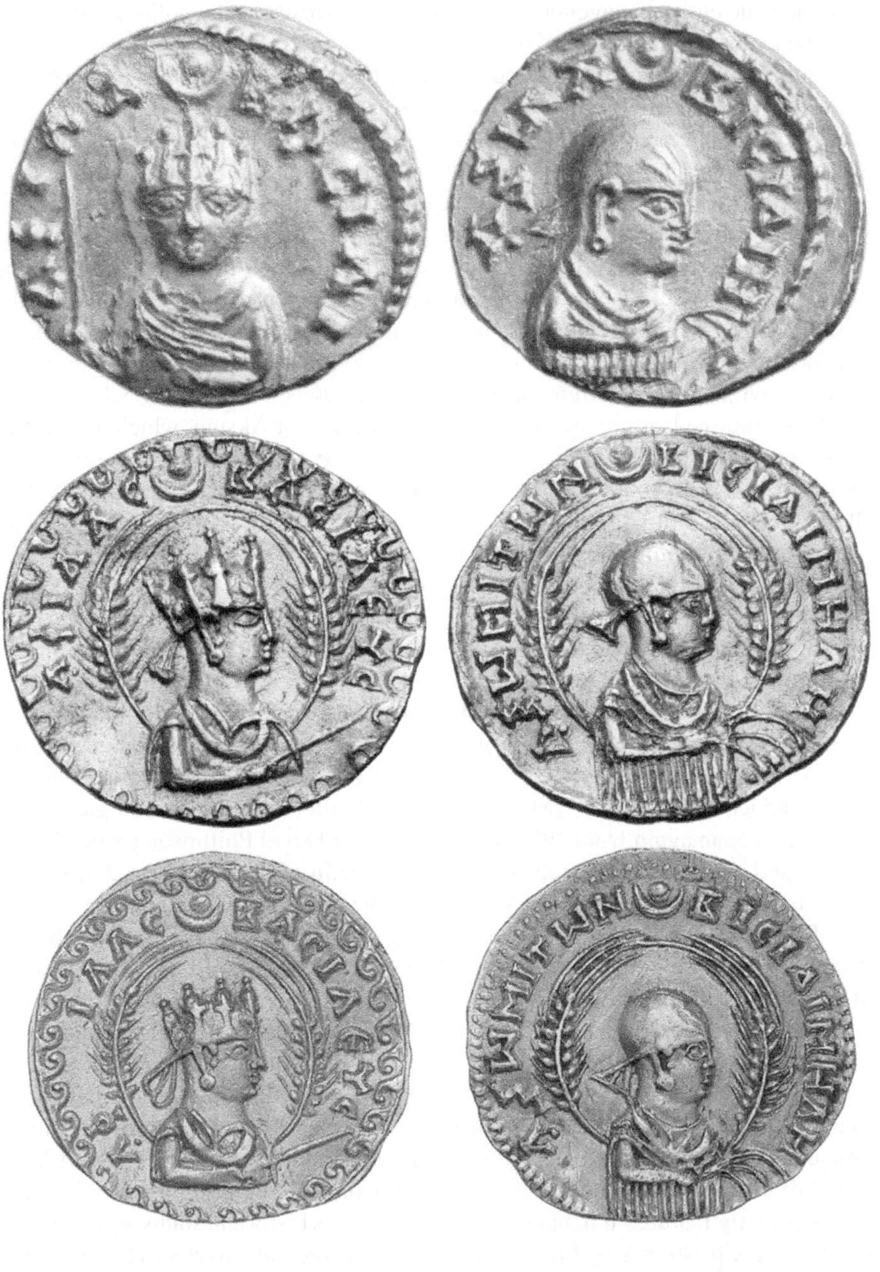

Fig. 6.2 Examples of Aksum coins from King Aphilas, dating to the early fourth century CE. *Sources* (from top to bottom) https://commons.wikimedia.org/wiki/File:Aphilas_front_gold_01.jpg; https://commons.wikimedia.org/wiki/File:Aphilas_tiara.jpg; and https://commons.wikimedia.org/wiki/File:Axum-_Aphilas_-_Münzkabinett,_Berlin_-_5556640.jpg

ensure their findings supported official narratives (Pankhurst 1999). Aksum's romanticised past thus served not only as a historical anchor for the Ethiopian state but also as a religious and ideological tool for legitimising political authority.

6.1.3 North Africa

Outside Egypt, for much of the twentieth century CE, North African historical research focussed on Romanisation (Quinn 2003, p. 7). However, earlier perspectives were marred by prejudicial views of indigenous African communities. One of the most detailed investigations was written by Thomas Boughton (1929, p. vii), *The Romanization of Africa Proconsularis,* who expressed doubt that local communities "had remained untouched by foreign influence if they would have evolved any advanced political or social organization". Studies prior to the 1960s were largely focussed on Phoenician, Punic, and Libyco-Punic cultures in the Mediterranean region of North Africa. They were also mostly examined through Near Eastern or Semitic research programmes in Europe and North Asia, detaching the region, to an extent, from sub-Saharan Africa (Hitchner 2022, p. 5).

From the 1960s and 1970s, archaeology in North Africa began to shift away from colonial frameworks, influenced by the wave of national independence, changing political agendas, and broader theoretical movements towards decolonisation (Hitchner 2022, p. 5). While colonial narratives were largely abandoned, traces of migrationist thinking persisted in some later works (e.g., Berg Briese and Lund 2000, p. 223). Alongside continued interest in Roman Africa, new attention was directed toward the Phoenicians in the western Mediterranean and to pre- and protohistoric North African cultures (Doak and López-Ruiz 2019). The 1956 excavation of the Punic town of Kerkouane, led by the newly formed Tunisian National Institute of Art and Archaeology with state support, marked an important moment in locally driven research tied to national unity (Hitchner 2022, p. 5). Likewise, the Save Carthage project, involving both local and foreign archaeologists, highlighted a more collaborative but nationally grounded approach to heritage (Hurst 1975, p. 197; Wells 1982). A major scholarly intervention came with Marcel Bénabou's (1978) *La Résistance Africaine à la Romanisation*, which challenged colonial-era narratives by proposing a more complex, interactive history shaped by both Africans and Romans. Though not universally accepted, Bénabou's (1978) critique disrupted the dominance of Romanisation as a historical lens and helped open the field to alternative interpretations of North Africa's past (Conant 2012). As such, the development of archaeology in the region has been deeply intertwined with local political contexts, and understandings of the past continue to evolve in dialogue with shifting national and scholarly priorities (Hitchner 2022, p. 8).

Along with this shift in research, interest in the Palaeolithic and Neolithic periods in North Africa increased and gained greater traction (Bazile 2002). Hominins followed by modern humans have lived in the Sahara for at least 300,000 years, and the region's occupation history includes significant shifts in material culture and social networks. Foraging groups still exist here and have aided in ethnographic reconstructions of past ways of living (Blench 2024). An excellent example is the work of the Palaeolithic-trained Cambridge University archaeologist and Royal Air Force Volunteer Reserve member, Charles McBurney (Clark and Wilkinson 1986). When he served from 1942 to 1943, McBurney traversed nearly 2000 km of the North African coastal region, from Egypt's Alexanderia to Libya's Tripoli. Across this expanse, he identified archaeological traces from the Stone Age and recovered plenty of artefacts from brief visits to sites (McBurney 1947). In 1946, once back in Cambridge, McBurney organised and expedition to take place in 1947 and 1948 under the Department of Archaeology and Anthropology to the Gebel Akhdar and northern coastal district of Cyrenaican. There, he excavated Haua Fteah (Fig. 6.3), a large karstic cave in the Cyrenaican district; the cave's opening is 50 m high with an interior roofed area of around 80 m and a depth of about 20 m (Douka et al. 2014). McBurney (1967) recovered an extensive sequence that included seven major cultural units, which are now known to begin at c. 73,000 BP and continue until at least c. 7000 BP (Barker et al. 2009; Douka et al. 2014). His findings are still widely referred to and they established a Stone Age sequence unlike most in Africa. What he also demonstrated was a rich and impressive archaeological sequence that predated this Mediterranean region's contacts with Europe and Asia. He titled one of his papers, *Libya before the Greeks*, in which he presented the archaeology of Libya from this period as it was known at the time (McBurney 1971).

Another early investigation into North African history came through rock art studies led by the French ethnographer Henri Lhote (Coulson and Campbell 2010). First introduced to the rock art of the Tassili n'Ajjer in the 1930s, Lhote later returned in the 1950s to undertake systematic surveys and documentation (Fig. 6.4). Guided by Tuareg collaborators, Lhote helped bring this rich visual record to wider scholarly and public attention. Photographs of the artwork were placed on display in the Louvre, Paris, and described as 'fine art' as opposed to something defamatory. Lhote's work promoted African art in a way that few other scholars had by that time, though his interpretations, often focusing on external influences and fantastical theories, have since been critically reassessed, and he and his team were even accused of faking images (Lajoux 1963; Soleilhavoup 1978; e.g., Hachid 1998; Keenan 2002). For example, Lhote interpreted some of the art as scenes from the lives of pastoral groups in the past, their rituals and cultural practices, and suggested some art may represent the migration of groups across the Sahara, such as the Fulani. He proposed these ideas based on the meticulous analysis of iconography and a desire to generate cultural narratives, but they were based on selective interpretations, personal visual observations, limited ethnography, and overall methodological weakness; the link between the art and Fulani was ultimately tentative (Le Quellec 2002). Despite this, Lhote's work attempted to push the limits of what one could say about rock art at a time when methodological frameworks and theoretical underpinnings themselves were yet to develop into a robust set of principles. Moreover, he sought to do so at a time when considering the history of African groups in depth and with detail was not necessarily something practiced by many and only emerging among scholars of history.

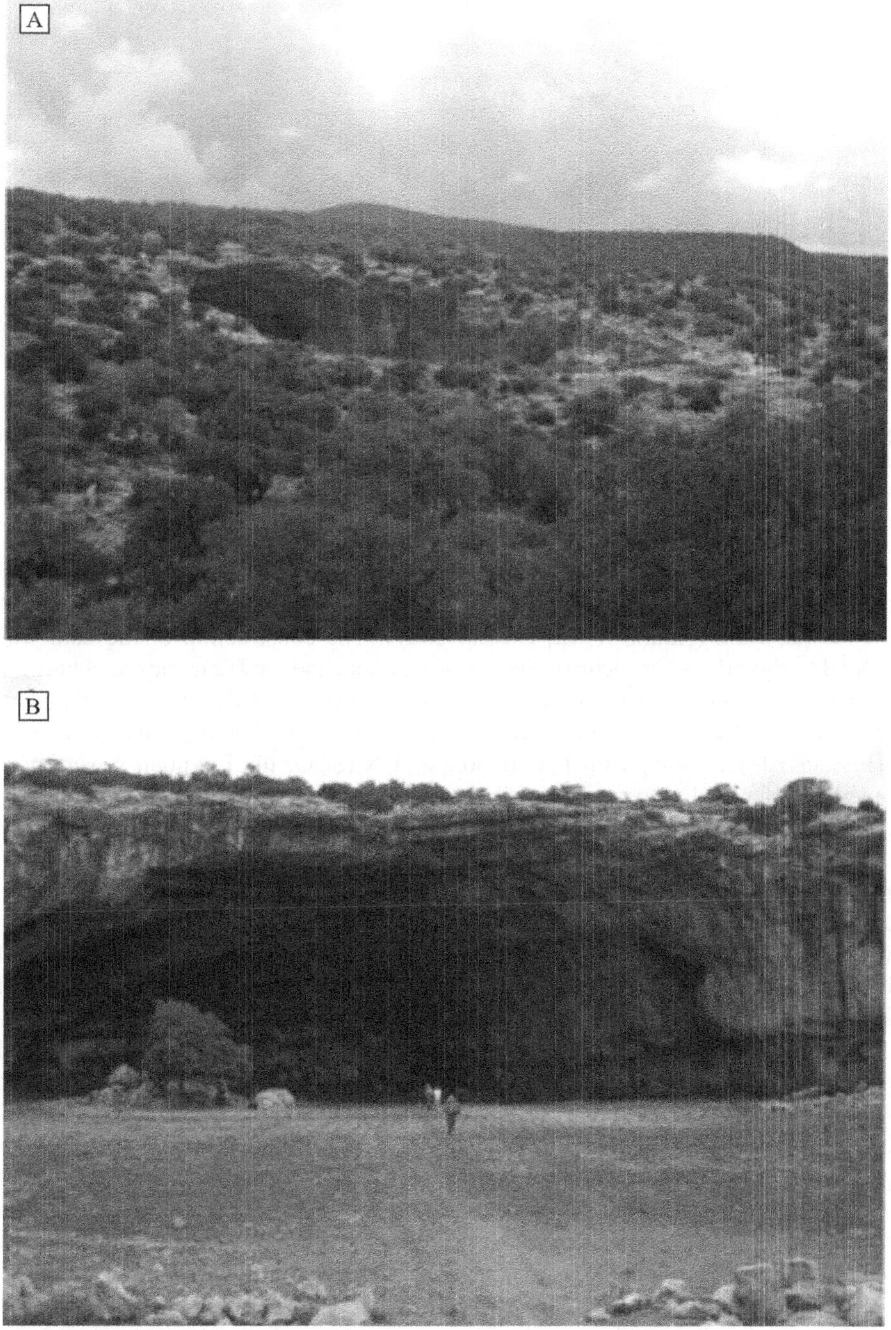

Fig. 6.3 (**A**) Looking southwest from the coastal plain to Haua Fteah, and (**B**) Looking south into the cave (c. 50 m wide and c. 20 m high) (photographs: Graeme Barker). *Source* https://commons.wikimedia.org/wiki/File:Haua_Fteah_cave.jpg

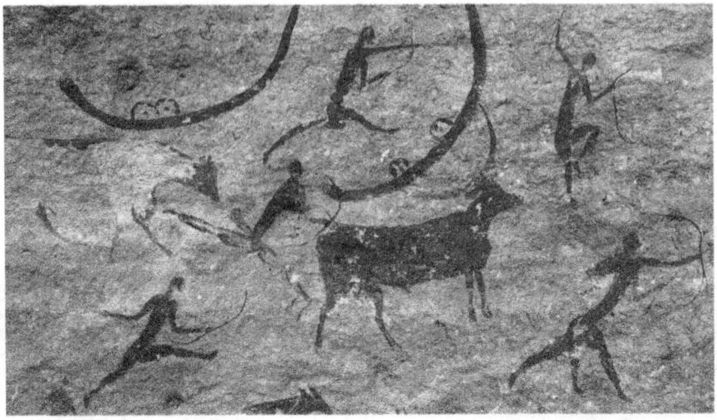

Fig. 6.4 An example of a rock art scene, including humans with acaccoutrements and a cow, from Algeria (photograph: Gruban). *Source*: https://commons.wikimedia.org/wiki/File:Algerien_Desert.jpg

Another important development that had global impact in terms of advancing the concept of 'world heritage' was the archaeological work carried out ahead of the Aswan Dam (Adams 1992; Hassan 2007). The construction of the dam was crucial to Egypt's water security, energy production, and land demands, and became a significant flood deterrent (Hassan 2007). These issues led to the establishment of the Aswan Dam development in 1960, following Egypt's independence in 1954 (Hussein 1981). Along with the support of UNESCO, the Egyptian government opted to safeguard all monuments that would be affected by the dam through an unprecedented mitigation programme. The massive undertaking led to the relocation of temples and monuments by an interdisciplinary team of archaeologists, architects, Egyptologists, engineers, and geologists. The work led to thousands of archived texts and academic publications – along with increased interest in Nubian archaeology – as well as educational products in a wide-sweeping public archaeology exercise, and it placed the Abu Simbel temples on tourist itineraries. Aswan and its associated activities and byproducts galvanised what world heritage meant in a changing, post-colonial African context; local heritage was often important on a scale that included the international community (Hassan 2007). The Egyptian president at the time, Gamal Abdel-Nasser, said that "the preservation of the legacy of mankind is no less important than the construction of dams, the erection of factories and the greater prosperity of the people" (Säve-Söderberg 1987, p. 90). Aswan was an important case that demonstrates the importance of preserving heritage, the extent one can take in doing so, and the global impact this may have. It also demonstrates the key shifts that took place in heritage management, preservation, and tourism, which were driven in part by African contexts.

6.1.4 West and Central Africa

In West and Central Africa, early archaeological investigations were closely tied to colonial agendas and narratives. A common theme was the portrayal of major cultural and technological developments as the result of external influences, rather than local innovation. These studies often aimed to depict the regions as lacking complexity or advancement prior to European contact. West and Central Africa are discussed together here because of these shared colonial assumptions, alongside a major mid-twentieth-century CE debate that spanned multiple regions: the theory of 'Bantu migrations', which came to influence interpretations not only in these areas, but also in East and southern Africa.

An early example of scholarship engaging critically with African history emerged from West Africa on the eve of independence. Kenneth Dike's (1956) book, *Trade and Politics in the Niger Delta 1830–1885,* examined processes by which British administration gradually supplanted local rulers. He argued that "commerce was the fundamental relationship that bound Africa to Europe" after five centuries of trade (Dike 1956, p. 1). While gold was initially the most coveted commodity, the trade in enslaved people came to dominate from the sixteenth century CE. The 1830 European discovery of the mouth of the Niger River opened a trade route into the interior, further enabled by steam-powered transport and, later, by the medical use of quinine from 1854, which reduced European mortality from malaria. British influence spread not through formal annexation but through strategic treaties with local rulers. Dike's (1956) work, written at a time when African historians were beginning to reshape narratives from within the continent, offered a locally grounded critique of colonial interference and established a foundation for postcolonial historiography (Watkins 1956).

A few years later, another powerful challenge to Eurocentric histories emerged from West Africa in a different form. Cheik Anta Diop's (1960, 1974, 1981) work drew on archaeology, linguistics, and historical interpretation to promote an African-centred understanding of the past, arguing that Egypt (Kemet) was not only the cradle of African civilisation but the origin of global civilisation itself. Like Dike (1956), Diop (1960, 1974) challenged European distortions of Africa's past, but whereas Dike (1956) focused on the political and economic history of British intervention, Diop's (1960, 1974) intervention was civilisational and pan-African in scope. Building on earlier thinkers like Anténor Firmin (1885, 2002 the 2002 reference was translated by Asselin Charles) and echoing contemporaries such as Léopold Sédar Senghor (1964), Diop (1960, 1974) articulated a vision of African diffusionism in which the Nile Valley was a centre from which populations and ideas spread across the continent. His bold assertions, while controversial, were instrumental in confronting deeply entrenched narratives that marginalised Africa's role in world history. Diop's (1960, 1974, 1981) influence extended beyond Africa, energising the Afrocentric movement in the United States (Asante 1980, 1987; Bernal 1987; Mazama 2001), and prompting renewed scrutiny of the political agendas embedded in Western scholarship (Asante 1990; Okafor 1991; Nantambu 1996; Falola 2017). Together, these scholarly interventions signalled a turning point, marking the emergence of African voices that not only contested colonial distortions but also asserted agency in shaping the continent's historical narrative, catalysing new research and excavation (Scerri 2017).

Diop's (1960, 1981) revision of African history has not withstood scrutiny (Lefkowitz and Rogers 1996; MacDonald 2003; North 2003). Most international scholars, as well as those from within Africa, argued that these conclusions were drawn from a limited dataset and were overly politicised. They also created a locally enchanting view of African identity and history as rooted in great wealth, ingenuity, and civilisations. However, such reconstructions nonetheless promoted a European view of Africa as a single entity, and equated 'race' and 'culture' across this vast and diverse region (Mitchell 2005a). Moreover, they disfigured African history into a unilinear, evolutionist perspective (Stahl 1999), as well as promoting a hyperdiffusionist model for African change (Appiah 1997). These perspectives, in this sense, are victim to the same mentality as Eurocentric views propagated during the colonial era of drawing broad conclusions on a limited understanding and generating preferred narratives. Unfortunately, it also echoed another European sentiment that Africa was mostly devoid of creativity other than in a few key areas, from which innovations diffused into other regions (Trigger 2006, p. 203).

Stone Age research in West Africa also saw considerable transformation. It received comparable attention to other regions in Africa during the first half of the twentieth century CE, but this changed when the 'Out of Africa' model came into favour and the continent's western regions were then treated as peripheral to human evolution (Scerri 2017). East Africa was instead favoured as a more profitable region for Stone Age research. To some extent, this perception has penetrated into the present day, despite important finds being made, such as the identification of the Kintampo Culture.

The Kintampo Culture was first identified by Oliver Davies (1962). He not only defined the material culture of the Kintampo Culture, but also its associated settlement patterns. Sites were typically found in central Ghana and initially located near to the town Kintampo, its namesake, but their identification was tricky due to dense vegetation, survey gaps, and the creation of Lake Volta, which drowned many sites (Watson 2010, p. 145). Following Davies, Colin Flight (1967, 1970, 1976) suggested a population replacement had taken place based on his excavations at Kintampo 6 Rock Shelter. He thought groups from the Sahel had moved into the central Ghanian region and replaced the earlier, local Punpun Culture, which sharply declined. Punpun was produced by mobile hunter-gatherers whereas Kintampo offered the earliest evidence of food production in the region and assemblages include grinding stones, ground axes and domestic caprines (Shaw 1977; Clark 1980; Watson 2005). Ann Stahl (1985, p. 146) examined the chronology and noted later dates in the northern reaches of the Kintampo region, suggesting an incursion from the north is unlikely as the dates should be older. Alternatively, Posnansky (1984, p. 150) proposed a dynamic context in which Kintampo-producers came into contact with northeners and integrated aspects of their material culture into the Kintampo culture, doing so variably, which accounted for regional differences. In such a scenario, and based on radiocarbon dates, this must have happened fairly rapidly between 3600 and 3200 BP (Watson 2005, 2010, pp. 142–143). However, contact alone is an insufficient motivation for change. Conversely, Derek Watson (2005) proposed a model in which Sahelian societies moved into the Kintampo region and re-adapted aspects of their material culture and economy to suit prevailing ecological conditions. Nonetheless, although the Kintampo Culture is subject to debate, all agree that it is unlike any preceding entity (Stahl 1985, p. 145).

The Kintampo Culture in the once thought of 'backwaters' of the Stone Age presents several striking contradictions to this perspective. Notably, it represents one of the earliest instances of food production in West Africa (Casey 2005), marking a shift away from a purely foraging society. This marks the adaptive strategies in early society to exploit natural and cultivatable resources, as well as demonstrating environmental adaptations. It also marks a shift in settlement patterns. Kintampo producers were less sedentary than the previous Punpun producers and lived in semi-permanent settlements. These residential camps demonstrate social organisation and specialisation within the community based on differences in site layouts and variations in tools, respectively. These findings significantly show that key innovations took place in Africa independently and without the need for external drivers. Crucial cultural traits present in Kintampo society – sedentism, food production, and social complexity – appeared long before the arrival of European colonists. The Kintampo Culture challenges Eurocentric models of African prehistory by demonstrating innovative change and historicism.

One of the great discussions in African archaeology, that ties together so many different regions in a dynamic fashion, is the so-called 'Bantu migration'. It presents a quandary that has exercised intellectual problem solving and approaches for decades (Ehret 2001). At its roots it refers to the peopling of Central, East and southern Africa from groups leaving parts of West Africa. When they began their migration, some have argued, they departed with the 'Iron Age package', including metallurgy, livestock and crop domestication, a specific worldview, and other socio-cultural traits that operated in tandem together. Where they settled, this package was often at odds with any cultural systems in those regions, and this brought about interesting, dynamic, and often poorly understood sets of interactions and reactions. The Bantu migration threads together multiple centuries as it does regions; it began some 5000–4000 years ago in West Africa and ended roughly by at least the mid-first millennium CE when Iron Age farmers eventually arrived and settled in the southern territories of eastern southern Africa (Greenberg 1972; de Maret 2013). It has been described as one of the most significant events in recent African history (Grollemund et al. 2015).

The use of the term Bantu comes from Bleek's work in the 1850s. He became interested in African languages before his arrival in South Africa, at which point he categorised them based on racial affinities. He defined the terms 'Hottentot' (a derogatory word not used any longer) and 'Bantu', the latter a Zulu word (*aba-ntu*) meaning 'men' (de Maret 2013, p. 301). His views were that each group represented different 'races', both of which were similar to an original form of humankind. He considered Europeans to be at an advanced and higher stage (Bleek 1858; Thornton 1983; Bank

1999). Bleek's work was followed by Carl Meinhof (1912), another German linguist, who further developed Bantu language studies. He classified African languages in his influential study, *Die Sprachen der Hamiten,* in which he controversially linked Bantu languages to the Hamites. He also developed a linguistic tree and placed the origin of Bantu languages in Central Africa. The British colonial administrator, Harry Johnston (1919) also examined the Bantu languages and published his study that integrated linguistics, cultural and physical anthropology to propose a cohesive narrative of Bantu origins and migrations. Likewise, he suggested Central Africa as the starting point and argued that Bantu groups absorbed local populations and technologies as they spread through Africa. In 1913 already, he read a paper at the Royal Anthropological Institute in London where he proposed a process of conquest with regard to the Bantu migration (Oliver 1966, p. 362). Diedrich Westermann (1911, 1939, 1952) advanced both Bleek and later Meinhof's theories by emphasising the dynamic relationships that emerged between Bantu and non-Bantu language speakers. He challenged diffusion theory and instead emphasised the complexity of cultural exchanges. Finally, Jospeh Greenberg (1949, 1972) refined the Bantu languages' origin region to the Nigeria-Cameroon border area. By the 1970s, 200–400 languages were considered Bantu (Vansina 1979, p. 291), but recent estimates suggest up to 600 (Vansina 1995, pp. 179–180). This outline is a simplified overview of a much more complex history of research but a thread that blends through most of them is the aim of classifying racial groups in Africa (De Filippo et al. 2012; De Maret 2013).

Linguistics played an important role in tracking Bantu movements, but archaeology is crucial in dating movements and determining what moved, if people, for example. Roland Oliver (1966) proposed population growth as a driver of expansion, rather than only migration and conquest, which he suggested would have taken place nonetheless. He based the initial occupation area, which he called the Bantu nucleus, in the Democratic Republic of Congo, and envisioned four stages of growth. These phases were based on linguistic evidence and archaeological finds, importantly ceramic facies, trade goods, and radiocarbon dates. However, the movement from the core area is debated (de Filippo et al. 2012). For example, two primary schools of thought emerged. Initially it was thought that the Bantu western and eastern branches split in the nucleus area (Coupez et al. 1975; Möhlig 1981; e.g., Bastin et al. 1999). The eastern branch migrated eastwards north of the central forest and made their way eventually to Kenya, and then to South Africa. However, the other approach argued that there was a southern movement through the forested zone when it receded due to climatic changes, followed by the splitting of a western and eastern branch (e.g., Henrici 1973; Ehret 2001). Little consensus on this emerged (e.g., Lwanga-Lunyiigo 1976; Gramly 1978; Vansina 1979, 1980; Möhlig 1981, 1989; Ehret 2001; Eggert 2005; De Maret 2013).

The archaeology alludes to a somewhat different set of outcomes. In the Nigeria-Cameroon region, archaeological work was conducted to identify the Eastern-Bantu language homeland, such as Pierre De Maret's (1982) work at Shum Laka, which produced a sequence dating from around 30,000 BP. Several sites have since been investigated that present evidence of early cultivation and livestock rearing (e.g., De Maret 1989; Essomba 1992; Mbida et al. 2000; Oslisly 2006; Meister 2007). Sites in the region include underground storage pits, pottery commonly with comb-stamping, charred plant remains, and polished stone axes or hoes dating from 2600–1500 BP. Stone tools also progressively disappear and may have been replaced with iron tools (Lavachery et al. 1996; Clist 2006). Faunal remains have not preserved well in the acidic soils, but from the evidence, hunting, fishing and caprine keeping have all been identified (Mbida et al. 2000). Plant remains such as yams have been identified (Neumann 2005), and while direct genomic evidence is limited, domestication of yams is widely believed to have occurred in the Niger River basin (Scarcelli et al. 2019). Evidence for early banana cultivation has also been found (Mbida et al. 2000; Mindzie and Vrydaghs 2020), but the chronology of its introduction to West and Central Africa remains contested (Vansina 2003; Neumann et al. 2012). Pearl millet has been found dating to 2350–2100 BP (de Maret 1992; Eggert et al. 2006) and ground nut c. 1750 BP (Eggert et al. 2006). These plants originate further north and are savannah and not forest species. It appears to indicate that the forest retreated around this time opening savannah-like patches that communities occupied and cultivated (Schwartz 1992; Maley and Brenac 1998; Maley 2004; Eggert et al. 2006). Similar sites have been found further south in Gabon (Clist 1995; Assoko Ndong 2002) coinciding with drier episodes and the opening of savannah tracts (Schwartz 1992). This southern spread is attested by additional sites and radiocarbon dates in the Congo (de Maret 1982), but Central Africa remains largely undated. The Great Lakes region of East Africa, however, also has early evidence of Iron Age farmers. In the Lake Victoria region, dimple-based ceramics were identified by Mary Leakey et al. (1948), and Posnansky (1961) and Jean Hiernaux (1962) proposed that they were characteristic of wares associated with the beginning of the Iron Age. These assemblages, known as Urewe (Posnansky 1967), became recognised as the parent branch of traditions spreading east and south, eventually reaching South Africa (Huffman 1970; Soper 1971; Phillipson 1976; Ashley 2010). The movement of these wares into new areas, along with associated iron tools, cultivated crops, and livestock, has been described by some as the 'Iron Age package' (Fig. 6.5) (Maggs 1984, p. 331). However, it seems increasingly more likely that certain traits were adopted after the initial expansion began.

The Bantu migration has not been accepted without contest. Phillipson (1976, p. 65) early on bemoaned that "[t]he correlation has frequently been made and, on occasion, somewhat acritically accepted, between the spread of the Iron Age culture… and the dispersal of the Bantu speakers". He noted that the assumption exists that indigenous groups living in areas prior to farmers could not have adopted an 'Iron Age package', and that a complex process was being oversimplified. For example, Phillipson (1976) examined over 400 radiocarbon dates that were available and challenged simplistic expansion frameworks from the west, eastwards, and south in various streams. However, when he examined the linguistic data, he noted that it was problematic because the observed linguistic homogeneity may, rather, have been the result of contact over a lengthy period rather than shared ancestry. Moreover, linguistics does not provide a stringent chronology, leading one to make the assumption that language spread with cultural material, which in this case is somewhat uniform within the various migratory streams. The archaeology itself

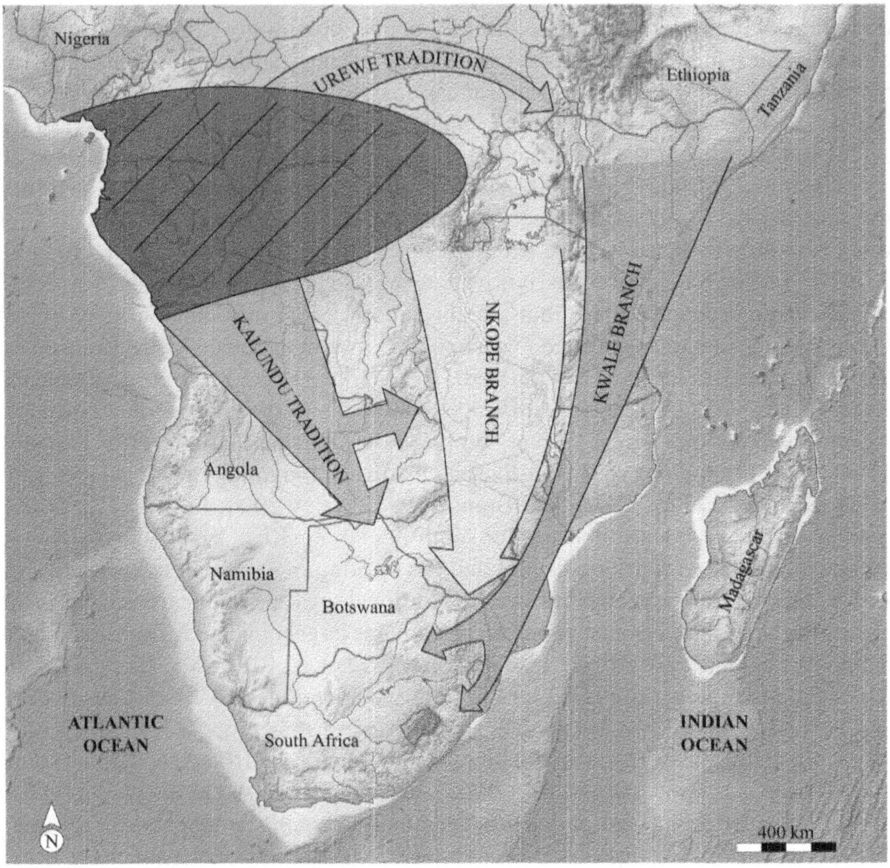

Fig. 6.5 An illustration of Bantu migration based on ceramic evidence (modified from Huffman 2005, p. 72)

does not allow for the spoken language to be determined, whether Bantu at all. He also critiqued the linguistic approach for placing overemphasis on vocabulary. Bantu studies for at least the period covered in this chapter, largely relied on linguistics and assumptions (de Maret 2013, p. 301). Instead, Phillipson (1976) proposed an initial movement of proto-Bantu groups beginning c. 5000 BP, followed by a later Bantu migration c. 2000 BP once the recognised 'Iron Age package' had been developed.

While Phillipson (1976) still supported the conclusion that a migration took place, Samwiri Lwanga-Lunyiigo (1976) suggested that 'migration mania' contributed to this idea. He argued that proto-Bantu speakers were more widely dispersed and not located in a core region from which they spread. Instead, he argued in favour of independent regional developments, diffusion and exchange, and a broader geographic and temporal context. Ultimately, he disregarded the linguistic evidence because it may be the result of contact and not migrations, and suggested that the archaeology of the interlacustrine region in East Africa (near the Great Lakes) was an area of independent development. The latter argument was based on early radiocarbon dates showing first millennium BCE metallurgy and skeletal evidence which showed the widespread distribution of proto-Bantu speakers.

Perhaps drawing the various perspectives together is the view that a single migration did not take place, but rather a variety of regional expansions, cross-cultural encounters, and economic, social and political exchanges resulted in the widespread distribution of the 'Iron Age package' and Bantu languages (Ehret 2001). In a more recent approach, Christopher Ehret (2001) adopted a dynamic model that developed a historical view of Bantu relations. Lane (2004) likewise highlighted variability in the spread of food production through Africa. He argued that the movement of agriculture and livestock herding could not be solely attributed to a single migration. As such, the notion of a 'package' spreading uniformly across sub-Saharan Africa lacks nuance and regional histories. De Maret (2013, p. 637) also implored scholars to consider associated traits of the migration, such as demographic movements and contact with hunter-gatherers along the expansion routes, comparative studies of myths and rituals, and technological features of material culture and production training. Only in doing so, he continued, can we determine if the 'Bantuization' was a process of "colonisation, migration, expansion, dispersal, or diffusion".

The study of the Bantu migration highlights how archaeological interpretation is deeply shaped by broader political and ideological contexts. Initially embedded in colonial narratives that emphasised conquest and racial hierarchies, the framework shifted in the post-independence era toward one that foregrounded African agency, innovation, and unity. This transformation reflected not only new methodological developments but also the influence of nationalism, Pan-Africanism, and efforts to reclaim the continent's past from Eurocentric distortions.

6.2 Colonial Legacies in Post-colonial Africa

A crucial shift in African archaeology occurred with the transition from colonial to post-colonial paradigms. Although African countries gained independence, the legacy of colonialism persisted (Gosden 2001; Green et al. 2003; Leone 2009). Its effects continued to shape economies, politics, representation, and the lives of people across the continent, and archaeology was no exception. The discipline witnessed a transformation in its character during the pre- and post-independence periods, influenced not only by broader political change but also by specific national contexts and local initiatives. Several key developments typify the archaeological landscape during this era.

Prior to the Second World War, archaeological interpretations were shaped by colonial ideologies that downplayed African agency. These narratives were not only the result of scholarly interpretation (Hall 1984; Pratt 1992; Shepherd 2002) but were also manipulated in national discourse to support colonial rule. The contested history of Great Zimbabwe exemplifies this, with the Rhodesia Front attributing its construction to foreign builders and condemning archaeologists who challenged this view as misguided or even traitorous (Garlake 1982). In response, post-war and especially post-independence scholars began reclaiming Africa's past. Steve Biko (1987, p. 95) remarked that colonialism sought to "disfigure and distort" African history, an observation that resonated with efforts to re-centre African perspectives. While Diop's (1960) diffusionist arguments have been debated, they helped dismantle colonial assumptions. Likewise, Ken Mufuka (1983) used oral traditions and archaeology to challenge colonial readings of Great Zimbabwe and reimagine it as a complex local state.

Yet, even as African nations gained independence, archaeology remained strongly Eurocentric (Segobye 2005, p. 34; Lane 2011, p. 8). Still, the early post-independence period brought a wave of optimism. Many countries invested in heritage institutions, established archaeology departments, and encouraged scholarship that reflected national pride and cultural identity (Shaw 1989; Posnansky 1996). In Nigeria, for example, a growing number of local historians and archaeologists emerged to reclaim the writing of African history from within. This intellectual and institutional growth was shaped by the political geography inherited from colonial rule. National borders often isolated scholars from one another and encouraged inward-looking research agendas. These borders also shaped how histories were constructed, as archaeologists worked within recently formed nations, what Benedict Anderson (2006) described as "imagined communities." The influence of nationalism encouraged historical narratives that legitimised the post-colonial state, often through selective engagement with the past (Kohl 1998). Celebrations of the Iron Age, for instance, not only provided deep historical roots for modern communities but also attracted state funding and scholarly interest (Robertshaw 1990, pp. 92–93). While archaeologists were often motivated by genuine scholarly concerns, they were also aware of the political value of their work. In the midst of this national reimagining of the past, some scholars voiced concern about the direction of the field. Bruce Trigger (1990, p. 309) acknowledged that archaeology was inherently political, but he warned that an overly relativistic approach could undermine its credibility. For him, archaeology's greatest contribution to African societies lay in its ability to present as objective an account of the past as possible.

By the late 1970s, however, the early enthusiasm invested in archaeological research began to fade. Funding dwindled, staff left or emigrated, and institutions shrank (Musonda 1990, p. 12; Posnansky 1996, p. 148; Robertshaw 2000, pp. 274–275). Foreign-led projects, often hampered by their own funding issues, frequently exported finds without building local capacity or knowledge-sharing structures. These challenges would continue to shape the field, even as renewed efforts sought to rebuild and decolonise African archaeology in the decades that followed.

References

Adams, W.M., 1992. Wasting the Rain: Rivers, people and planning in Africa. *Minneapolis: University of Minnesota Press.*

Adamu, A. Y. 2013. Diversity in Ethiopia: A historical overview of political challenges. *International Journal of Community Diversity* 12:17–27.

Adamu, M. M. 2009. The legend of Queen Sheba, the Solomonic Dynasty and Ethiopian history: An analysis. *African Research Review* 3 (1): 468–482.

Alexander, J. 1837. *Narrative of a voyage of observation among the colonies of Western Africa, in the flagship Thalia: And of a campaign in Kaffir-Land, on the staff of the commander-in-chief, in 1835*. London: Colburn.

Anderson, B. 2006. *Imagined communities: Reflections on the origin and spread of nationalism*. London: Verso.

Appiah, K. A. 1997. Europe upside down: Fallacies of the new Afrocentrism. In *Perspectives on Africa: A reader in culture, history, and representation*, ed. R. R. Grinker and C. B. Steiner, 728–731. Oxford: Blackwell.

Asante, M. K. 1980. *Afrocentricity*. Trenton: Africa World Press.

Asante, M. K. 1987. *The Afrocentric idea*. Philadelphia: Temple University.

Asante, M. K. 1990. *Kemet, Afrocentricity and knowledge*. Trenton: Africa World Press.

Ashley, C. Z. 2010. Towards a socialised archaeology of ceramics in Great Lakes Africa. *African Archaeological Review* 27:135–163.

Assoko Ndong, A. 2002. Synthèse des données archéologiques récentes sur le peuplement à l'Holocène de la réserve de faune de la Lopé, Gabon. *L'Anthropologie* 106:135–158.

Atwood, R. 2011. The Nok of Nigeria. *Archaeology* 64 (4): 34–38.

Bahn, P. G. 2010. *Prehistoric rock art: Polemics and progress*. Cambridge: Cambridge University Press.

Barker, G., Antoniadou, A., Barton, H., Brooks, I., Candy, I., Drake, N., Farr, L., Hunt, C., Ibrahim, A.A., Inglis, R., Jones, S., Morales, J., Morley, I., Mutri, G., Rabett, R., Reynolds, T., Simpson, D., Twati, M., and White, K., 2009. The Cyrenaican Prehistory Project 2009: The third season of investigations of the Haua Fteah cave and its landscape, and further results from the 2007–2008 fieldwork. *Libyan Studies, 40*, 55–94.

Bank, A. 1999. Anthropology, race and evolution: Rethinking the legacy of Wilhelm Bleek. *Journal of Southern African Studies* 25 (3): 387–409. https://phambo.wiser.org.za/files/seminars/Bank%20On%20Bleek.pdf. Accessed on 23 Jan 2025.

Barrow, J. 1801. *An account of travels into the interior of Southern Africa in the years*. London: Cadell and Davies.

Bastin, Y., A. Coupez, and M. Mann. 1999. *Continuity and divergence in the Bantu languages from a Lexicostatistic study*. Tervuren: Royal Museum for Central Africa.

Bazile, F., 2002. Gabriel Camps (1927-2002). PALEO. *Revue d'Archéologie Préhistorique*, (14), 9–10.

Beach, D. N. 1983. Oral history and archaeology in Zimbabwe. *Zimbabwean Prehistory* 19:8–11.

Bénabou, M. 1978. *La Résistance Africaine à la Romanisation*. Paris: Maspero.

Berg Briese, M., and J. Lund. 2000. The late and neo-punic periods. In *Africa Proconsularis: Historical conclusions*, ed. P. Ørsted, L. Ladjimi Sabai, and H. Ben Hassen, 217–224. Aarhus: Copenhagen.

Bernal, M. 1987. *Black Aihena: The Afroasiatic roots of classical civilization (The fabrication of ancient Greece 1785–1985)*. Brunswick: Rutgers University Press.

Biesele, M. 1974. A note on the beliefs of modern Bushmen concerning the Tsodilo Hills. *Newsletter SWA Scientific Society* 15 (3–4): 1–3.

Biko, S. 1987. *I write what I like: A selection of his writings*. Oxford: Heinemann.

Binford, L. R. 1962. Archaeology as anthropology. *American Antiquity* 28 (2): 217–225.

Bishop, W. W., and D. Clark. 1967. *Background to evolution in Africa*. Chicago: University of Chicago Press.

Bleek, W. H. I. 1858. South African philology. *Cape Monthly Magazine* 3:23–24.
Bleek, W. H. I., and L. Lloyd. 1911. *Specimens of Bushman folklore*. London: G. Allen Limited.
Blench, R. 2015. The uses of the past: Indigenous ethnography, archaeology, and ethnicity in Nigeria. In *Ethnic ambiguity and the African past: Materiality, history, and the shaping of cultural identities*, ed. F. G. Richard and K. C. MacDonald, 145–171. Walnut Creek: Left Coast Press.
Blench, R. 2024. The evolution of foraging and the tranistion to pastoralism in the Sahara. In *Landscapes and landforms of the Central Sahara*, ed. J. Knight, S. Merlo, and A. Zerboni, 161–171. Cham: Springer International Publishing.
Boughton, T. R. S. 1929. *The romanization of Africa Proconsularis*. New York: Greenwood.
Breunig, P., and N. Rupp. 2010. Outline of a new research project on the Nok culture of Central Nigeria, West Africa. *Nyame Akuma* 73:46–54.
Butzer, K. W. 1964. *Environment and archaeology: An introduction to Pleistocene geography*. Chicago: Aldine Publishing.
Casey, J., 2005. Holocene occupations of the forest and savanna. In: A.B. Stahl, ed. *African Archaeology: A critical introduction*. Oxford: Blackwell, 225–248.
Chidester, D. 2002. Credo Mutwa, Zulu Shaman: The invetion and appropriation of indigenous authenticity in African folk religion. *Journal for the Study of Religion* 15 (2): 65–85.
Clark, J. D., ed. 1957. *Third Pan-African congress on prehistory: Livingstone 1955*. London: Chatto and Windus.
Clark, J. D. 1960. Human ecology during Pleistocene and later times in Africa south of the Sahara. *Current Anthropology* 1 (4): 307–324.
Clark, J. D. 1964. The prehistoric origins of African culture. *Journal of African History* 5 (2): 161–183.
Clark, J. D. 1970. *The prehistory of Africa*. London: Thames & Hudson.
Clark, J. D. 1979. Radiocarbon dating and African archaeology. In *Radiocarbon dating*, ed. R. Berger and H. E. Suess, 7–31. Berkeley: University of California Press.
Clark, J. D. 1980. Human populations and cultural adaptations in the Sahara and Nile during prehistoric times. In *The Sahara and the Nile*, ed. M. A. J. Williams and H. Faure, 527–582. Rotterdam: Balkema.
Clark, J. D. 1981. The prehistory of southern Africa. In *Harmondsworth, England*, ed. J. Ki-Zerbo, 487–529. Paris: Heinemann.
Clark, J. D. 1994. Digging on: A personal record and appraisal of archaeological research in Africa and elsewhere. *Annual Review of Anthropology* 23:1–23.
Clark, J. D., and L. P. Wilkinson. 1986. Charles Brian Montagu McBurney (1914–1979): An appreciation. In *Stone Age prehistory: Studies in memory of Charles McBurney*, ed. G. N. Bailey and P. Callow, 7–25. Cambridge: Cambridge University Press.
Clist, B.-O. 1995. *Gabon: 100 000 ans d'histoire*. Libreville: Sépia.
Clist, B.-O. 2006. Mais où se sont taillées nos pierres en Afrique Centrale entre 7.000 et 2.000 bp. In *Grundlegungen: Beiträge zur europäischen und afrikanischen Archäologie für Manfred KH Eggert*, ed. H.-P. Wotzka, 291–302. Tübingen: Francke.
Cole, S. 1954. *The prehistory of East Africa*. Harmondsworth: Penguin.
Cole, S. 1964. *The prehistory of East Africa*. Harmondsworth: Penguin.
Conant, J. 2012. *Staying Roman: Conquest and identity in Africa and the Mediterranean, 439–700*. Cambridge: Cambridge University Press.
Coquery-Vidrovitch, C. 1969. Recherches sur un mode de production africain. *La Pensée* 144:61–78.
Coulson, D., and A. Campbell. 2010. Rock art of the Tassili n Ajjer, Algeria. *Adoranten* 2010:24–38.
Coupez, A., E. Evrard, and J. Vansina. 1975. Classification d'un échantillon de langues Bantoues d'après la lexicostatistique. *Africana Linguistica* 6:131–158.
Cruz Berrocal, M. 2011. Analogical evidence and shamanism in archaeological interpretation: South African and European Palaeolithic rock art. *Norwegian Archaeological Review* 44 (1): 1–20.

Darling, P. 2004. Migrants, millenialists and mayhem: Kari-Kari, Ningi, Gwari, Kebbi, Kwatarkwashi and Zuru 'enclaves' in northern Nigeria. *Azania: Archaeological Research in Africa* 39 (1): 90–109.

Darling, P. J. 2000. The rape of Nok and Kwatakwashi: The crisis in Nigerian antiquities. *Culture Without Context, The Newsletter of the Illicit Antiquities Research Centre* 6:15–20.

Davies, O. 1962. Neolithic cultures of Ghana. In *Acres, IVe Congrès Panafricain de Préhistoire et de l'Etude du Quaternaire*, ed. G. Mortelmans and J. Nenquin, 291–302. Musée Royal de l'Afrique Centrale: Tervuren.

De Filippo, C., K. Bostoen, M. Stoneking, and B. Pakendorf. 2012. Bringing together linguistic and genetic evidence to test the Bantu expansion. *Proceedings of the Royal Society B: Biological Sciences* 279 (1741): 3256–3263.

De Maret, P. 1992. Sédentarisation, agriculture et métallurgie du Sud-Cameroun: synthèse des recherches depuis 1978. In *L'Archéologie au Cameroun: Actes du premier colloque international de Yaoundé (6–9 Janvier 1986)*, ed. J.-M. Essomba, 247–262. Paris: Karthala.

De Maret, P. 1982. From the Stone Age to the Iron Age. In *The archaeology of Central Africa*, ed. F. Van Noten, 59–67. Graz: Akademische Druck-und Verlagsanstalt.

De Maret, P. 1989. Le contexte archéologique de l'expansion bantu en Afrique centrale. In *Les Peuples Bantu: Migration, expansion et identité culturelle*, ed. T. Obenga, 118–138. Paris: L'Harmattan.

De Maret, P. 2013. Archaeologies of the Bantu expansion. In *The Oxford handbook of African archaeology*, ed. P. J. Mitchell and P. J. Lane, 627–643. Oxford: Oxford University Press.

Deacon, H. J. 1972. A review of the post-Pleistocene in South Africa. *South African Archaeological Society Goodwin Series* 1:26–45.

Dike, K. O. 1956. *Trade and politics in the Niger delta, 1830–1885*. Oxford: Clarendon Press.

Diop, C. A. 1960. *L'Afrique Noire Précoloniale: Étude comparée des systèmes politiques et sociaux de l'Europe et de l'Afrique eoire, de l'antiquité à la formation des états modernes*. Paris: Présence Africaine.

Diop, C. A. 1974. *The African origin of civilization: Myth or reality?* Chicago: Laurence Hill.

Diop, C. A. 1981. Origins of the ancient Egyptians. In *UNESCO general history of Africa: Ancient civilizations of Africa*, ed. G. Mokhtar, 10–38. Paris: UNESCO.

Doak, B. K., and C. López-Ruiz. 2019. Introduction. In *The Oxford handbook of the Phoenician and Punic Mediterranean*, ed. C. López-Ruiz and B. K. Doak, 3–8. Oxford: Oxford University Press.

Douka, K., Z. Jacobs, C. Lane, R. Grün, L. Farr, C. Hunt, R. H. Inglis, T. Reynolds, P. Albert, M. Aubert, V. Cullen, E. Hill, L. Kinsley, R. G. Roberts, E. L. Tomlinson, S. Wulf, and G. Barker. 2014. The chronostratigraphy of the Haua Fteah cave (Cyrenaica, northeast Libya). *Journal of Human Evolution* 66:39–63.

Eggert, M. K. 2005. The Bantu problem and African archaeology. In *African archaeology: A critical introduction*, ed. A. B. Stahl, 301–326. Oxford: Oxford University Press.

Eggert, M. K., A. Höhn, S. Kahlheber, C. Meister, K. Neumann, and A. Schweizer. 2006. Pits, graves and grains: Archaeological and archaeobotanical research in southern Cameroun. *Journal of African Archaeology* 4 (2): 273–298.

Ehret, C. 2001. Bantu Expansions: Re-envisioning a central problem of early African history. *International Journal of African Historical Studies* 34 (1): 5–41.

Ekholm, K. 1972. *Power and prestige: The rise and fall of the Kongo Kingdom*. Uppsala: Skriv Service.

Emeni, F. C., and J. E. Nukueye. 2019. A concise analysis of innovation, culture, history/archaeology education for national integration. *Journal of Resourcefulness and Distinction* 17 (1): 1–17.

Essomba, J.-M., ed. 1992. *L'Archéologie au Cameroun: Actes du premier colloque international de Yaoundé (6–9 Janvier 1986)*. Paris: Karthala.

Fagg, A. 2014. Discovery and early research on the Nok culture in Nigeria. In *Nok: African sculptures in archaeological contexts*, ed. P. Breunig, 81–92. Frankfurt: Africa Magna Verlag.

Fagg, B. 1956. An outline of the Stone Age of the Plateau Minesfield. In *Proceedings of the Third International West African Conference Ibadan*, ed. B. Fagg, 41–50. Nigerian Museum: Lagos.

Fagg, B. 1977. *Nok terracottas*. Lagos: The Nigerian Museums.

Fagg, B. E. 1959. The Nok culture in prehistory. *Journal of the Historical Society of Nigeria* 1 (4): 288–293.

Falola, T., ed. 2017. *Africanizing knowledge: African studies across the disciplines*. New York: Routledge.

Fanon, F. 1967. *The wretched of the earth*. Harmondsworth: Penguin Books.

Finneran, N. 2003. The persistence of memory: National identity and migrationism. A case study from African and Ethiopian archaeology. *Studies in Ethnicity and Nationalism* 3:21–37.

Finneran, N. 2013. Lucy to Lalibela: Heritage and identity in Ethiopia in the twenty-first century. *International Journal of Heritage Studies* 19:41–61.

Firmin, A. 1885. *De l'égalité des Races Humaines*. Paris: Fischbacher.

Firmin, A., 2002. *The equality of the human races*, trans. Asselin Charles. Urbana: University of Illinois Press.

Flight, C. 1967. Kintampo 1967. *West African Archaeological Newsletter* 8:15–20.

Flight, C. 1970. Excavations at Kintampo. *West African Archaeological Newsletter* 12:71–72.

Flight, C. 1976. The Kintampo culture and its place in the economic prehistory of West Africa. In *West African culture dynamics*, ed. B. K. Swartz and R. E. Dumett, 91–100. The Hague: De Gruyter Mouton.

Fontein, J. 2006. *The silence of great Zimbabwe: Contested landscapes and the power of heritage*. London: Routledge.

Franke, G. 2016. A chronology of the central Nigerian Nok culture–1500 BC to the beginning of the common era. *Journal of African Archaeology* 14 (3): 257–289.

Gabel, C. 1985. Archaeology in sub-Saharan Africa. *International Journal of African Historical Studies* 18 (2): 241–264.

Gallinaro, M., and S. Biagetti. 2016. The role of mobility in Saharan archaeological research (1960-present). *Azania: Archaeological Research in Africa* 51 (4): 435–452.

Garlake, P. S. 1982. Prehistory and ideology in Zimbabwe. *Africa* 52:1–19.

Garlake, P.S., 1984. Ken Mufuka and Great Zimbabwe. *Antiquity, 58*(223), 121.

Giblin, J. 2013. Politics, ideology, and indigenous perspectives. In *The Oxford handbook of African archaeology*, ed. P. J. Mitchell and P. J. Lane, 253–265. Oxford: Oxford University Press.

Good, C. M. 1972. Salt, trade, and disease: Aspects of development in Africa's northern Great Lakes Region. *International Journal of African Historical Studies* 5 (4): 543–586.

Goodwin, A. J. H. 1953. *Method in prehistory*. Claremont: South African Archaeological Society.

Gosden, C. 2001. Postcolonial archaeology: Issues of culture, identity and knowledge. In *Archaeological theory today*, ed. I. Hodder, 241–261. Oxford: Blackwell.

Gramly, R. M. 1978. Expansion of Bantu-speakers versus development of Bantu language and African culture in situ: An archaeologist's perspective. *South African Archaeological Bulletin* 33 (128): 107–112.

Green, L. F., D. R. Green, and E. G. Neves. 2003. Indigenous knowledge and archaeological science: The challenges of public archaeology in the Reserva Uaça. *Journal of Social Archaeology* 3:366–398.

Greenberg, J. H. 1949. Studies in African linguistic classification: I. The Niger-Congo family. *Southwestern Journal of Anthropology* 5:79–100.

Greenberg, J. H. 1972. Linguistic evidence regarding Bantu origins. *Journal of African History* 13:189–216.

Grollemund, R., S. Branford, K. Bostoen, A. Meade, C. Venditti, and M. Pagel. 2015. Bantu expansion shows that habitat alters the route and pace of human dispersals. *Proceedings of the National Academy of Sciences* 112:13296–13301.

Grove, A. T., and A. Warren. 1968. Quaternary landforms and climate on the south side of the Sahara. *Geographical Journal* 134 (2): 194–208.

Hachid, M. 1998. *Les Tassili des Ajjer. Cinquante Siècles avant les pyramides*. Paris: Paris Mediterranée.
Hall, M. 1984. The burden of tribalism: The social context of Southern African Iron Age studies. *American Antiquity* 49:455–467.
Hall, M. 1987. *The changing past: Farmers, kings and traders in southern Africa, 200–1860*. Cape Town: David Philip.
Hall, M. 1990. Hidden history: Iron Age archaeology in Southern Africa. In *A history of African archaeology*, ed. P. Robertshaw. London: James Currey Ltd: 59–77.
Hance, W. A. 1970. *Population, migration, and urbanization in Africa*. New York: Columbia University Press.
Henrici, A. 1973. Numerical classification of Bantu languages. *African Language Studies* 14:82–104.
Hassan, F.A., 2007. The Aswan high dam and the international rescue Nubia campaign. *African Archaeological Review, 24*, 73–94.
Hiernaux, J. 1962. Le début de l'âge des métaux dans la région des Grands Lacs africains. In *Actes IVe Congrès Panafricain de Préhistoire et de l'étude du Quaternaire III: Préhistoire et protohistoire*, ed. G. Mortelmans and J. Nenquin, 381–389. Tervuren: Musée Royal de l'Afrique Centrale Tervuren.
Hitchner, R. B. 2022. The historiography of North Africa in antiquity: An overview. In *A companion to North Africa in antiquity*, ed. R. B. Hitchner, 3–8. Wiley-Blackwell: Hoboken.
Horton, M. C. 1987. Early Muslim trading settlements on the East African coast: New evidence from Shanga. *Antiquaries Journal* 67:290–233.
Huffman, T. N. 1970. The Early Iron Age and the spread of the Bantu. *South African Archaeological Bulletin* 25 (97): 3–21.
Huffman, T. N. 1986. Iron Age settlement patterns and the origins of class distinction in southern Africa. In *Advances in world archaeology*, ed. F. Wendorf and E. Close, 291–338. New York: Academic.
Huffman, T.N., 2005. The stylistic origin of Bambata and the spread of mixed farming in southern Africa. Southern African Humanities, 17 (1), 57–79.
Huntingford, G. W. B. 1933. The Azanian civilization of Kenya. *Antiquity* 7:153–165.
Hurst, H. 1975. Excavations at Carthage 1974: First interim report. *Antiquaries Journal* 55 (1): 11–40.
Hussein, F., 1981. Dams, People, and Development: The aswan high dam case. New York: Pargamon Press.
Inskeep, R. R. 1961. The present state of archaeology in South Africa. *South African Museums Association Bulletin* 7:225–227.
Jemkur, J. 1986. Recent results of thermoluminescent (TL) tests on Nok Terracottas and sherds. *West African Journal of Archaeology* 16:165–168.
Johnston, H. 1919. *A comparative study of the Bantu and Semi-Bantu languages*. New York: AMS Press.
Jolly, P. 1996. Symbiotic interaction between black farmers and south-eastern San: Implications for southern African rock art studies, ethnographic analogy, and hunter-gatherer cultural identity. *Current Anthropology* 37 (2): 277–305.
Junod, S. M. 1963. A note on pottery from Tsodilo, Bechuanaland. *South African Archaeological Bulletin* 18 (69): 20.
Keenan, J. 2002. The lesser gods of the Sahara. *Public Archaeology* 2:131–150.
Kidane, Girma, and R. Wilding. 1977. *The Ethiopian cultural heritage*. Addis Ababa, Ethiopia: Ministry of Culture, Ethiopian Tourist Organisation and Institute for Ethiopian Studies.
King, R. 2015. 'A Loyal liking for fair play': Joseph Millerd Orpen and knowledge production in the Cape Colony. *South African Historical Journal* 67 (4): 410–432.
Kohl, P. L. 1998. Nationalism and archaeology: On the constructions of nations and the reconstructions of the remote past. *Annual Review of Anthropology* 27 (1): 223–246.

Kristiansen, K. 1993. 'The strength of the past and its great might': An essay on the use of the past. *Journal of European Archaeology* 1 (1): 3–32.
Lajoux, J.-D. 1963. *Merveilles du Tassili n'Ajjer*. London: Thames & Hudson.
Lane, P. J. 2004. The 'moving frontier' and the transition to food production in Kenya. *Azania: Archaeological Research in Africa* 39 (1): 243–264.
Lane, P. J. 2011. Possibilities for a postcolonial archaeology in sub-Saharan Africa: Indigenous and usable pasts. *World Archaeology* 43 (1): 7–25.
Lavachery, P., E. Cornelissen, J. Moeyersons, and P. De Maret. 1996. 30,000 ans d'occupation, 6 mois de fouilles: Shum Laka, un site exceptionnel en Afrique centrale. *Anthropologie et Préhistoire* 107:197–211.
Le Quellec, J.-L. 2002. Henri Lhote et le Lootori. *Cahiers de l'AARS* 7:141–156.
Leakey, L. S. B. 1935. *The Stone Age races of Kenya*. London: Oxford University Press.
Leakey, L. S. B. 1950. Part II: The crania. In *Excavations at the Njoro River Cave*, ed. M. D. Leakey, 41–73. Oxford: Clarendon Press.
Leakey, L. S. B., and M. D. Leakey. 1945. Notes on the skulls and skeletal remains from hyrax hill (Report on the excavations of Hyrax Hill, Nakuru, Kenya Colony, 1937–1938). *Transactions of the Royal Society of South Africa* 30:271–409.
Leakey, M. D., W. E. Owen, and L. S. B. Leakey. 1948. *Dimple-based pottery from Central Kavirondo, Kenya Colony*. Nairobi: Coryndon Memorial Museum Nairobi.
Lefkowitz, M. and Rogers, G.M., 1996. *Black Athena Revisited*. Chapel Hill: University of North Carolina Press.
Leone, M. 2009. Making historical archaeology postcolonial. In *International handbook of historical archaeology*, ed. T. Majewski and D. Gaimster, 159–168. London: Springer.
Lewis-Williams, J. D. 1972. The syntax and function of the Giant's castle rock paintings. *South African Archaeological Bulletin* 27:49–65.
Lewis-Williams, J. D. 1981. *Believing and seeing: Symbolic meaning in Southern San rock paintings*. London: Academic.
Lewis-Williams, J. D. 1984. The empiricist impasse in southern African rock art studies. *South African Archaeological Bulletin* 39 (139): 58–66.
Lewis-Williams, J. D. 2002. *Mind in the cave: Consciousness and the origins of art*. London: Thames & Hudson.
Lewis-Williams, J. D. 2006. The evolution of theory, method and technique in southern African rock art research. *Journal of Archaeological Method and Theory* 13 (4): 341–375.
Lewis-Williams, J. D., and T. A. Dowson. 1990. *Images of power: Understanding San Rock Art*. Cape Town: Struik.
Loubser, J. 1991. The ethnoarchaeology of Venda-speakers in South Africa. *Navorsinge van die Nasionale Museum (Bloemfontein)* 7:146–464.
Lucas, G. 2006. Archaeology at the edge. An archaeological dialogue with Martin Hall. *Archaeological Dialogues* 13 (1): 55–67.
Lwanga-Lunyiigo, S. 1976. The Bantu problem reconsidered. *Current Anthropology* 17 (2): 282–286.
MacDonald, K.C., 2003. Cheikh Anta Diop and *Ancient Egypt in Africa*. In: D. O'Connor and D.A.M. Anderson, eds. Ancient Egypt in Africa. London: UCL Press, 93 106.
Maggs, T. M. 1984. The Iron Age south of the Zambezi. In *Southern African prehistory and palaeoenvironments*, ed. R. G. Klein, 329–360. Rotterdam: A. A. Balkema.
Maley, J. 2004. Les variations de la végétation et des paléoenvironnements du domaine forestier africain au cours du Quaternaire récent. In *L'Évolution de la Végétation depuis deux Millions d'Années*, ed. A.-M. Sémah and J. Renault-Miskovsky, 143–178. Paris: Éditions Artcom'-Errance.
Maley, J., and P. Brenac. 1998. Vegetation dynamics, palaeoenvironments and climatic change in the forests of Western Cameroon during the last 28,000 years BP. *Review of Palaeobotany and Palynology* 99:157–187.

Matenga, E. 1998. *The soapstone birds of great Zimbabwe: Symbols of a nation*. Harare: African Publishing Group.

Mazama, A. 2001. The Afrocentric paradigm: Contours and definitions. *Journal of Black Studies* 31 (4): 387–405.

Mbida, C. M., W. Van Neer, H. Doutrelepont, and L. Vrydaghs. 2000. Evidence for banana cultivation and animal husbandry during the first millennium BC in the forest of southern Cameroon. *Journal of Archaeological Science* 27 (2): 151–162.

McBurney, C. B. M. 1947. The Stone Age of the Libyan littoral: The results of a war-time reconnaissance. *Proceedings of the Prehistoric Society* 13:56–84.

McBurney, C. B. M. 1967. *The Haua Fteah (Cyrenaica) and the Stone Age of the South-East Mediterranean*. Cambridge: Cambridge University Press.

McBurney, C. B. M. 1971. Libya before the Greeks. *Libyan Studies* 2 (1): 19–25.

McCall, G. S. 2007. Add shamans and stir? A critical review of the shamanism model of forager rock art production. *Journal of Anthropological Archaeology* 26 (2): 224–233.

McIntosh, R. J., and S. K. McIntosh. 1981. The Inland Niger Delta before the empire of Mali: Evidence from Jenné-jeno. *Journal of African History* 22:1–22.

McIntosh, S. K., and R. J. McIntosh. 1983. Current directions in West African prehistory. *Annual Review of Anthropology* 12:215–258.

Meinhof, C. 1912. *Die Sprachen der Hamiten*. Hamburg: L. Friederrichsen & Co.

Meister, C. 2007. Recent archaeological investigations in the tropical rain forest of southwest Cameroon. In *Dynamics of forest ecosystems in Central Africa during the Holocene: Past–present–future*, ed. J. Runge, 43–57. London: Taylor & Francis.

Mindzie, C. M., and L. Vrydaghs. 2020. Nkang: Early evidence for banana cultivation on the African continent. In *Encyclopedia of global archaeology*, ed. C. Smith, 7780–7782. Cham: Springer International Publishing.

Mitchell, P. J. 2005a. *African connections: An archaeological perspective on Africa and the wider world*. Oxford: AltaMira Press.

Mitchell, P. J. 2005b. Why hunter-gatherer archaeology matters: A personal perspective on renaissance and renewal in southern African Later Stone Age research. *South African Archaeological Bulletin* 60 (182): 64–71.

Möhlig, W. J. 1981. Stratification in the history of the Bantu languages. *Sprache und Geschichte in Afrika* 3:251–316.

Möhlig, W. J. 1989. Sprachgeschichte, kulturgeschichte und archäologie: Die kongruenz der forschungsergebnisse als methodologisches problem. *Paideuma* 35:189–196.

Mufuka, K. 1983. *Dzimbahwe: Life and politics in the Golden Age, 1100–1500*. Harare: Harare Publisher.

Munro-Hay, S. C. 1989. *Excavations at Aksum: An account of research at the ancient Ethiopian capital directed in 1972–74 by the late Dr Neville Chittick*. London: British Institute in Eastern Africa.

Munro-Hay, S. C. 1991. *Aksum: An African civilisation of late antiquity*. Edinburgh: Edinburgh University Press.

Murdock, G. P. 1959. *Africa: Its peoples and their culture history*. New York: McGraw-Hill.

Musonda, F. 1990. African archaeology: Looking forward. *African Archaeological Review* 8:3–22.

Mutwa, V. C. 1964. *Indaba, my children: African tribal history, legends, customs and religious beliefs*. Edinburgh: Canongate Books.

Nantambu, K. 1996. *Egypt and Afrocentric politics: Essays on European supremacy*. Kent: Imhotep Publishing Company.

Ndlovu-Gatsheni, S. J., and W. Willems. 2009. Making sense of cultural nationalism and the politics of commemoration under the Third Chimurenga in Zimbabwe. *Journal of Southern African Studies* 35 (4): 945–965.

Neumann, K. 2005. The romance of farming: Plant cultivation and domestication in Africa. In *African archaeology: A critical introduction*, ed. A. B. Stahl, 249–275. Oxford: Blackwell.

Neumann, K., K. Bostoen, A. Höhn, S. Kahlheber, A. Ngomanda, and B. Tchiengué. 2012. First farmers in the Central African rainforest: A view from southern Cameroon. *Quaternary International* 249:53–62.
North, J.A., 2003. Attributing colour to the ancient Egyptians: Reflections on Black Athena. In: D. O'Connor and D.A.M. Anderson, eds. *Ancient Egypt in Africa*. London: UCL Press, 31–38.
Nldovu-Gatsheni, S. 2012. Rethinking Chimurenga and Gukurahundi in Zimbabwe: A critique of partisan national history. *African Studies Review* 55:1–26.
Nyakatura, J. W. 1973. *Anatomy of an African kingdom: A history of Bunyoro-Kitara*. New York: Anchor Press-Doubleday.
Okafor, V. O. 1991. Diop and the African origin of civilization: An Afrocentric analysis. *Journal of Black Studies* 22:252–268.
Oliver, R. 1953. A questions about the Bacwezi. *Uganda Journal* 17:135–137.
Oliver, R. 1966. The problem of the Bantu expansion. *Journal of African History* 7:361–376.
Orpen, J. 1874. A glimpse into the mythology of the Maluti Bushmen. *Cape Monthly Magazine* 9:1–13.
Oslisly, R. 2006. Les traditions culturelles de l'Holocène sur le littoral du Cameroun entre Kribi et Campo. In *Grundlegungen: Beiträge zur europäischen und afrikanischen Archäologie für Manfred KH Eggert*, ed. H.-P. Wotzka, 303–317. Francke: Tübingen.
Pankhurst, R. 1999. Ethiopia, the Aksum obelisk, and the return of Africa's cultural heritage. *African Affairs* 98 (391): 229–239.
Parkington, J. E. 1980. Time and place: Some observations on spatial and temporal patterning in the later stone age sequence in southern Africa. *South African Archaeological Bulletin* 35:73–112.
Passarge, S. 1907. *Die Buschmanner der Kalahari*. Berlin: Dietrich Reimer, Ernst Vohsen.
Pearce, D. G. 2012. Ethnography and history: The significance of social change in interpreting rock art. In *Working with rock art: Recording, presenting and understanding rock art using indigenous knowledge*, ed. B. W. Smith, K. Helskog, and D. Morris, 135–145. Johannesburg: Wits University Press.
Phaladi, S. G. G. 1998. The organisation of archaeology. In *Ditswa Mmung: The archaeology of Botswana*, ed. P. J. Lane, A. Reid, and A. Segobye, 233–239. Gaborone: Pula Press and the Botswana Society.
Phillipson, D. W. 1976. Archaeology and Bantu linguistics. *World Archaeology* 8 (1): 65–82.
Phillipson, D. W. 2000. *Archaeology at Aksum, Ethiopia, 1993–7*. London: British Institute in Eastern Africa.
Phillipson, D. W. 2003. Aksum. *Azania: Archaeological Research in Africa* 38:1–68.
Phillipson, D. W. 2012. *Foundations of an African civilisation. Aksum and the northern horn 1000 BC-AD 1300*. Woodbridge: James Currey Ltd.
Plumb, J. H. 1969. *The death of the past*. London: MacMillan & Co.
Posnansky, M. 1961. Pottery types from archaeological sites in East Africa. *Journal of African History* 2 (2): 177–198.
Posnansky, M. 1966. Kingship, archaeology and historical myth. *Uganda Journal* 30:1–12.
Posnansky, M. 1967. The Iron Age in East Africa. In *Background to evolution in Africa*, ed. W. Bishop and J. D. Clark, 629–649. Chicago: Chicago University Press.
Posnansky, M. 1969. *Bigo bya Mugenyi. Uganda Journal* 33:125–150.
Posnansky, M. 1982. African archaeology comes of age. *World Archaeology* 13:345–358.
Posnansky, M. 1984. Early agricultural societies in Ghana. In *From hunters to farmers: The causes and consequences of food production in Africa*, ed. J. D. Clark and S. Brandt, 147–151. Berkley: University of California Press.
Posnansky, M. 1996. Coping with collapse in the 1990. In *Plundering Africa's Past*, ed. P. R. Schmidt and R. J. McIntosh, 143–163. Bloomington: Indiana University Press.
Pratt, M.-L. 1992. *Imperial eyes: Travel writing and transculturation*. London: Routledge.
Quinn, J. 2003. Roman Africa? *Digressus Supplement: Romanization?* 1:7–34.
Reid, A., 1991. The role of cattle in the later Iron Age communities of southern Uganda. PhD thesis, University of Cambridge, Cambridge.

Renfrew, C., and P. Bahn. 2020. *Archaeologies: Theories, methods, and practice*. 8th ed. New York: Thames & Hudson.

Robbins, L. H. 1993. The future of African archaeology: Anthropological archaeology. *African Archaeological Review* 13:21–23.

Robertshaw, P. 1990. The development of archaeology in East Africa. In *A history of African archaeology*, ed. P. Robertshaw, 78–94. Oxford: James Currey Ltd.

Robertshaw, P. 1994. Archaeological survey, ceramic analysis, and state formation in western Uganda. *The African Archaeological Review* 12 (1): 105–131.

Robertshaw, P. 1996. Knowledge and power. *African Archaeological Review* 13:7–9.

Robertshaw, P. 1997. Munsa earthworks: A preliminary report on recent excavations. *Azania: Archaeological Research in Africa* 32 (1): 1–20.

Robertshaw, P. 2000. Sibling rivalry? The intersection of archaeology and history. *History in Africa* 27:261–286.

Robertshaw, P. 2002. The ancient earthworks of western Uganda: Capital sites of a Cwezi empire? *Uganda Journal* 48:17–32.

Robertshaw, P. 2003. Explaining the origins of the state in East Africa. In *East African archaeology: Foragers, potters, smiths and traders*, ed. C. M. Kusimba and S. B. Kusimba, 149–166. Philadelphia: University of Philadelphia Press.

Robertshaw, P. 2010. Beyond the segmentary state: Creative and instrumental power in western Uganda. *Journal of World Prehistory* 23:255–269.

Robertshaw, P., and D. Taylor. 2000. Climate change and the rise of political complexity in western Uganda. *Journal of African History* 41 (1): 1–28.

Rudner, I. 1965. Archaeological report on the Tsodilo Hills, Bechuanaland. *South African Archaeological Bulletin* 20 (78): 51–70.

Säve-Söderberg, T., 1987. Temples and Tombs of Ancient Nubia. London: Thames & Hudson.

Scarcelli, N., P. Cubry, R. Akakpo, A.-C. Thuillet, J. Obidiegwu, M. N. Baco, E. Otoo, B. Sonké, A. Dansi, G. Djedatin, C. Mariac, M. Couderc, S. Causse, K. Alix, H. Chaïr, O. François, and Y. Vigouroux. 2019. Yam genomics supports West Africa as a major cradle of crop domestication. *Science Advances* 5 (5): eaaw1947.

Scerri, E. 2017. The Stone Age archaeology of West Africa. In *Oxford research encyclopedia of African history*, ed. T. Spear. Oxford: Oxford University Press. https://ora.ox.ac.uk/objects/uuid:1442d1c1-7f76-454d-97db-8fd52a4c6c1e

Schmidt, P. R. 1990. Oral traditions, archaeology and history: A short reflective history. *A History of African Archaeology* 1990:252–270.

Schmidt, P. R. 2009. *Postcolonial archaeologies in Africa*. Santa Fe: School for Advanced Research Press.

Schmidt, P. R. 2014. Deconstructing archaeologies of African colonialism: Making and unmaking the subaltern. In *Rethinking colonial pasts through archaeology*, ed. N. Ferris, R. Harrison, and M. V. Wilcox, 445–465. Oxford: Oxford University Press.

Schwartz, D. 1992. Assèchement climatique vers 3.000bp et expansion Bantu en Afrique centrale atlantique: quelques réfl exions. *Bulletin de la Société Géologique de France* 163:353–361.

Segobye, A. 2005. The revolution will be televised: African archaeology education and the challenge of public archaeology—Some examples from southern Africa. *Archaeologies* 1:33–45.

Selden, D. 2013. How the Ethiopian changed his skin. *Classical Antiquity* 32 (2): 322–377.

Senghor, L. S. 1964. *On African socialism*. New York: Frederick A. Praeger.

Shaw, T. 1963. Field research in Nigerian archaeology: A brief survey and discussion of policy. *Journal of the Historical Society of Nigeria* 2 (4): 449–464.

Shaw, T. 1967. *West African archaeological newsletter*, 9–43. Institute of African Studies, University of Ibadan.

Shaw, T. 1968. Radiocarbon dating in Nigeria. *Journal of the Historical Society of Nigeria* 4 (3): 453–465.

Shaw, T. 1977. Hunters, gatherers and first farmers in West Africa. In *Hunters, gatherers and first farmers beyond Europe*, ed. J. V. S. Megaw, 69–125. Leicester: Leicester University Press.

Shaw, T. 1981. The Nok sculptures of Nigeria. *Scientific American* 244 (2): 154–167.

Shaw, T. 1989. African archaeology: Looking back and looking forward. *African Archaeological Review* 7 (1): 3–31.

Shepherd, N. 2002. The politics of archaeology in Africa. *Annual Review of Anthropology* 31:189–209.

Shepherd, N. 2003. State of the discipline: Science, culture and identity in South African archaeology, 1870–2003. *Journal of Southern African Studies* 29 (4): 823–844.

Shinnie, P. 1960. Excavations at Bigo 1957. *Uganda Journal* 24:16–29.

Skotnes, P. 1994. The visual as a site of meaning: San parietal painting and the experience of modern art. In *Contested images: Diversity in southern African rock art research*, ed. T. A. Dowson and J. D. Lewis-Williams, 315–329. Johannesburg: Witwatersrand University Press.

Smith, I. 1997. *Bitter harvest: The great betrayal*. London: Blake Publishing.

Soleilhavoup, F. 1978. *Les Oeuvres Rupestres Sahariennes Sont-Elles Menacées? Algiers: L'Office du Park national du Tassili*. Algiers: UNESCO.

Solomon, A. 1998. Ethnography and method in southern African rock art research. In *The archaeology of rock art*, ed. P. S. C. Taçon and C. Chippindale, 268–284. Cambridge: Cambridge University Press.

Solomon, A. 2006. Roots and revolutions: A critical overview of early and late San rock art research. *Afrique & Histoire* 6 (2): 77–110.

Solomon, A. 2008. Myths, making, and consciousness differences and dynamics in San rock arts. *Current Anthropology* 49:59–86.

Soper, R. 1971. A general review of the Early Iron Age of the southern half of Africa. *Azania: Archaeological Research in Africa* 6:5–38.

Stahl, A. B. 1985. Reinvestigation of Kintampo 6 rock shelter, Ghana: Implications for the nature of culture change. *African Archaeological Review* 3:117–150.

Stahl, A. B. 1999. Perceiving variability in time and space: The evolutionary mapping of African societies. In *Beyond chiefdoms: Pathways to complexity in Africa*, ed. S. K. McIntosh, 39–55. Cambridge: Cambridge University Press.

Steyn, H. C. 2003. Where New Age and African religion meet in South Africa: The case of credo mutwa. *Culture and Religion* 4 (1): 67–158.

Sutton, J. E. 1993. The antecedents of the interlacustrine kingdoms. *Journal of African History* 34 (1): 33–64.

Thondhlana, T. P., S. S. Chitima, and S. Chirikure. 2021. Nation branding in Zimbabwe: Archaeological heritage, national cohesion, and corporate identities. *Journal of Social Archaeology* 21:283–305.

Thornton, R. J. 1983. "This dying out race" W.H.I. Bleek's approach to the languages of southern Africa. *Social Dynamics* 9 (2): 1–10.

Tobias, P. V. 1985. The life and times of Emeritus Professor Raymond A. Dart. *South African Medical Journal* 67 (4): 134–138.

Trigger, B. G. 1990. The history of African archaeology in world perspective. In *A history of African archaeology*, ed. P. Robertshaw, 303–319. Oxford: James Currey Ltd.

Trigger, B. G. 2006. *A history of archaeological thought*. 2nd ed. Cambridge: Cambridge University Press.

Van Der Beken, C. 2007. Ethiopia: Constitutional protection of ethnic minorities at the regional level. *Afrika Focus* 20:105–151.

van der Post, L. 1958. *The lost world of the Kalahari*. Harmondsworth: Penguin.

Vansina, J. 1979. Bantu in the crystal ball, I. *History in Africa* 6:287–333.

Vansina, J. 1980. Bantu in the crystal ball, II. *History in Africa* 7:293–325.

Vansina, J. 1995. New linguistic evidence and 'The Bantu Expansion'. *Journal of African History* 36:173–195.

Vansina, J. 2003. Bananas in Cameroun c. 500 BCE? Not proven. *Azania: Archaeological Research in Africa* 28:174–716.

Vinnicombe, P. 1967. The recording of rock paintings: An interim report. *South African Journal of Science* 63 (7): 282.

Vinnicombe, P. 1976. *People of the Eland: Rock paintings of the Drakensberg Bushmen as a reflection of their life and thought*. Johannesburg: Wits University Press.

Watkins, M. H. 1956. Review of trade and politics in the Niger Delta, 1830–1885. *Journal of Negro History* 41 (3): 260–263.

Watson, D. J. 2005. Under the rocks: Reconsidering the origin of the Kintampo tradition and the development of food production in the savanna-forest/forest of West Africa. *Journal of African Archaeology* 3:3–25.

Watson, D. J. 2010. Within savanna and forest: A review of the Late Stone Age Kintampo tradition, Ghana. *Azania: Archaeological Research in Africa* 45:141–174.

Wells, C. M. 1982. Recent excavations at Carthage: A review article. *American Journal of Archaeology* 86 (2): 293–296.

Wendorf, F. 1992. The impact of radiocarbon dating on North African archaeology. In *Radiocarbon after four decades*, ed. R. E. Taylor, A. Long, and R. S. Kra, 310–323. New York: Springer New York.

Westermann, D. 1939. The study of African languages: Present results and future needs. *Africa* 12 (1): 12–26.

Westermann, D. 1952. African linguistic classification. *Africa* 22 (3): 250–256.

Westermann, D. D. 1911. *Die Sudansprachen: Eine sprachvergleichende studie*. Hamburg: L. Friederrichsen & Co.

Wrigley, C. C. 1958. Some thoughts on the Bacwezi. *Uganda Journal* 22:11–17.

Chapter 7
Archaeology's Diaspora Across Africa

Abstract Covering the late twentieth century CE and the democratic wave, this chapter describes a dispersed yet increasingly networked field. It surveys how archaeology proliferated across universities, NGOs, CRM firms, and museums; how new laboratories and dating facilities broadened archaeological datasets; and how digital catalogues, GIS, and remote sensing altered scales of analysis. The chapter tracks shifting thematic emphases, from hunter-gatherer societies and pastoralism to Indian Ocean worlds, Sahelian urbanisms, Saharan connectivity, and rainforest lifeways. The chapter also examines policy and politics at the millennium's turn: heritage laws, restitution debates, illicit trafficking, and the public life of archaeology in new democracies. It argues that "diaspora" captures both spread and hybridity: African archaeology now circulates through multiple institutions and publics, generating new alliances and frictions that redefine expertise, ethics, and impact.

The 3000 kilometre coastal region spanning from Mogadishu in southern Somalia to Ilha de Moçambique in northern Mozambique includes four mainland countries – Somalia, Kenya, Tanzania, and Mozambique – as well as the island nations of the Comoros, Madagascar and Seychelles (Fig. 7.1). While it would be a mistake to see this vast area as culturally, economically, or politically uniform – its internal diversity, layered histories, and varying expressions of agency are significant – certain common features recur across the region. Chief among these is its long-standing connection to distant lands through Indian Ocean trade, which dates back to the mid-first millennium CE. In the second millennium, towns emerged that were typically built in stone or coral, with coral construction being a distinctive regional practice. The spread of Islam also left a deep imprint, visible in mosques, tombs, and inscriptions that speak both to the integration of Islamic values and to the presence of Muslim communities. This interconnected cultural and historical landscape is often referred to as the Swahili world (Wynne-Jones and LaViolette 2018).

The Swahili coast is linked by a network of urban centres, ports, and trading hubs, many of which are still inhabited, that emerged and flourished from the late

T. Forssman, *Archaeology in Africa: Why the Past Matters*, Archaeology of Africa,
https://doi.org/10.1007/978-3-032-13365-6_7

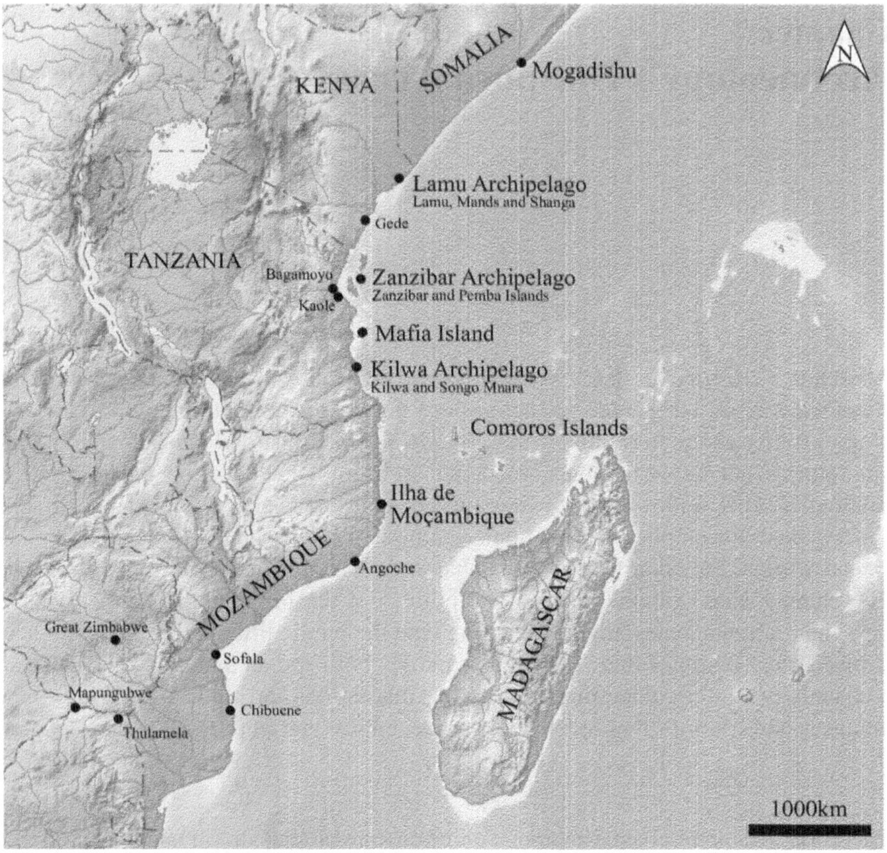

Fig. 7.1 The Swahili coast and important sites shown and the six countries listed in the text marked (modified from Wynne-Jones and LaViolette 2018: p. xxii)

first century CE (Wynne-Jones 2007). The Swahili littoral includes several well-known sites, such as Lamu, Gede, Manda, and Shanga in Kenya; Ilha de Moçambique and Angoche in Mozambique; and in Tanzania, Zanzibar's Stone Town, Pemba Island, Bagamoyo, Kaole, Songo Mnara, and Kilwa. These reflect a deeply connected trade system and a rich tapestry of Islamic and African traditions, spanning multiple chronologies from the precolonial through to the contemporary period that includes Islamic, Portuguese Omani, Yemen, and British influences during different periods (Brielle et al. 2023: p. 867). Among them, the longest history of research is at Kilwa, an island within an inlet 33 km long and 26 km wide. West of Kilwa, rivers merge to form an estuary with mangroves, mudflats, and river channels, whereas on the eastern, ocean-exposed side are wave-cut coral limestone cliffs (Pollard et al. 2025: p. 8). By the fourteenth century CE, Kilwa was the most powerful city in the Swahili world, playing a dominant role in coastal trade and serving as a gateway to interior networks in southern Africa. Its Great Mosque is the oldest mosque in East Africa, being built

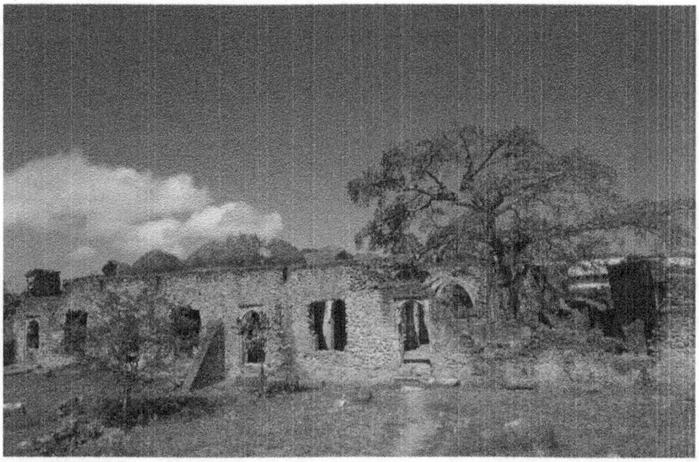

Fig. 7.2 The great mosque at Kilwa Kisiwani (photograph: CosiMapi). *Source* https://commons.wikimedia.org/wiki/File:Kilwa-Kisiwani-ruins-tanzania.jpg)

first in the twelfth century CE (Horton 2017), with large extensions added between 1200 and 1290, including vaulted or domed roofing (Fig. 7.2) (Horton et al. 2022; Purdy 2024). The town was visited by Ibn Battuta (Dunn 2012), who commented on the trade taking place through Kilwa, and noted the exchange of cultural and artistic items (Purdy 2024: p. 659). Later Portuguese accounts compared Kilwa to a Spanish town with high buildings (Fig. 7.3), mentioning rich merchants, gold, silver, amber, musk and pearls (or beads), and describing the people as adorned in fine cotton and silk among other accoutrements (Grenlee 1938: cf. Purdy 2024). Also in the Kilwa Archipelago are Songo Mnara to the south and Sanja ya Kati to the west (Pollard 2008a). The medieval towns on these islands were likely connected through broader spatial and social networks between not only themselves but the mainland as well (Pollard et al. 2012).

Perhaps Kilwa is best known as a trading centre. From the eleventh to sixteenth centuries CE, trading activities, facilitated by monsoon winds that reverse direction twice a cycle (Datoo 1974), boomed (Ichumbaki and Pollard 2019). Control of the extensive Indian Ocean trading network was largely orchestrated by those ruling at Kilwa. Gold from the Zimbabwe Plateau was brought to Kilwa via land links to Sofala (Chirikure 2014), and then north by seafaring traders (Horton and Middleton 2000: p. 101). By the late thirteenth century CE, or soon after, Kilwa had secured a trade monopoly (Chittick 1974: pp. 239–240), leading to further growth within the town and in the surrounding hinterland (Wynne-Jones 2005: p. 116). Housing reflected socio-economic differentiation, with the sultan's palace at Husuni Kubwa the pinnacle. Stone built, wooden private, wattle-and-daub and grass-on-wood-frame houses were erected to home people depending on their status and economic position (Wynne-Jones 2007: p. 368). Peoples' consumption patterns further demonstrate this stratification (Kirkman 1966: p. 24). Higher status dwellings include glazed wares in

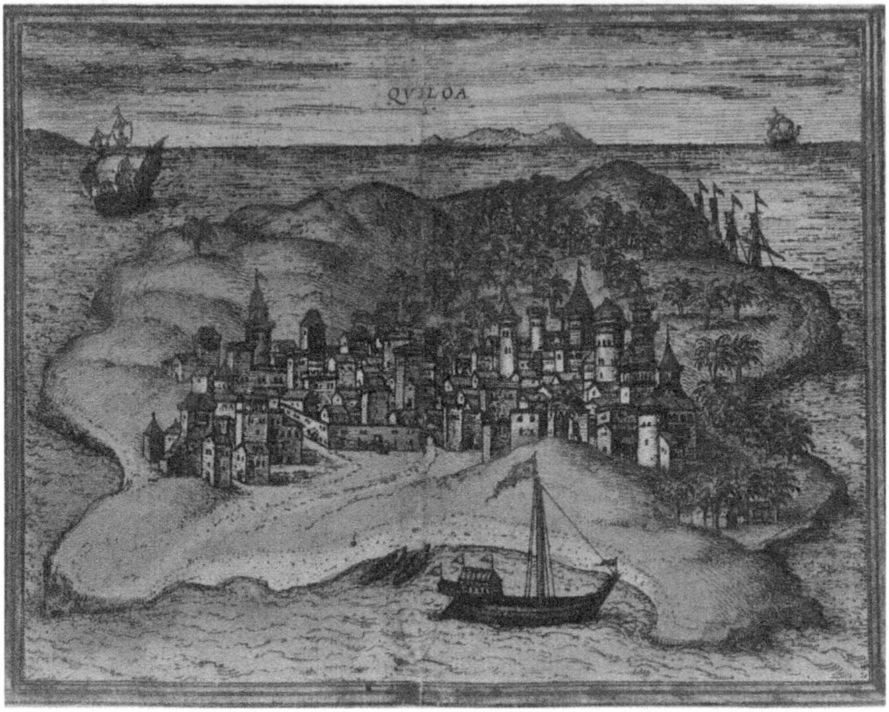

Fig. 7.3 A bird's-eye view of Quiloa (Kilwa) by George Braun, 1572. *Source* https://commons.wikimedia.org/wiki/File:City_of_Kilwa,_1572.jpg.

their confines, and these individuals or families are likely those to have been adorned in various items and fine cloth (Pollard 2008b: p. 266).

Kilwa was first excavated in the 1950s, before Tanzanian independence (1961 for the mainland and 1964 for Zanzibar), when narratives of African development were still deeply tied to external influence (Holl 1990; Robertshaw 1990: p. 84). Neville Chittick's (1974) early excavations interpreted the site as initially occupied by marine fishing communities in the late first millennium CE, followed by a period of abandonment. He proposed that Shirazi Persian settlers later colonised the island, establishing Kilwa's stone town, which was then taken over by the Mahdali Dynasty in the thirteenth century. Chittick's (1974) four-phase model aligned with mid-century views that positioned foreign influence as the driver of African advancement.

From the 1980s, however, scholars increasingly challenged this framework. Archaeologists argued for the indigenous development of Swahili stone towns (Horton 1984, 1996; Abungu 1989; Chami 1994), and recognised that Kilwa's growth was embedded in a much longer, 1500-year sequence predating Muslim and European involvement (Chami 1998). Felix Chami's (2006) later excavations revealed inland ceramic connections, indicating longstanding regional ties. Earlier dynastic histories are now understood as political myths emphasised to legitimise rule (Wynne-Jones 2007: p. 370), and greater attention has been paid to oral traditions and cultural analogies (Allen 1981, 1993; Nurse and Spear 1985). This shift brought greater focus on African agency but also introduced a hesitancy to acknowledge the complexity of local and foreign interactions. As Stephanie Wynne-Jones (2007, p. 371) noted, Swahili towns are now seen as African in origin; although shaped by Arabic influence, they are rooted in local society.

Over time, archaeological interest expanded beyond monumental ruins and elite narratives, which had dominated earlier work by Chittick (1965, 1974) and Peter Garlake (1966, p. 19). Recent research examines subsistence strategies, economic practices, and the lives of non-elite groups (Horton and Middleton 2000; Breen and Lane 2004; Wynne-Jones 2007). Studies of mainland communities across from Kilwa, for instance, highlight their interdependence with island populations (Wynne-Jones 2018: p. 258). New techniques in archaeological science have enhanced interpretations, such as high-resolution dating using Bayesian models to refine Kilwa's occupational sequence (Horton et al. 2022), while numismatic studies, once central, are approached with caution due to issues of mixing and reuse (Purdy 2024). Material culture, including symbolic forms linked to social status, has received more interpretative attention, aided by collaborations with local scholars and student training (Sutton 2018). The development of DNA studies has also aided in tracing intercontinental connections. Recently, 80 individuals were sampled from six towns spanning the medieval period until the recent past (1250–1800 CE) that demonstrated increasing inter-mixing of African and Asian populations, mostly Persian and Indian, from 1000 CE when Islam was more widely adopted. By 1500 CE, Asian ancestry was mainly Persian, consistent with the oldest history local reported, the Kilwa Chronicle (Brielle et al. 2023).

The archaeology of the Swahili world encapsulates many of the broader transformations that have defined African archaeology since the 1980s. It reflects a decisive move away from earlier, colonial-era frameworks that prioritised elite narratives and monumental architecture, towards more inclusive approaches that foreground everyday lives, inland–coastal interactions, and local agency. The Swahili case is particularly instructive because it demonstrates how African societies were not passive recipients of external influence but actively shaped their own histories in dialogue with wider Indian Ocean networks. These shifts mirror wider disciplinary trends: archaeologists increasingly challenged diffusionist models, explored indigenous histories with greater confidence, and integrated oral traditions, local histories, and collaborations with descendant communities into their interpretations. Methodologically, Swahili archaeology exemplifies how archaeological science has enriched African studies, from high-resolution dating and material sourcing to advanced remote sensing techniques like LiDAR and drone surveys. Importantly, research has extended beyond national borders, recognising the transregional dynamics of trade and culture, and embracing collaborative, often international, scholarship. In this sense, the Swahili World is not only a case study of a vibrant coastal civilisation, but a lens through which to view the evolution of African archaeology itself:

its methodological maturation, its critical engagement with history, and its growing integration into global archaeological conversations.

7.1 Archaeology at the End of the Millennium

In 2006, South African President Thabo Mbeki spoke of an "African naissance" and envisioned the third millennium as "Africa's millennium," a time of renewed optimism across the continent (Maggs 2000). By then, colonialism had formally ended, and even the last strongholds of white minority rule – Namibia, Zimbabwe, and South Africa – had transitioned to democracy. Despite this, archaeology continued to reflect many of its earlier patterns. A significant proportion of archaeologists working in Africa were still based at institutions abroad. Operating from a distance, it was easy for the nuances, rhythms, and lived experiences of African communities to become muted. Research agendas were often shaped by priorities rooted in the scholars' home institutions, priorities that were then brought to the continent through large, externally funded teams. As a result, many projects pursued questions generated in European or North American academic settings (Pikirayi 2015: p. 3), rather than arising from local histories, interests, or collaborations. John Giblin (2013: p. 260) put this into perspective quite bluntly: "African archaeology in the postcolonial era typically remained an elite, white endeavour in which foreign academics with their own interests continued to appropriate the past, largely for the benefit of a non-indigenous audience".

The pessimism expressed in Giblin's (2013) quote, to a large extent, had its roots in the 1970s and 1980s. Nicholas David (1983: p. 2), as editor of the *African Archaeological Review*, in the first pages to ever be printed in the journal, commented that archaeology in Africa was "in a state of regression, unduly affected by the political and economic problems of the continent". Ray Inskeep's (1961) comments in the late 1960s about the decline in South African archaeology once again come to mind as they also related to governance and identity building, although in this case involving the National Party and apartheid regime. However, from the 1970s, African countries were grappling with pressing issues, such as decoupling from the colonial vice, legitimising new identities and leadership regimes, coming to terms with managing foreign nations and created communities, and stemming the upsurge of corruption and governance issues that began to pervade administrations (Ebegbulem 2012; Mlambo et al. 2023). Archaeology was seen as a luxury discipline that obtains useful results but at great financial cost (David 1983; Shaw 1989). The economic climate hindered archaeological research, affecting the availability of funding but also university courses, training, conference attendance, publications and the conservation of collections. However, while the difficulties and challenges were numerous, growth was to come from the 1980s and increasingly more due to the influence of the Cold War when archaeological projects entwined with geopolitics (Luke and Meskell 2023).

Publications are a useful measure of growth, although not without their own problems. Cameron Gokee and Akin Ogundiran (2023: p. 3) showed that in the *African Archaeological Review* there has been an increase in publications since its establishment in 1983. In their first five years, 57 publications went to print, followed by a few declining intervals, but overall a strong increase to 203 between 2018 and 2022. Peter Mitchell and Jakub Seneši (2023) examined publications in the *South African Archaeological Bulletin* from 1980 to 2019 and noted consistency in the number of papers published per decade before 2010 (135.5/decade), which then rose to 168 in the decade that followed. Mitchell et al. (2024) also looked at publications in the *Journal of Archaeological Science* and found an increase in papers on African archaeology from about 1982, but with a large proportion from Egypt and South Africa. From a macro-perspective, these findings suggest that archaeological research remained at least steady throughout this period, but on the whole seem to have grown, despite the aspersions made by David (1983) and others. This of course does not cast doubt or delegitimise the negative perspectives and more than likely shows that archaeology, as David (1983) further noted, was being driven by motivated individuals in spite of the difficult context they operated within.

Archaeology's character was being challenged and reshaped from the 1980s. Post-processualism contested the foundational tenets of processualim, influencing the aims, goals, and aspirations of archaeological research. In Africa, archaeology's character was also upended, partly following the emerging North American frameworks but also responding to local contexts (Ashley et al. 2016). In East Africa, for example, an emphasis on historical sources gave way from 1980 to greater importance placed on archaeological remains that would provide independent evidence for written and oral accounts (Abungu 1989; Kusimba 1999). Studies sought to investigate subsistence and economic patterns (Horton and Mudida 1993; Kusimba 1993; Wynne-Jones 2007), religious and social transformations (Horton 1996), human-environment impacts (Breen and Lane 2004), and pre-cursors to the Swahili world (LaViolette et al. 1989, 1999; Kessy 1997; Chami 1998; Helm 2000). Notably, as described above, emphasis on African origins in the Swahili world became a focal point, whether archaeological or linguistic in nature (Nurse and Hinnebusch 1993; Chami 1998). The field shifted temporally as well as topically; recent pasts became the focus along with material studies and culture-making processes (Stahl 2009: p. 244). Archaeologists began to consider how material remains provided insights into identities and social histories. It is no straightforward correlation (see Carr and Neitzel, 1995; Conkey and Hastorf, 1990; David et al., 1991; Hegmon, 1992, 1998; Hodder, 1982; MacEachern, 1998; Shennan, 1989).

It was recognised that identity is not an entity but rather a process, and these are materialised in archaeological assemblages (Gosselain 2000). The growing emphasis in African archaeology, and archaeology generally, on this process led to studies into gender, class division and enclaves, domination versus resistance, social relations and contact, and migration. However, the materials to study these are often unconvincing, low in frequency, discrete, or mundane, rather than the conspicuous finds or categories that tend to dominate material analyses. This is partly so because the incorporation of social traits into material items is not necessarily a conscious process. Additionally, things may have multiple meanings influenced by their own social lives that have distinct strategies and networks (Appadurai 1986; Hoskins 1998; Gosden and Marshall 1999). Not only is finding these histories a great challenge in the archaeological record, but they accumulate to tell multiple stories and histories about people (Leroi-Gourhain 1965; Tixier 1967): meaning and materials combine to form palimpsests. Olivier Gosselain's (1995, 1998) examination of ceramic production in Cameroon illustrates this. He found multiple layers of group identifications within the chain of operations. Processing clay was distinct within a specific community, whereas vessel fashioning was conducted in the same manner as a larger community, and an even larger group produced the same motifs and ornamental tools. Each of these layers is expressed variably in the final product, of which an archaeologist might see only a fraction. Whether such an approach reflects regular patterns, differences between people, artefacts or even single artefact categories, is debatable, along with the resolution of these social lives that we can reliably read from the artefacts (Gosselain 2000).

A sentiment that appeared in the 1980s was Africa's ethnographic value. John Atherton (1983) referred to this as 'living archaeology'. He was particularly enthusiastic about the lack of western influence found among many groups on the continent, and hoped to "preserve an enormous amount of data pertinent to traditional material culture" (Atherton 1983: p. 93). However, not all scholars were as enchanted by ethnographic potential. David Phillipson (1989) expressed grave concern in the potential of such approaches in creating timelessness among indigenous communities and ignoring major social changes that have taken place in the past. He proposed banishing the ethnographic present as misleading. Kofi Agorsah (1990) pessimistically referred to Africa as the testing ground for ethnoarchaeological ideas that were produced elsewhere. Like Phillipson (1989), Agorsah (1990) expressed concern that ethnography would ignore the "fluidity and multidimensionality" of human societies.

These developments point to a discipline in transformation. While challenges persisted, especially around equity, authorship, and access, archaeology in Africa increasingly embraced collaborative, locally rooted, and methodologically diverse approaches. The growth of African-led institutions and centres (Shepherd 2002; Ashley and Bouakaze-Khan 2011; Thondhlana et al. 2022), the expansion of community archaeology (Chirikure and Pwiti 2008; Posnansky 2017; Schmidt and Arthur 2018), and the integration of new technologies reshaped the field (Rüther and Palumbo 2012; Campana 2017; Davis and Douglass 2020; Lombard et al. 2020). At the same time, calls for decolonisation continued to urge archaeologists to rethink not only what they study, but how and for whom. As the discipline moved forward, it must remain attuned to the multiplicity of African pasts, and the people whose lives those pasts continue to shape.

7.1.1 Southern Africa

> As South Africa changes, its history is being reviewed. Old emphases are giving way to new interests. Old explanations and evaluations of the past are being questioned. Old stereotypes of indigenous people and, indeed, of the whole sweep of African history are being challenged as a new history is constructed. The nature of this new southern African history implicates archaeology; it also poses a fundamental question: What is archaeology? (Lewis-Williams 1993: 45)

Although writing in a paper about South African archaeology nearing the end of apartheid, David Lewis-Williams (1993) aptly summed up two fundamental challenges that faced archaeology at this juncture across Africa. The continent was well into a phase of rewriting history and revaluating accepted narratives that dominated political and social discourse. While this did not take place at the same time in each of Africa's countries, South Africa, for example, witnessed this more generally only in the 1990s when apartheid ended, its character was largely the same: archaeology had the ability to redress the garbs draped over the continent's history and people. With this in mind, Lewis-Williams (1993) proposed another challenge: defining archaeology. Though, was this really necessary? Archaeology was advancing but even in post-colonial contexts it was serving the same goal – using the past in the present to suit agendas, frameworks, and politics.

At 1983's meeting of the Southern African Association of Archaeologists in Gaborone, Botswana, delegates from Mozambique tabled a motion requesting the association to condemn apartheid and the discrimination taking place in South Africa. Most archaeologists were not actively involved in politics, and many opposed the country's racial policies. The motion was not put to vote. In protest, Mozambiquen and Zimbabwean archaeologists resigned from the association (Hall 1990). Two years later at the same organisation's meeting in Grahamstown, South Africa, news arrived that the South African and Namibian archaeologists were banned from the 1986 World Archaeological Congress in Southampton (Ucko 1990). The banning came while the country was in a state of emergency and battling to resist the majority of the population's protest to apartheid laws, combining to weaken the local currency. Mitchell (2005b: p. 64) commented that the discussions between archaeologists inside the halls of the conference intersected with the political developments outside. Notably, he referred to Lewis-Williams' call to introduce social theory into archaeology, who described much of the work that was being carried out as 'technicist' with an over-emphasis on subsistence economies and typologies. He argued, instead, for historical materialism, suggesting that it would transform southern African archaeology into social enquiry. Taking up the call fairly soon after Lewis-Williams' comments was Lyn Wadley (1987) and Aron Mazel (1989) who applied a historical materialist approach to understanding their finds, notably settlement patterns (aggregations and dispersal camps, and gift-giving), and social groupings and relations (using stone scrapers among other features), respectively. These studies began a shift in Later Stone Age archaeology, and more generally, from a 'people-to-nature' approach to one of 'people-to-people' (Mazel 1987). Deeply intertwined in this social shift was the Kalahari Debate, which became one of the key debates to have taken place from the 1980s in southern Africa with ramifications around the world (Sylvain 2015; Forssman 2022).

The Kalahari Debate's roots press back into the 1950s, at least, but it began quietly in 1978 (Wilmsen 1978) and then escalated in the 1980s (Wilmsen 1989a; Solway and Lee 1990; Wilmsen and Denbow 1990; Lee and Guenther 1991). Come the mid-1990s, battle-worn archaeologists and anthropologists gyrated around agreement and found little ground in common (Kent 1992; Barnard 2007). Frustrated with the outcome of the debate, some wrote of their willingness to seek consul outside of the field for assistance (Lee and Guenther 1995). From then, the debate fractured with irregular although sterling contributions and studies moving broadly apart from one another (Sadr 1997; Wilmsen 2002; Sylvain 2015). The debate was taken from the desert to the mountains and into river valleys where its various tenets were considered against archaeological and anthropological datasets (Mitchell et al. 2008; Forssman 2022). It was also interestingly positioned at the intersection of colonial and post-colonial contexts, which in the case of Namibia and South Africa included oppressive government regimes, as well as a shift in archaeological schools of thought. Much of the debate, therefore, reflected contemporary ideologies and approaches to examining the present and using it to understand the past.

The wide-ranging Kalahari Debate addressed issues relating to identity, history and status. It drew on the discord between the way San groups were being portrayed in the Kalahari region of Botswana and the information gathered at archaeological sites. The Kalahari School of Ethnographers had, from the 1950s until the 1970s, spent a considerable amount of time living among ! Kung groups in Botswana's Dobe, Nyae Nyae, Ghanzi, Kalahari and Boteti regions (Lee 1979; Tanaka 1980; Silberbauer 1981). The decision to study these groups was partly motivated by the notion that such people provided reliable taxa for Stone Age, 'early man' lifeways (Murdock 1968; Morgan 1982 [1877]). Richard Lee's initial descriptions of the San were angled with this in mind: they were "taken to imply a state of isolation and 'original affluence' nowadays almost unique in the world" (Barnard 1990: p. 122). Elsewhere he said that they "represent the original condition of humankind (and)… a basic human adaptation" (Leacock and Lee 1982: p. 5). As such, Kalahari Bushmen became archetypes (Lee and DeVore 1968) that preserved long-lost human ways of living and being. These notions would persist for three decades in archaeological, anthropological and historical fields (e.g., Sahlins 1972; Wadley 1987; Haviland 1990; Van Doornum 2005; Pearce 2012). Summarised briefly, the image that was formed of the San was that they were a peaceful, egalitarian society that were highly mobile, lived in kin groups, made decisions collectively, and subsisted by hunting and gathering (Thomas 1959; Lee and DeVore 1968; Silberbauer 1981; Cashdan 1984). Central to their identity was their way of living, which integrated multiple survival strategies (Hitchcock 2012).

Primarily in the 1980s, a revisionist perspective emerged. Archaeologists and other scholars queried the autochthony of San groups using historical and archaeological evidence collected at sites in Botswana. Most classically is a single, but now lost, cow (*Bos taurus*) tooth found at a San camp at /Xai /Xai that signalled far longer interactions with farmer groups than had been recognised (Wilmsen 1989b). Revisionists instead argued for a long period of social interactions between largely disparate groups that resulted in the appearance of contemporary San society (Parkington 1984; Schrire 1984a; Wilmsen 1989a, 2003; Wilmsen and Denbow 1990). In this social network, Ed Wilmsen (1989a: p. 3) argued that the San's "appearance as foragers is a function of their relegation to an underclass". Robert Gordon (1992: p. 6) echoed these sentiments arguing that the terms used for these groups, such as hunter-gatherer, were sociopolitical, which Carmel Schrire (1980, 1984b) interpreted as failed pastoralism. For example, prior to the rinderpest epidemic in the nineteenth century CE, many San groups owned livestock (Wilmsen 1997) and oral history also indicated the possession of domestic stock (Robbins et al. 2008). A considerable shortcoming of the revisionist's argument as it is made from archaeological remains is the paucity of evidence signalling distinct disruption or change to their lifeways; very few cultural items appear in forager contexts that were obtained from social relations with farmers (Sadr 1997).

Both approaches to understanding San identity were vastly different from one another: isolated and affluent versus integrated and underclass. In some respects, they could not oppose one another more. Revisionists placed a great amount of emphasis on historical processes and culture-making sequences whereas traditionalists did not consider contact to be so impactful and instead interpreted San culture as a resilient and largely constant entity (Kent 1992). The perspectives are firmly grounded in their own contextual, historic positionality, which was influenced by developments within the fields of archaeology and anthropology, and political machinations that were transforming the academies at the time.

The traditionalist perspective was heavily impacted by colonial ethnography. The main aim was to document 'pure' indigenous people and way of living, hence the notion of the pristine, primordial hunter-gatherers who were isolated, self-sufficient and at harmony with nature. These views were supported by ecological anthropological perspectives at a time when structural-functionalism dominated the field. Hence, of interest was diet, foraging behaviour, and self-sufficiency within an ecological system (Robins 2001; Barnard 2006). However, the revisionists appeared at a time of post-colonial and post-modern revolution and instead accepted the premise that the San had for many centuries been a part of a broader economic and political systems (Kuper 1992). The approach was aligned with a political economy model from the 1980s. Their views were proposed during a time when the romanticised view of a 'noble savage' was being challenged by scholars rejecting the hegemonic traits of Eurocentric perspectives. To them, produced knowledge was tied to colonial legacies (Kuper 1992; Widlok 1994). Casting these views into further disrepute was the emergence of indigenous rights movements and indigenous sovereignty. Indigenous communities preferred traditionalists perspectives that presented them as pristine, which supported land rights. However, revisionists argued that while not pristine, indigenous groups were still the subject of historic injustice, but groups saw this as undermining legal claims amidst other land and sustainability concerns (Robins 2001; Segobye 2006; Sylvain 2015; Thomas and Sporton 2002). What became clear from the 1990s was the sense that the 'community', as it was presented, was not as cohesive as portrayed. Conflict, homicide, alcohol abuse and various afflictions and disagreements appeared in the ≠Khomani San community after a successful land claim in South Africa. Within this and other examples, it became clear the distinction between 'traditional' and 'integrationist' and how this intersected with 'indigenous' or 'community' was far more dynamic, nuanced, and layered than previously acknowledged (Robins 2001). The Kalahari Debate highlighted, over time, the deeply influencing roots of disciplinary processes and the impact of unfolding political, economic and social change in a national framework.

The Kalahari Debate has considerable ramifications in understanding the past. If contemporary San groups are considered to be archetypal and primordial, then constructing their identity as an entity is justified. In so doing, archaeologists have access to a San cultural compendium to interpret finds against. This has variably been done across southern Africa. One of the earliest attempts was by Wadley (1987), as briefly mentioned, who interpreted two sites in South Africa's Magaliseberg region, Jubilee Shelter and Cave James, to represent aggregation and dispersal occupation phases, respectively; an occupation cycle that was recorded ethnographically in the Kalahari Desert and in its neighbouring areas (Brooks and Yellen 1987). Her identification of these site types was based on the recovered archaeological assemblage from each. At Jubilee, a wide diversity of finds were made that indicated a broad set of activities at the site, a large faunal assemblage suggesting a large group occupied the substantially-sized shelter, and symbolic items such as crystals suggested rituality. At James, it was more or less the inverse: a small site with a limited set of activities and a constrained faunal record. By associating an archaeological site with an ethnographic phenomenon the assumption that follows is that the contemporary meaning and values attached to that feature in the contemporary era were similarly present in the past. As such, at aggregation sites the archaeological traces would not only mark a wide range of activities and higher food consumption patterns but also multiple bands converging at a site, group hunting activities and feasting, ritual performances including the trance dance and marriage ceremonies, and craft production for the purposes of *hxaro* (delayed, reciprocal gift giving with the aim of forming social and kin alliances). As such, with ethnography, it is possible to generate far greater interpretive depth (Barnard 2019; McGranaghan 2017; Pearce 2012).

If ethnography is so compelling, Karim Sadr (1997) quipped, then we may as well abandon excavations at Later Stone Age sites since all of the answers are already at hand. Mitchell (2003) also expressed concern and argued that identifying *hxaro* in the archaeological record is particularly tricky when we cannot show that these goods were traded in the first place or produced for personal use. Other scholars have expressed trepidation in the wholesale adoption of ethnography when one considers the varied and diverse sets of social relations and outcomes that existed over the past 1500 years (Forssman 2020; Jolly 1996; Parkington 1984). Further complicating the matter of analogy are differences in rock art and buried sequences. Whereas the latter appears to match less neatly, rock art is argued to more convincingly be contiguous with San spiritual and cosmological beliefs (Pearce 2012). Although only briefly summarised, the importance of the Kalahari Debate is not only in how we construct indigenous identities but how that information is deployed in understanding the past, justifying the present, and making reparations going forward.

7.1.2 East Africa

Across most of Africa, transitions remained a key archaeological topic. While not the only theme that has seen considerable attention, it is one that appears regularly. In East Africa, over the last thirty years, it has featured in discussions and studies examining pastoralist shifts (Crowther et al. 2018; Hilderbrand et al. 2022; Prendergast 2020; Robertshaw 2021), long-distance, maritime trade and connections with foreign trading centres (Horton et al. 2021; Stahl 2014; Wood et al. 2017), the involvement of extant communities in studying the contemporary past (Pollard et al. 2025; Schmidt and Arthur 2018), and urban transitions (LaViolette and Fleisher 2005; McIntosh and McIntosh 1993; Monroe 2013). A key early development that transformed landscapes and social systems was the appearance of ceramics and associated shifts in ways of living.

The earliest ceramics in East Africa are associated with a hunter-gatherer economy that included delayed return and a focus on aquatic resources (Prendergast 2010; Seitsonen 2010). The ceramic facies is known as Kansyore and dates to between 8000 and 2000 BP (Ashley and Grillo 2015: p. 461). Sites are found in western Kenya, northern Tanzania, southern Uganda, and possibly South Sudan—where the facies is known as Lokabulo. Another facies known as Nderit appears from c. 4500 BP and is likely associated with pastoralists (Grillo and Hildebrand 2013) due to its association with cattle and caprine remains (Hildebrand and Grillo 2012: p. 344). This emerged following the African Humid Period (c. 15–5.5 ka), after which changing landscapes likely suited herding practices, driving the shift from hunting and gathering (Hildebrand et al. 2022). However, Nderit might instead be associated with foragers with domestic animals (Gifford-Gonzalez 2011: p. 37). Sites containing Nderit ceramics are found in Kenya as well as northern Tanzania (Gifford-Gonzalez 1998) and eventually appear in Kansyore areas in a later phase called the Pastoral Neolithic (Bower 1991; Marshall et al. 2011). Nderit ceramics have also been identified at four megalithic pillar sites, which are standing-stone constructions in various spatial organisations typically associated with seasonality (Wandibba 1980; Nelson 1995). Other wares associated with pastoralists include Remnant (Elmenteitan), Narosura (Wandibba 1980) and Akira (Prendergast et al. 2014), but scholars debate how these should be grouped (Ambrose 1998; Collett and Robertshaw 1983; Lane 2011b). The geographic convergence of these two facies associated with different subsistence approaches are also considered proxies for language groups and migrations (Nelson 1995; Lane 2004: p. 247). Hence, the occurrence and spread of Kansyore and Nderit wares signal a dynamic interchange of cultures, but also the movement or transition of foodways prior to the Bantu migration (Chami and Kwekason 2003). Although these ceramic traditions require better understanding, they demonstrate a dynamic interplay between people showing a degree of complexity not previously considered.

The interplay between Kansyore and Pastoral Neolithic wares was succeeded by the appearance of Urewe ceramics (Ashley and Grillo 2015). Urewe assemblages have received more interest than any other ceramic facies in East Africa, having first been described by Mary Leakey (Leakey et al. 1948), and as a result of focussed research have a strongly supported chronology of 500 BCE to 800 CE (Clist 1987; Stewart 1993; Ashley 2010b). Significantly, Urewe signals the arrival of Bantu-language speakers and the 'Iron Age package' (Ashley 2010b: p. 144), leading to the spatial overlap of multiple subsistence groups and associated responses to contact. It appears, though, that Urewe producers were mixed farmers who placed greater emphasis on farming than herding, although evidence for both is scarce (Karega-Munene 2002). For example, at Usenge 3 in Nyanza, Kenya, ceramics superficially resembling Urewe have been identified (Dale and Ashley 2010); they have similar decorations but in lower frequencies (4% are decorated compared to c. 66–85%). However, they lack the emphasis on quality and finish typical of Urewe ceramics and possess a heavy temper. Chronologically this localised tradition falls within the fifth and sixth centuries CE (Ashley 2010b: p. 148). The emphasis on wild fauna and continuity in stone tool production in the Urewe levels is much like those in the Kansyore levels below, leading some to suggest that the two occupations are related (Lane et al. 2007; Dale and Ashley 2010; Seitsonen 2010). The Contact Urewe, as they have been called, have been thought to represent hunter-gatherers 'imperfectly' emulating the Urewe ceramics of their neighbours during a 'moving frontier' phase in the region's occupation sequence (Lane 2004). This example is but one on a landscape characterised by varied transitions played out by several agents and mechanisms (Lane 2004: p. 254).

Pinpointing the beginning of social relations between hunter-gatherers and farmers, or more broadly, between foragers and food producers, is not as straightforward as the clear differences between Kansyore and Urewe ways of life might suggest. As elsewhere in Africa (e.g., Sadr 2003, 2015), the transition is gradual and varied. On Kenya's Laikipia Plateau, for example, the earliest evidence of domesticates appears in Later Stone Age forager contexts, such as rock shelters (Lane 2004). At Enkapune ya Muto, livestock were adopted by foragers around 3000 BP (Marean 1992), possibly through exchange, theft, or other means (Gifford et al. 1980). Across the region, sites yielded ceramics from multiple traditions – Kansyore, Pastoral Neolithic and Urewe – suggesting sustained, long-term contact between different subsistence groups (Lane 2004). These ceramics, once assumed to signal distinct cultural or economic identities, appear increasingly fluid. At Gogo Falls, for example, Elementeitan levels show evidence of both cattle husbandry and wild resource use, indicating a mixed subsistence strategy (Marshall 1991: p. 178). In contrast, eastern sites associated with the same tradition show less diversity, perhaps due to ecological constraints or inter-group competition (Marshall 1994: p. 32). Interpretations of Urewe layers at Gogo Falls vary: Peter Robertshaw (1991) cautioned that agricultural activity may have disturbed assemblages, while James Karega-Munene (2002: pp. 128–139) argued instead for continuity between the Elementeitan and Urewe periods. This continuity, he suggested, supports a more flexible understanding of ceramic use and identity. Taken together, the evidence points to a mosaic of interactions and transitions, shaped by local conditions, where material culture and lifeways were not rigidly tied to ethnic or economic boundaries, but reflected a dynamic and interconnected landscape (Kusimba and Kusimba 2005, 2017).

7.1.3 North Africa

Of the many themes that pervade the North African archaeological landscape, one that has grown in stamina since 1990 is addressing how colonialism has shaped local archaeological sequences (Mattingly 1996; Fenwick 2007; Lemos 2022). From this renewed perspective, a focus on post-colonial nation building arose, specifically around the accommodation of diversity in opposition to ethnic division-based systems of governance (Hassan 1999). As part of this movement was a desire to acknowledge technological and societal advances that are archaeologically visible. However, this was not only through using archaeological methods, but as in other parts of Africa, it was through inter-disciplinary approaches that would also aid in approaching grand challenges, such as urbanism, water shortages, ecological instability, and poverty (e.g., Samuels 2009). The, at times, divergent narrative of colonial and post-colonial approaches have created blind spots in the missing middle, such as migration, which some have argued is an important but now neglected driver in Africa's past (Ashley *et al.* 2016). A North African example is Algeria and its Roman history (Mahjoubi 1997; Mattingly 1996).

David Mattingly (1996: pp. 49–50) demonstrated how "modern and ancient colonialism have become interwoven, and how this has affected the development of Roman archaeology in the independent countries of the Maghreb" in his study of the Roman occupation in Algeria. His work confronted the "self-justifying perspective of the nineteenth- and early-twentieth-century" antiquarians views that were perpetuated in French and Italian claims to inheritance of North Africa because of Roman rule. This view justified a European presence in the region. When the Italians were preparing to invade Libya in 1911, their press claimed that Italy had every right to do so, and a legal-historical claim, as they were descendants of the Roman Empire (Segré 1974). Part of this process, however, was the disinheritance of North Africa from local people, which was achieved by emphasising inferiority and separation through various means, including architectural and iconographic approaches. Colonists, in this framing, introduced civilisation and upliftment into the region (Anderson 2006; Hassan 1999; Mattingly 1996; Fenwick 2007). French generals, for example, were compared to legendary Roman commanders who defeated local rebels. Commemorative monuments and inscriptions produced by the French, or the Italian museum in Tripoli's old Turkish castle, imitated Roman counterparts. The French army even busied themselves with antiquarian work in their free time to uncover Roman remains. In the post-colonial era, the over-emphasis of Roman occupation and military exploits has led to a now stigma attached to Roman archaeology (Mattingly 1996: p. 55).

Locals, to the contrary, were viewed as savages, ungoverned, bands of nomadic groups, and invaders in the case of those with Muslim roots (Fenwick 2007: p. 78).

Independence brought with it new claims to legitimate rule. An early challenge to the Romancentric approach came from within North Africa in the form of *L'histoire du Maghreb* (Abdallah 1970), which rejected the European hijacking of Maghreb history. However, in Algeria the National Liberation Front glossed over ethnic differences and inculcated pure Islam in national discourse where it dealt with the past (Silverstein 2004, pp. 67–68). In this rendering, the nation's foundation originated from the Muslim occupation of the region beginning in the seventh century CE. The Berber past was not explicitly mentioned (Fenwick 2007: p. 80). Moreover, authorities saw the Eurocentric perspectives of the Berber as interwoven with European occupations predating the arrival of Muslim groups as an attempt to distance Berber from Asian histories (McDougall 2006). As the French and Italians had done before them, the new government installed artworks and symbols in anthems and flags to materialise national identity (Anderson 2006). Over time, Berbers vociferously expressed discontent with this narrative. Berber identity has appeared contiguously across North Africa in many regions where it is often expressed as *Amazigh*, a term ascribed to Africanus in the sixteenth century CE meaning 'free man'. It is used to refer to the imagined, transnational community that feel disenfranchised within their national contexts (Maddy-Weitzman 2006).

The role of archaeology in North Africa has long been shaped by competing narratives and political agendas, with tensions persisting between colonial legacies, nationalist ideologies, and marginalised identities such as the Berber (Fenwick 2007: p. 83). Corisande Fenwick (2007: p. 83) questioned whether archaeology in North Africa will serve to legitimate one structure or the other. Ian Hodder (1999, 2003) acknowledged this but argued that it is the archaeologist's job to defend the past from its adverse use in the present using evidence. It is also argued that there is a need to make archaeology anti-colonial and deploy it in building nations and identities through engaging the past and reshaping concepts of others (Hassan 1999: p. 396). However, nationalist agendas of any nature in Africa reinforce European boundaries and crystalise essentialist constructions of the African landscape. Beyond the focus on European colonialism there is another that has taken place in North Africa, and this is the 'Egyptification' of the region.

Narratives for much of northeast Africa's past is centred around Egyptian histories developed from the perspective offered in their texts (Smith 2003: pp. 113–124). These result in the dispossession of the past on behalf of colonised people, such as in Nubia (Carruthers 2013). Egypt colonised Nubia in two principal phases: first in the Middle Kingdom (c. 2050–1650 BCE), when control extended into Lower Nubia, and later more extensively during the New Kingdom (c. 1550–1070 BCE), reaching as far south as the Fifth Cataract. In the early Eighteenth Dynasty, Egyptian forces reoccupied Middle Kingdom fortresses along the Middle Nile (Davies 2004; Gabolde 2012). This was followed, from the mid-Eighteenth Dynasty onward, by the construction of new settlements and temples (Rocheleau 2008; Thill 2017; Budka 2018; Gabolde 2020). Cemeteries were also established and burials included material items that travelled from Egypt into the occupied territory. Other items of material culture present in the colony include ceramics, burial containers, funerary masks, weapons, tools, cosmetic items, and more (Lemos 2020). The typical perspective of this history is that at the centre existed the powerful coloniser and in the periphery the colonised (Stein 1999: pp. 16–17). Such a perspective aligns with World Systems Theory in which the centres became wealthy and the peripheries poor (Wallerstein 2004). Such a modelling of the Nubian landscape shaped archaeological reconstructions (Lemos 2022).

Post-colonial theory, however, unpacks this dichotomy by emphasising local agency and textured cultural interactions (Kaps and Komlosy 2013; Sulas and Pikirayi 2020). Rennan Lemos (2022: p. 26) attempted to reconfigure this power network and focus on "centres of other experiences". An examination of Tomb 3-P-50, located at the periphery, showed that both Egyptian (coloniser) and Nubian (colonised) material culture was present. The co-occurrence of these finds draws into the frame Nubian experiences, Nubian ways of engaging Egyptian material culture, and may also suggest that foreign items had their materiality altered. These new orientations created alternate versions of those material things that performed tasks within new, in this case colonised, contexts. For example, shabtis (figurines placed in a tomb) have been modified to include Nubian decorative elements and names (Lemos 2020); originally it was thought that the Egyptian producers had left blank spaces for Nubians to add their inscriptions (Steindorff 1937: p. 75). These sets of interplay demonstrate complexity in the archaeological record and diversity that a coloniser perspective does not afford the past, and it provides the basis to examine colonial inequalities (Van Pelt 2013; Lemos 2020, 2022).

The work at Jebel Moya, Sudan, is an example of the transformative contributions archaeological sequences in regions long ignored may provide. Jebel Moya is the largest massif in the southern Gezira Plains and was initially excavated by Henry Wellcome from 1911 to 1914 (Addison 1949). Despite a remarkable archaeological sequence, which included 3136 human burials, little work was carried out at the site (although see Clark 1984) until an international collaboration began new excavations in 2017 (Brass et al. 2019). The aim of the new study intended to understand past ways of living in the arid to semi-arid region, which included economic, identity, health, and mobility dynamics. Jebel Moya has a lengthy sequence that can be divided into four phases: 1 (Late Mesolithic; late sixth millennium BCE), 2 (c. 2750–2250 BCE), 3 (c. mid-second millennium BCE), and 4 (c. 700 BC – 2000 years ago). Of interest is domestic sorghum found in Phase 2 dating to c. 2500 BCE. This chronology places it as the second oldest domesticated sorghum currently known, contributing significantly to our understanding of Africa's Neolithic phase. Moreover, at Jebel Moya, trade took place with the Merotic state that was supported by a mobile residential component used seasonally by the occupants (Brass *et al.* 2019). The findings keenly show the need to consider the archaeology present in landscapes beyond key research areas, such as East Africa or South Africa.

A feature of Africa's colonialism is how the past is re-enacted in the present (Lemos 2020: p. 29). This is well illustrated in the construction of the Merowe Dam at the Fourth Cataract and the groundwork that took place ahead of its development. The idea to build such a dam appeared in the 1940s, but serious planning only began in the 1980s (Failer et al. 2006: p. 68). Merowe is one of the largest developments to have taken place in Sudan. It was built primarily as a hydroelectric power plant to provide electricity to northern Sudan, doubling the country's power output, but also to aid in irrigation schemes, flood protection, and the reduction of sedimentation (Failer et al. 2006: p. 70). It was envisaged to directly benefit the nation's economic growth. Construction started in 2003 and was completed in 2008 (Hildyard 2008). Over 180 km of the landscape were flooded and the lives of at least 50,000 people practicing small-scale farming in the area were impacted. The community at large was promised a resettlement package, but this was seen by the different groups as wholly inadequate (Askouri 2004; Bosshard and Hildyard 2005; McDonald et al. 2009). Internal and external observers were concerned with human rights violations that began surfacing with the responsibility placed on developers and companies involved, but none of the contractors or the Sudanese state accepted responsibility, who largely withdrew into a position of neutrality (Askouri 2004; Hildyard 2008).

The archaeology community become deeply concerned about the dam's development as it was situated in *terra incognita* (Kleinitz and Näser 2011). Assessments in the early stages of dam planning indicated that the area was relatively rich in cultural remains, although it lacked monumental sites like those found along other stretches of the Nile. Additionally, ethnographic work was not carried out but its importance was noted in the original report to UNESCO (Leclant 1990). A later report supported the earlier archaeological findings and recommended mitigation steps, including establishing a documentation centre in Khartoum, Sudan's capital (Grzymski 2010). A decade passed by with little action before another report was produced ahead of dam construction, which included worryingly little cultural information (cf. Kleinitz and Näser 2011: p. 257). After development started, more and more archaeological teams began in earnest to record the cultural heritage before it was lost or irreparably damaged. These attempts were plagued with issues, including a lack of funding and access, but one that became problematic was the lack of concern for local communities affected by the dam. In 2006, community relations directly resulted in a demand that archaeologists leave the region, despite their intentions to limit the destruction and work with communities (Welsby 2008). Archaeologists had hoped their presence might help delay the flooding, raise international awareness, and offer a degree of protection should armed conflict erupt (Askouri 2007; Kleinitz and Näser 2011: p. 262). In many cases, archaeologists left the area without their finds; instead, sorted artefacts were stored in bags and entrusted to local custodians for safekeeping (Kleinitz and Näser 2011: p. 264). It is important to recognise that it was not the local communities that invited archaeologists into the region, and their vision of the past is vastly different to the one constructed through archaeological approaches (Kleinitz and Näser 2011). Consequently, part of the underlying problem is the power dynamic between core and periphery, where the core directs decisions without the periphery being involved. In this example, archaeologists who did not do everything correctly and arguably appropriately (Hildyard 2008) were caught between communities and government, livelihoods and development, and indigenous groups and political entities. Additionally, they opted to be neutral in this encounter, but as has been shown in numerous contributions listed here, archaeology is everything but neutral.

7.1.4 West Africa

The late 1980s and early 1990s was an exciting time in West African archaeology (McIntosh 1994: pp. 165–166). The field became more dynamic and evolved further, taking on board a range of topics, themes, and theoretical frameworks. In the years prior, site recording, inventories, and chronologies dominated, with a focus on regional settlement systems and environmental archaeology. While still important topics, the field was moving in new directions. Previous studies also focussed on linear progressions at single sites: change was viewed from an evolutionary model rather than heterarchical models (McIntosh 1998). Narrow descriptive parameters gave way to more explicitly articulated archaeological theory (e.g., Holl 2006a; Insoll 1996; Gosselain 2008; Haour 2013). Questions involving economies, settlement dynamics, social organisation and so on arose with multi-site comparisons and interdisciplinary methods leading the new approaches (e.g., D'Andrea et al. 2006; Fuller and Stevens 2018; Haour and Christie 2019; Killick 2016; MacDonald 2011a). Additionally, a movement to refute European generalisations using empirical evidence gradually grew in focus and strength (Trigger 1990). These various studies led to the recognition of diverse pathways in the archaeological past that led to key outcomes such as urbanism (McIntosh and McIntosh 1984) or pastoralism (Holl 1998). A useful example of this is the lack of centralisation in the appearance of certain West African states.

The dominant notion pervading West Africa until the 1980s was that urbanism post-dated the Muslim penetration from North Africa (Mitchell 2005a). However, work in several regions dispelled this notion. Centuries of continuous occupation in the Niger Delta's inland region led to the emergence of an urban landscape in the first millennium CE (McIntosh 2020). Focussed research in the region examined, to various extents, 65 mounds surrounding Jenné-jeno and Djenné. A large number of radiocarbon dates ($N = 75$) were obtained that date an extensive cultural sequence retrieved from several largescale and focussed excavations. They showed that Jenné-jeno expanded in the first century BCE and grew two about two-thirds of its overall size, which measures about 2 km in circumference, by 500 CE, and then all districts were occupied by 900 CE. The entire settlement was surrounded by a massive wall that enclosed approximately 3000 people, but between 6000 and 13,000 people lived around Jenné-jeno based on analyses at mounds within 1 km from the settlement (McIntosh 2024). Jenné-jeno did not meet the expectations of a standard city's outline, with a central urban agglomeration, but rather comprised a mosaic of satellite sites atop mounds (McIntosh 2021). The Jenné-jeno landscape, and others, were home to cosmopolitan towns and political regimes (Bedaux et al. 2001; Gokee 2012; Togola 1996).

What generally supports urbanism is the centralisation of wealth, ritual landscapes, authority, and other social traits that relate to socio-political differentiation (Trigger 2003; Linares-Matás 2022), but that appears not to be the case at Jenné-jeno. To examine this, what has been asked is why did local society disperse across disconnected mounds? The Jenné-jeno society has been described as heterogenous, with different subsistence practices (e.g., rice, millet, wild plants, and fishing) and craft specialisation between mounds occupations. In spite of this, wealth and power differentials did not vary; burial rituals and prestige goods, for example, were comparable across the investigated sites. What appears absent are leadership hierarchies that typically accompany population increases and political development. The lack of centralised leadership and the impact of its absence may have been mitigated by the spatial organisation of settlement patterns. Additionally, a horizontal decision-making system appears to have assisted in the form of secret societies and the sort (McIntosh 1999). Although it is not clear why society spread across mounds, they relied on trade and exchange to support growth due to a lack of critical resources (Dueppen 2024). This included local trade into the northern, drier reaches of nearby rivers supplying provisions as well as more extensive trade into the Sahara Desert for copper and salt (McIntosh and McIntosh 1995). Jenné-jeno's trade network appears earlier than later Muslim trade routes and drew in important and locally unavailable resources to the urban landscape (McIntosh and McIntosh 1981: p. 612).

Jenné-jeno demonstrates African originality. It is characterised by a heterarchal system that can be summarised as a city without a citadel (McIntosh and McIntosh 1993; McIntosh 2021). Such a system lacks the socio-political hierarchy that is found at many other sites, most classically perhaps Great Zimbabwe (Huffman 2015b). The Jenné-jeno innovation, as well as others like it, challenges perspectives on the past in multiple ways. First, it dispels the notion that Muslim's introduced advancement into the region. Such an approach leans heavily on earlier notions of external forces to especially sub-Saharan Africa advancing change along the 'linear pathway' from village to kingdom. Instead, this happened before their arrival in West Africa and independently. Second, the establishment of such urban landscapes was not based on the same pillars as many other state-level societies. To the contrary, it emerged as a cosmopolitan entity drawing on local opportunities and establishing widespread connections co-ordinated by a host of interlocking but disconnected settlements. The urban landscape relied heavily on trade entrepôts that acted as hubs for long-distance and local trade, and in some instances were involved in craft specialisation (Dueppen 2024). Jenné-jeno, therefore, diverges from traditional hierarchal models of urbanism. It forces archaeologists to rethink urban development in Africa rather than relying on urbanism paradigms developed at a few centres or that rely on deeply embedded Eurocentric views (McIntosh 2015).

Another example that demonstrates the nuanced historical sequences of West Africa took place on Tichitt-Oualata escarpments in modern-day Mauritania where non-state complexity appeared even before Jenné-Jeno. The sites here were known from before the mid-twentieth century CE (Laforgue 1924; Laforgue and Mauny 1939; Mauny 1951, 1951; Verneau 1920) but the first focussed work was carried out in the late 1960s (Munson 1971). Communities here settled around an endorheic (disconnected from oceans) lake basin from between 2900 and 1900 BCE. At this stage, local communities hunted and gathered and lived in small, temporary camps. This phase was followed by the appearance of pearl millet cultivation along with high mobility. From at least 1600 BCE, however, settlements comprising conjoined stone-walled clusters appear (Fig. 7.4) (MacDonald 2015). Livestock, fish reserves and shellfish were all important at this time (Holl 2009). Local communities might also have been involved in long-distance trade in various goods, including luxury and food items (Amblard-Pison 2006; Holl 2009; MacDonald 1998). The largest Tichitt Tradition settlement is Dakhlet el Atrous, being around 80 ha (Dueppen 2024). Settlements can further be divide into neighbourhood districts and are also associated with funerary tumuli. Recent work has argued that status and power differences existed between residences, indicating scalar hierarchies (Linares-Matás 2022).

It is debated whether the Tichitt Tradition included social complexity, such as being characterised by socio-political hierarchies. Susan McIntosh and Roderick McIntosh (1988) argued that the lack of prestige wealth items, as reported by Sylvie Amblard (1984, p. 273), suggests a lack of socio-political complexity. Augustin Holl (1985), conversely, sees the small number of items as evidence for consolidation of wealth by elite members of society, and their control of trade networks. There are other metrics that may indicate that complexity was present. For example, asymmetric living space sizes and storage facilities potentially provide indices that individuals

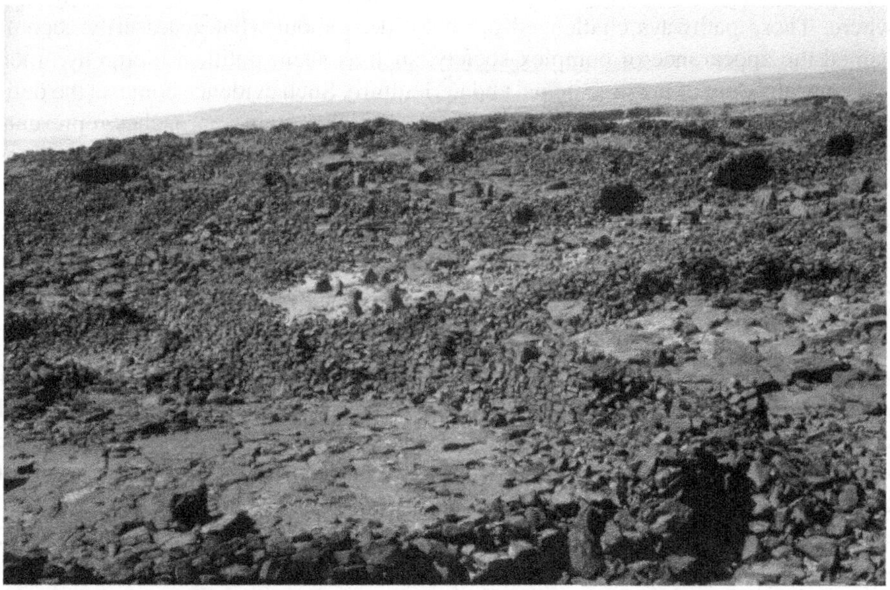

Fig. 7.4 Conjoined stone walls at village v.72 in Dhar Tichitt (see Amblard-Pison 2014) (photograph: Sylvie Amblard-Pison). *Source* https://commons.wikimedia.org/wiki/File:Un_aspect_du_village_v.72,_Dhar_Tichitt-Oualata.jpg.

within the residential area or neighbourhoods organised themselves into social hierarchies (Linares-Matás 2022). Moreover, several endogenous factors appear to differentiate households. Some settlements exhibit multi-tiered settlement hierarchies (Holl 1993), demarcated space through stone compounds (Munson 1971), differences in tumuli size and clustering (Amblard-Pison 2006; MacDonald 2015), and variable proportions of decorated ceramics (MacDonald 2011b). Additionally, although challenged by a lack of robust chronology, spatial symmetries within settlements and even between them may reflect social organisations (Holl 2006b).

Of interest in the Tichitt-Oualata escarpment is the emergence of complex society among mostly pastoral, mobile groups with limited cultivation. The early Tichitt Tradition phase includes higher levels of mobility than those that followed, and it appears that millet cultivation appeared earlier than initially thought (MacDonald 2015). Despite this, expansions into new territories existed with mobile groups moving into neighbouring regions, such as Nema and Mena, during the second and third millennium BCE (Dueppen 2024). During these phases, pastoral lineages existed between family compounds in nearby neighbourhoods (Holl 1993; Linares-Matás 2022; MacDonald 1998). Mobility, thus, was an important feature of Tichitt Tradition ways of living and relating to one another as well as the landscape, but it gradually declined when more permanent settlements were established by the early first millennium BCE (MacDonald 2015: p. 60).

The Tichitt-Oualata and Jenné-jeno examples demonstrate that there existed multiple trajectories to complexity in Africa that are not necessarily reflected elsewhere. These pathways challenged pre-held ideas about what necessarily accompanied the appearance of complex society, such as socio-political hierarchy, trade and centralisation of prestige items, and agriculture. Such evidence contests the definitions used for town, village, and chieftain. The change in approaches represents a move from a derivative to a generative mode of archaeological reconstructions (McIntosh 1994: p. 167).

7.1.5 Central Africa

Archaeological progress in Central Africa has moved at a slower pace than in other African regions. There are several reasons why, some of which include environmental challenges, political instability, conflict, and historical neglect (e.g., Denbow 2014; De Matos et al. 2021). As a result, Central Africa is often left out of archaeological conversations regarding other regions even though it connects the northern, western, eastern and southern domains (Padilla-Iglesias et al. 2022). However, since the 1990s, progress has been made, and it is increasing. Integral to this growth are shifts in perspectives. Narratives focussed on widescale migrations have been replaced with regional histories that consider adaptive processes and cultural blending (Vansina 1990, 2004). Similarly, shifts in metallurgy and technology perspectives have moved on from diffusionist ideas and examined local, indigenous innovations (Schmidt and Mapunda 1997).

Important shifts taking place in Central Africa as well as to the east and south were advances in metallurgical studies. Peter Schmidt and Bertram Mapunda (1997) challenged previous diffusionist models and demonstrated technological ingenuity in ironworking in the Congo Basin and Great Lakes region by adopting a cognitive approach (e.g., Huffman 2015a). It was in this region, specifically Burundi and Rwanda, that smelting appeared in the second millennium BCE (Van Grunderbeek 1992) – earlier than elsewhere in West Africa where it appeared in the mid-first millennium BCE. Schmidt and Mapunda (1997) were interested in life histories as they related to smelting and smithing. Whereas some studies considered similarities in smelting and smithing technologies (e.g., Miller and Van Der Merwe 1994), they were more concerned with variability and what this might say about thoughts, beliefs, and cultural logics. It is well acknowledged that cosmological beliefs and ideologies are linked to metal, and ritual performances are usually associated as well (Childs and Herbert 2005; Childs and Killick 1993; Chirikure 2015; Herbert 1993; Kusimba 1993). In Schmidt and Mapunda's (1997: p. 75) view, the underlying "symbolic armatures" may link iron technologies more closely than technological processes themselves. They examined metallurgy across central and East Africa using several examples to demonstrate cross-cultural regularities.

As an example, the trade of copper is worth considering in detail. It has been extracted since at least the mid-first millennium CE in Zambia's Copperbelt region (Bisson 1976), where copper is locally abundant and remains of significant economic value, and in Zimbabwe from the early second millennium CE, though possibly earlier based on seventh- to eighth-century copper objects (Swan 2007). Its value is widely recognised – sometimes referred to as "red gold" because of its importance (Herbert 1984). From at least the ninth century CE, burials at Ingombe Ilede in the Upemba Depression attest to its cultural significance (Fagan 1969; De Maret 1992), where it was used to produce status symbols, decorative items, and ingots that likely functioned as currency (Bisson 1975). Michael Bisson (2000) traced copper exchange networks across Central Africa and beyond using historical sources, identifying distinctive forms such as *croisettes*—cross-shaped ingots (De Maret 1995). One such type, the HIH croisette, appears to connect the Copperbelt and Upemba Depression with the Zambezi River and possibly Great Zimbabwe between the ninth and fourteenth centuries CE (Nikis and Livingstone Smith 2017). These networks are further supported by Muslim and European accounts, which document copper's circulation over vast areas, including across the Sahara (Martin 1972). Copper, along with other traded goods, played a key role in the emergence and consolidation of political formations, and by the nineteenth century, the distribution of copper ingots strongly correlated with centres of political power (Zeebroek 2015).

Beyond exchange or trade, smelting and smithing practices are argued by many to be deeply symbolic. The social construction of these technologies often orientates around power dynamics and gender. Commonly, smelting is associated with an elite class who may oversee the production process or be involved (Calabrese 2000), and symbolically the royal class were seen as being 'forged' into new roles (Childs and Killick 1993; Herbert 1993). It is also in some instances linked to the ancestors. Among the Shona in Zimbabwe, for example, it is believed that spirits provided the information needed for smelting and could influence the smithing process (Dewey 1985, 1991). There is also a strong link between fertility and smelting, with the furnace representing the female that gives birth to the bloomery or child (Fig. 7.5) (Dewey 1990). Due to the association with what is a private activity, furnaces were located away from public or village areas. However, these ethnographic findings are not entirely congruent with the archaeological record. Shadreck Chirikure and Thilo Rehran (2006) studied two villages and their associated ironworking practices, revealing complexities in interpreting past metallurgy. At Baranda, dated to between 1500 and 1700 CE, evidence of smelting was found within the village itself, an unexpected finding, as ethnographic accounts typically place smelting outside domestic spaces. Moreover, furnaces often lack diagnostic features, such as symbolic markings, that are used to link them to specific social roles, such as those of women or wives (Killick 2009). These issues highlight the difficulty of relying solely on ethnographic analogies, particularly when they are applied uncritically across time. Interpreting smelting, smithing, and metallurgical activities requires sensitivity to both historical change and the limitations of ethnographic models.

What emerges from these studies is a research focus that forefronts historical and archaeological sequences in collaborative narratives. Importantly, in doing so, the historical sequence can be pushed back by about a millennium (Nikis and Livingstone Smith 2017). These attempts are nevertheless hindered by large, unexplored regions of Central Africa, a problem that still challenges many regions of the continent. Furthermore, many of the known smelting sites are yet to be dated, and these dates may impact our understanding of metallurgy and its appearance in Central Africa (Killick 2009: p. 405). Understanding the symbolic role of metallurgy and metal items hinges on direct historical connections, some that archaeologists accept in almost all

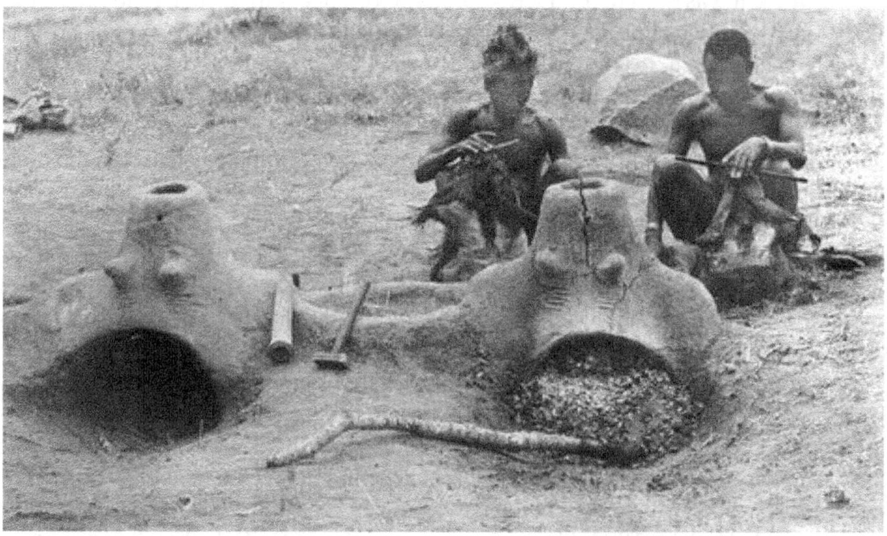

Fig. 7.5 Two men smelt using furnaces resembling female bodies (Schmidt 2009: p. 269)

cases (e.g., Huffman 2007), but in other instances the use of ethnography proceeds with a great degree of caution (Childs 1991; Killick 2009). What many of these studies importantly do is challenge assumptions held regarding Central Africa (and more broadly African) innovation, historic variability, ethnographic applicability, and semiotics. Moreover, they show the important role Central Africa played in metallurgical technological advances and trade that impacted a far wider region.

7.2 Archaeology in the Time of Democracy

> Despite the end of colonial rule and the subsequent implicit support of nationalist aims by some archaeologists, African archaeology retained elements of colonialism in purpose, practice, and interpretation (Giblin 2013: pp. 259–260).

After independence, archaeology across much of Africa began to reorient itself, seeking to liberate the continent's past from colonial legacies and to emphasise African agency and innovation (Mapunda 1991; Stahl 2009: p. 244). This shift marked a move from studying static cultural entities to examining the processes of culture-making and local development. Metallurgy, among other subjects, became a key area through which scholars explored Africa's technological histories, economic networks, and long-distance connections, not as derivatives of foreign influence but as achievements rooted in African contexts. These shifts reflected a broader realignment in archaeological frameworks toward more locally grounded interpretations.

Mitchell's (2005a) *African Connections* offered a timely synthesis of Africa's global entanglements, emphasising the continent's active role in shaping world history. This perspective has encouraged studies that trace African agency across long-distance trade and colonial interactions (e.g., Coutu et al. 2016; Delius et al. 2024; Wood et al. 2017). Work on the trans-Atlantic trading system, particularly in West Africa, has grown significantly (e.g., DeCorse 2001; Kelly 1997). Christopher DeCorse's (1992, 1996) archaeological investigations at Elmina (Fig. 7.6), combining excavation, documentary sources, and local histories, highlighted African-European interaction and continuity in worldviews and practices despite the transformations of colonialism and global trade. His work helped shift attention from European-built heritage to African experiences embedded within the trans-Atlantic world. On Africa's eastern coast, the archaeology of slavery had long been neglected, often due to the difficulty of identifying enslaved lives in the material record without textual support (Alexander 2001; Handler and Lange 2006). Yet, in recent decades, archaeologists have turned renewed attention to slavery's legacies, investigating sites associated with slaving and bonded labour in Zanzibar, Pemba, and the Great Lakes region (Lane 2021: p. 31), alongside earlier work in Cape Town (Mbeki et al. 2017; Schrire 1990). As in West Africa, these studies increasingly foreground African experiences and challenge inherited narratives through new theoretical and methodological approaches.

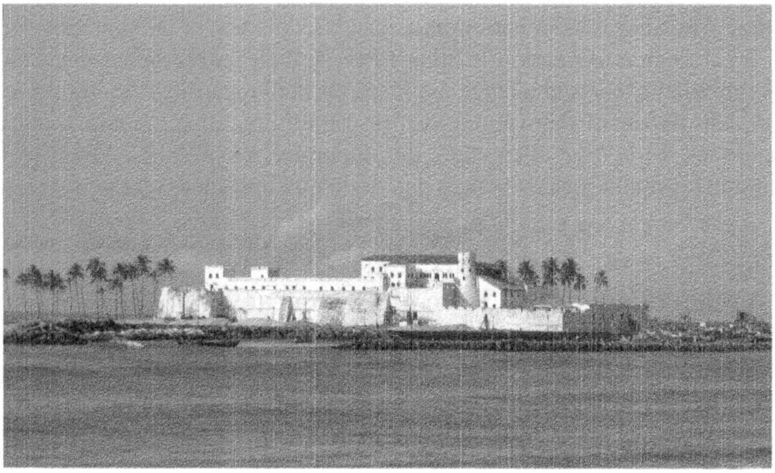

Fig. 7.6 Looking torwards Fort São Jorge de Mina, known also as Elmina Castle, across the Benya River (photograph: Francisco Anzola). *Source* https://commons.wikimedia.org/wiki/File:Elmina_Castle_(3,587,077,829).jpg

Alongside these developments, there has been a growing emphasis on the relevance of archaeology in contemporary contexts. Two broad models have emerged, one of which is the 'usable past' approach (Giblin 2013: p. 260). This model promotes archaeology as a tool to confront ongoing coloniality and contribute to present-day issues such as human rights, environmental change, and social justice (Lane 2011a; Schmidt 2009; Stump 2010;). It also emphasises meaningful engagement with local communities, while raising concerns about the potential for archaeology to be appropriated into nationalist agendas. The usable past has become an increasingly vital lens through which to consider archaeology's future. As this and the previous chapters have explored, the discipline in Africa contends not only with its history, but with the political, social, and ethical challenges of the present.

References

Abdallah, L. 1970. *L'histoire du Maghreb: Un essai de synthèse*. Paris: François Maspéro, Textes à l'Appui.

Abungu, G. O. 1989. *Communities on the River Tana, Kenya: An archaeological study of relations between the delta and the river basin, AD 700–1890*. PhD Thesis. Cambridge: University of Cambridge.

Agorsah, E. K. 1990. Ethnoarchaeology: The search for a self-corrective approach to the study of a past human behaviour. *African Archaeological Review* 8:189–208.

Alexander, J. 2001. Islam, archaeology and slavery in Africa. *World Archaeology* 33:44–46.

Allen, J. D. V. 1993. *Swahili Origins: Swahili culture and the Shungwaya phenomenon*. London: James Currey Ltd.

Amblard, S. 1984. *Tichitt-Walata, République islamique de Mauritanie. Civilisation et industrie lithique*. Paris: ADPF.

Amblard-Pison, S. 2006. *Communautés villageoises néolithiques des dhars Tichitt et Oualata (Mauritanie)*. Oxford: British Archaeological Reports.

Ambrose, S. H. 1998. Chronology of the Later Stone Age and food production in East Africa. *Journal of Archaeological Science* 25:377–392.

Anderson, B. 2006. *Imagined communities: Reflections on the origin and spread of nationalism*. London: Verso.

Appadurai, A. 1986. *The social life of things: Commodities in cultural perspective*. Cambridge: Cambridge University Press.

Ashley, C., and D. Bouakaze-Khan. 2011. Conservation and management of archaeological sites in Sub-Saharan Africa. *Conservation and Management of Archaeological Sites* 13:95–102.

Ashley, C. Z. 2010. Towards a socialised archaeology of ceramics in Great Lakes Africa. *African Archaeological Review* 27:135–163.

Ashley, C. Z., A. Antonites, and P. D. Fredriksen. 2016. Mobility and African archaeology: An introduction. *Azania: Archaeological Research in Africa* 51:417–434.

Ashley, C. Z., and K. M. Grillo. 2015. Archaeological ceramics from eastern Africa: Past approaches and future directions. *Azania: Archaeological Research in Africa* 50:460–480.

Askouri, A. 2004. A culture drowned: Sudan dam will submerge historically rich area, destroy Nile communities. *World Rivers Review* 19:8–9.

Askouri, A. 2007. China's investment in Sudan: Displacing villages and destroying communities. In *African perspectives on China in Africa*, ed. F. Manji and S. Marks, 71–86. Oxford: Fahamu.

Atherton, J. 1983. Ethnoarchaeology in Africa. *African Archaeological Review* 1:75–104.

Barnard, A. 1990. Comment on foragers: Genuine or spurious? Situating the Kalahari San in history by J.S. Solway and R. B. Lee. *Current Anthropology* 31:122–123.

Barnard, A. 2006. Kalahari revisionism, Vienna and the 'indigenous peoples' debate. *Social Anthropology* 14:1–16.

Barnard, A. 2007. *Anthropology and the Bushman*. Oxford: Berg.

Barnard, A. 2019. *Bushmen: Kalahari hunter-gatherers and their descendants*. Cambridge: Cambridge University Press.

Bedaux, R. M., K. C. MacDonald, A. Person, J. Polet, K. Sanogo, A. Schmidt, and S. Sidibé. 2001. The Dia archaeological project: Rescuing cultural heritage in the Inland Niger Delta (Mali). *Antiquity* 75:837–848.

Bisson, M. S. 1975. Copper currency in central Africa: The archaeological evidence. *World Archaeology* 6 (3): 276–292.

Bisson, M. S. 1976. *The Prehistoric copper-mines of Zambia*. PhD Thesis. Los Angeles: University of California.

Bisson, M. S. 2000. Precolonial copper metallurgy: Sociopolitical context. In *Ancient African Metallurgy: The sociocultural context*, ed. J. Vogel, 83–146. Walnut Creek: AltaMira Press.

Bosshard, P., and N. Hildyard. 2005. *A critical juncture for peace, democracy, and the environment: Sudan and the Merowe/Hamadab Dam project*. London: International Rivers Network and Corner House.

Bower, J. 1991. The pastoral neolithic of East Africa. *Journal of World Prehistory* 5:49–82.

Breen, C., and P. J. Lane. 2004. Archaeological approaches to East Africa's changing seascapes. *World Archaeology* 35 (3): 469–489.

Brielle, E. S., J. Fleisher, S. Wynne-Jones, K. Sirak, N. Broomandkhoshbacht, K. Callan, E. Curtis, L. Iliev, A. M. Lawson, J. Oppenheimer, L. Qiu, K. Stewardson, J. N. Workman, F. Zalzala, G. Ayodo, A. O. Gidna, A. Kabiru, A. Kwekason, A. Z. P. Mabulla, F. K. Manthi, E. Ndiema, C. Ogola, E. Sawchuk, L. Al-Gazali, B. R. Ali, S. Ben-Salem, T. Letellier, D. Pierron, C. Radimilahy, J.-A. Rakotoarisoa, R. L. Raaum, B. J. Culleton, S. Mallick, N. Rohland, N. Patterson, M. A. Mwenje, K. B. Ahmed, M. M. Mohamed, S. R. Williams, J. Monge, S. Kusimba, M. E. Prendergast, D. Reich, and C. M. Kusimba. 2023. Entwined African and Asian genetic roots of medieval peoples of the Swahili coast. *Nature* 615 (7954): 866–873.

Brooks, A. A., and J. E. Yellen. 1987. The preservation of activity areas in the archaeological record: Ethnoarchaeological and archaeological work in northwest Ngamiland, Botswana. In *Method and theory for activity area research: An ethnoarchaeological approach*, ed. S. Kent, 63–106. New York: Columbia University Press.

Budka, J. 2018. Addressing the gods home away from home: Case studies from New Kingdom Nubia. In *Across the Mediterranean – Along the Nile: Studies in Egyptology, Nubiology and Late Antiquity dedicated to László Török on the occasion of his 75th birthday*, ed. T. A. Bács, Á. Bollók, and T. Vida, 379–390. Budapest: Hungarian Academy of Sciences.

Calabrese, J. A. 2000. Metals, ideology and power: The manufacture and control of materialised ideology in the area of the Limpopo-Shashe confluence, c. AD 900 to 1300. *South African Archaeology Society Goodwin Series* 8:100–111.

Campana, S. 2017. Drones in archaeology. *State-of-the-art and future perspectives. Archaeological Prospection* 24 (4): 275–296.

Carr, C. and Neitzel, J. (eds.) 1995. *Style, Society, and Person: Archaeological and ethnological perspectives*. Plenum: New York.

Carruthers, W. 2013. Records of dispossession: Archival thinking and UNESCO's Nubian Campaign in Egypt and Sudan. *International Journal of Islamic Architecture* 9:287–314.

Cashdan, E. 1984. Territoriality among human foragers: Ecological models and an application to four Bushmen groups. *Current Anthropology* 24:47–66.

Chami, F. 1998. A review of Swahili archaeology. *African Archaeological Review* 15 (3): 199–218.

Chami, F. 2006. The archaeology of Pre-Islamic Kilwa Kisiwani (Island). In *The African archaeology network: Research in progress*, ed. J. Kinahan and J. Kinahan, 119–150. Dar es Salaam: Dar es Salaam University Press.

Chami, F., and A. Kwekason. 2003. Neolithic pottery traditions from the islands, coast and the interior of East Africa. *African Archaeological Review* 20:65–80.

Childs, S. T. 1991. Style, technology, and iron smelting furnaces in Bantu-speaking Africa. *Journal of Anthropological Archaeology* 10 (4): 332–359.

Childs, S. T., and E. Herbert. 2005. Metallurgy and its consequences. In *African Archaeology: A critical introduction*, ed. A. B. Stahl, 276–300. Oxford: Blackwell.

Childs, S. T., and D. Killick. 1993. Indigenous African Metallurgy: Nature and culture. *Annual Review of Anthropology* 22:317–337.

Chirikure, S. 2014. Land and sea links: 1500 years of connectivity between southern Africa and the Indian Ocean rim regions, AD 700 to 1700. *African Archaeological Review* 31 (4): 705–724.

Chirikure, S. 2015. *Metals in past societies: A global perspective on indigenous African Metallurgy*. New York: Springer.

Chirikure, S., and G. Pwiti. 2008. Community involvement in archaeology and cultural heritage management: An assessment from case studies in southern Africa and elsewhere. *Current Anthropology* 49 (3): 467–485.

Chirikure, S., and T. Rehren. 2006. Iron smelting in pre-colonial Zimbabwe: Evidence for diachronic change from Swart Village and Baranda, northern Zimbabwe. *Journal of African Archaeology* 4 (1): 37–54.

Chittick, H. N. 1965. The "Shirazi" colonization of East Africa. *Journal of African History* 6:275–294.

Chittick, H. N. 1974. *Kilwa: An Islamic trading city on the East African coast*. Nairobi: British Institute in Eastern Africa.

Clist, B.-O. 1987. A critical reappraisal of the chronological framework of the Early Iron Age Urewe Industry. *Muntu* 6:35–62.

Collett, D., and P. T. Robertshaw. 1983. Pottery traditions of early pastoral communities in Kenya. *Azania* 18:107–125.

Conkey, M. W. T and Hastorf, C. (eds.) 1990. *The Uses of Style in Archaeology*. Cambridge: Cambridge University Press.

Coutu, A. N., G. Whitelaw, P. Le Roux, and J. Sealy. 2016. Earliest evidence for the ivory trade in southern Africa: Isotopic and ZooMS analysis of seventh–tenth century AD ivory from KwaZulu-Natal. *African Archaeological Review* 33:411–435.

Crowther, A., M. E. Prendergast, D. Q. Fuller, and N. Boivin. 2018. Subsistence mosaics, forager-farmer interactions, and the transition to food production in eastern Africa. *Quaternary International* 489:101–120.

D'Andrea, A. C., A. L. Logan, and D. J. Watson. 2006. Oil palm and prehistoric subsistence in tropical West Africa. *Journal of African Archaeology* 4 (2): 195–222.

Dale, D., and C. Z. Ashley. 2010. Kansyore hunter-fisher-gatherers: New Research from Western Kenya. *Azania: Archaeological Research in Africa* 45:24–48.

Datoo, B. A. 1974. Influence of monsoons on movement of dhows along the East African coast. *East African Geographical Review* 12:23–33.

David, N. 1983. Editorial. *African Archaeological Review* 1:1–2.

Davies, W. V. 2004. Statue of Amenhotep I. In *Sudan: Ancient treasures*, ed. D. Weslby and J. Anderson, 102–103. London: British Museum Press.

Davis, D. S., and K. Douglass. 2020. Aerial and spaceborne remote sensing in African archaeology: A review of current research and potential future avenues. *African Archaeological Review* 37 (1): 9–24.

David, N., Gavua, K., MacEachern, A. S., and Sterner, J. 1991. Ethnicity and material culture in North Cameroon. *Canadian Journal of Archaeology*15: 171–177.

De Maret, P. 1992. *Fouilles Archéologiques dans la Vallée du Haut-Lualaba, Zaïre: Kamilamba, Kikulu, et Malemba Nkulu, 1975*. Tervuren: Musée Royal de l'Afrique Centrale.

De Maret, P. 1995. Histoires de croisettes. In *Objets-signes d'Afrique*, ed. L. De Heusch, 133–145. Musée Royal de l'Afrique Centrale: Tervuren.

De Matos, D., A. C. Martins, J. C. Senna-Martinez, I. Pinto, A. G. Coelho, S. S. Ferreira, and L. Oosterbeek. 2021. Review of archaeological research in Angola. *African Archaeological Review* 38 (2): 319–344.

de V., Allen, J. 1981. Swahili culture and the nature of east coast settlement. *International Journal of African Historical Studies* 14:306–334.

DeCorse, C. R. 1992. Archaeological research at Elmina. *Archaeology in Ghana* 3:23–27.

DeCorse, C. R. 1996. Culture contact and change in West Africa. In *Aspects of African Archaeology: Papers from the 10th Congress of the Pan-African association for prehistory and related studies*, ed. G. Pwiti and R. Soper, 681–686. Harare: University of Zimbabwe Publications.

DeCorse, C. R. 2001. *An Archaeology of Elmina: Africans and European on the Gold Coast, 1400–1900*. Washington: Smithsonian Institution Press.

Delius, P., L. Chewins, and T. Forssman. 2024. Turning South African history upside down: Ivory and gold production, the Indian Ocean trading system and the shaping of southern African society, 600–1900 AD. *Journal of Southern African Studies* 50 (3): 499–520.

Denbow, J. R. 2014. *The Archaeology and Ethnography of Central Africa*. Cambridge: Cambridge University Press.

Dewey, W. J. 1985. Shona ritual axes. Insight: The Magazine of the National Gallery of Zimbabwe 1: 1-5.

Dewey, W. 1990. *Weapons for the Ancestors*. Iowa City: University of Iowa Video Production Unit.

Dewey, W. J. 1991. *Pleasing the Ancestors: The traditional art of the Shona people of Zimbabwe*. Unpublished PhD. Thesis. Bloomington: Indiana University.

Dueppen, S. 2024. Reconnecting the forest, savanna, and Sahel in West Africa: The sociopolitical implications of a long-networked past. *Journal of Archaeological Research* 33:1–68.

Dunn, R. E. 2012. *The adventures of Ibn Battuta: A Muslim traveler of the 14th century*. Berkley: University of California Press.

Ebegbulem, J. C. 2012. Corruption and leadership crisis in Africa: Nigeria in focus. *International Journal of Business and Social Science* 3 (11): 221–227.

Fagan, B. M. 1969. Excavation at Ingombe Ilede, 1960–62. In *Iron Age Cultures in Zambia*, ed. B. M. Fagan and S. G. H. Daniels, 55–161. London: Chatto and Windus.

Failer, E., M. Mutaz, and A. El Tayeb. 2006. Merowe: The largest water resources project under construction in Africa. *International Journal on Hydropower & Dams* 13 (6): 68.

Fenwick, C. 2007. Archaeology and the search for authenticity: Colonialist, nationalist, and Berberist visions of an Algerian past. In *TRAC 2007: Proceedings of the seventeenth annual theoretical roman Archaeology conference*, ed. C. Fenwick and M. Wiggins, 75–88. Oxford: Oxford Books.

Forssman, T. 2020. Southern Africa's Later Stone Age and hunter-gatherer ethnography. In *Oxford Research Encyclopedia of Anthropology*, ed. M. S. Aldenderfer. Oxford: Oxford University Press.

Forssman, T. 2022. An archaeological contribution to the Kalahari Debate from the middle Limpopo Valley, southern Africa. *Journal of Archaeological Research* 30 (3): 447–495.

Fuller, D. Q., and C. J. Stevens. 2018. Sorghum domestication and diversification: A current archaeobotanical perspective. In *Plants and People in the African Past*, ed. A. M. Mercuri, A. C. D'Andrea, R. Fornaciari, and A. Höhn, 427–452. Cham: Springer International Publishing.

Gabolde, L. 2012. Réexamen des jalons de la présence de la XVIIIe dynastie naissante à Saï. *Cahiers de Recherches de l'Institut de Papyrologie et d'Égyptologie de Lille* 29:115–137.

Gabolde, L. 2020. The Amun cult and its development in Nubia. In *The Oxford Handbook of Ancient Nubia*, ed. G. Emberling and B. Williams, 343–368. Oxford: Oxford University Press.

Garlake, P. S. 1966. *The early Islamic architecture of the East African coast*. Nairobi: Oxford University Press.

Giblin, J. 2013. Politics, ideology, and indigenous perspectives. In *The Oxford handbook of African Archaeology*, ed. P. J. Mitchell and P. J. Lane, 253–265. Oxford: Oxford University Press.

Gifford, D., G. Isaac, and C. Nelson. 1980. Evidence for predation and pastoralism at Prolonged Drift: A Pastoral Neolithic site in Kenya. *Azania* 15:57–108.

Gifford-Gonzalez, D. 1998. Gender and early pastoralists in East Africa. In *Gender in African Prehistory*, ed. S. Kent, 115–137. Walnut Creek: AltaMira Press.

Gifford-Gonzalez, D. 2011. East African pastoralism: Routes, outcomes, questions. In *People and animals in Holocene Africa: Recent advances in archaeozoology*, ed. H. Jousse and J. Lesur, 27–42. Frankfurt: Africa Magna Verlag.

Gokee, C. D. 2012. Interregional exchange and local distinction: An Archaeological view from Diouboye, Senegal, AD 1000-1400. In *Proceedings of the SAfA/PAA conference 2012*. Dakar: IFAN.

Gokee, C. D., and A. Ogundiran. 2023. The African Archaeological review turns forty: Some reflections on the past, present, and future. *African Archaeological Review* 40 (1): 1–19.

Gordon, R. J. 1992. *The Bushman myth and the making of a Namibian underclass*. Westview: Boulder.

Gosden, C., and I. Marshall. 1999. The cultural biography of objects. *World Archaeology* 31:169–178.

Gosselain, O. 1995. *Identités Techniques. Le Travail de la Poterie au Cameroun Méridional*. PhD Thesis. Brussels: University of Brussels.

Gosselain, O. 1998. Social and technical identity in a clay crystal ball. In *The Archaeology of social boundaries*, ed. M. Stark, 78–106. Washington: Smithsonian Institution Press.

Gosselain, O. 2000. Materializing identities: An African perspective. *Journal of Archaeological Method and Theory* 7:187–217.

Gosselain, O. 2008. Inherited and transformed traditions in southwestern Niger. In *Cultural transmission and material culture: Breaking down boundaries*, ed. M. T. Stark, B. J. Bowser, and L. Horne, 150–177. Tucson: University of Arizona Press.

Grenlee, W. B. 1938. *The Voyage of Pedro Álvares Cabral to Brazil and India: From contemporary documents and narratives*. New Delhi: Asian Education Services.

Grillo, K. M., and E. A. Hildebrand. 2013. The context of early megalithic architecture in eastern Africa: The Turkana Basin c. 5000–4000 BP. *Azania: Archaeological Research in Africa* 48:193–217.

Grzymski, K. 2010. The 1989–1992 Merowe Dam feasibility study, an Archaeological perspective. In *Proceedings of the international conference 'The fourth Cataract Archaeological Salvage project 1996–2009'. Gdańsk, 2–4 July, 2009*, ed. H. Paner, S. Jakobielski, and J. R. Anderson, 67–70. Gdańsk: Gdańsk Archaeological Museum and Heritage Protection Fund African Reports 7.

Hall, M. 1990. Hidden history: Iron Age archaeology in Southern Africa. In *A history of African Archaeology*, ed. P. Robertshaw, 59–77. London: James Currey Ltd.

Handler, J.S. and Lange, F.W., 2006. On interpreting slave status from archaeological remains. *The African Diaspora Archaeology Newsletter*, June.

Haour, A. 2013. *Outsiders and strangers: An archaeology of liminality in West Africa*. Oxford: Oxford University Press.

Haour, A., and A. Christie. 2019. Cowries in the archaeology of West Africa: The present picture. *Azania: Archaeological Research in Africa* 54 (3): 287–321.

Hassan, F. A. 1999. African archaeology: The call of the future. *African Affairs* 98 (392): 393–406.

Haviland, W. A. 1990. *Cultural Anthropology*. Sixth ed. New York: Holt, Rinehart, and Winston.

Hegmon, M. 1992. Archaeological research on style. *Annual Review of Anthropology*21: 517–36.

Hegmon, M. 1998. Technology, style and social practices: archaeological approaches. In: Stark, M. (ed.), *The Archaeology of Social Boundaries*. Washington, DC: Smithsonian Institution Press, pp. 264–79.

Helm, R. M. 2000. *Conflicting histories: The archaeology of the iron-working, farming communities in the central and southern coast region of Kenya*. PhD Thesis. Bristol: University of Bristol.

Herbert, E. W. 1984. *Red gold of Africa: Copper in precolonial history and culture*. Madison: University of Wisconsin Press.

Herbert, E. W. 1993. *Iron, gender, and power: Rituals of transformation in African societies*. Bloomington: Indiana University Press.

Hildebrand, E. A., and K. M. Grillo. 2012. Early herders and monumental sites in eastern Africa: Dating and interpretation. *Antiquity* 86:338–352.

Hildyard, N. 2008. Neutral? Against what? Bystanders and human rights abuses: The case of Merowe Dam. *Sudan Studies* 37:19–38.

Hitchcock, R. K. 2012. The contributions of Richard B. Lee to anthropology, ethnoarchaeology, and Indigenous peoples' studies. *Classics Review* 4:226–260.

Hodder, I. 1982. *Symbols in Actions: Ethnoarchaeological studies of material culture*. Cambridge: University Press, Cambridge.

Hodder, I. 1999. *Archaeological process. An introduction*. Oxford: Blackwell.

Hodder, I. 2003. Archaeological reflexivity and the "local" voice. *Anthropological Quarterly* 76:55–69.

Holl, A. F. C. 1985. Background to the Ghana Empire: Archaeological investigations on the transition to statehood in the Dhar Tichitt region (Mauritania). *Journal of Anthropological Archaeology* 4:73–115.

Holl, A. F. C. 1990. West African archaeology: colonialism and nationalism. In *A history of African Archaeology*, ed. P. Robertshaw, 296–308. Oxford: James Currey Ltd.

Holl, A. F. C. 1993. Late Neolithic cultural landscape in southeastern Mauritania: An essay in spatiometrics. In *Spatial boundaries and social dynamics*, ed. A. F. C. Holl and T. A. Levy, 95–133. New York: Berghahn Books.

Holl, A. F. C. 1998. Livestock husbandry, pastoralisms, and territoriality: The West African record. *Journal of Anthropological Archaeology* 17 (2): 143–165.

Holl, A. F. C. 2006a. *West African early towns: Archaeology of households in urban landscapes*. Ann Arbor: University of Michigan Museum of Anthropology.

Holl, A. F. C. 2006b. *West African early towns: Archaeology of households in Urban landscapes*. Ann Arbor: University of Michigan Press.

Holl, A. F. C. 2009. Coping with uncertainty: Neolithic life in the Dhar Tichitt-Walata, Mauritania, (ca. 4000–2300 BP). *Comptes Rendus. Géoscience* 341 (8–9): 703–712.

Horton, M. 1996. *Shanga: The archaeology of a Muslim trading community on the coast of East Africa.* Nairobi: British Institute in Eastern Africa.

Horton, M. C. 2017. Islamic architecture of the Swahili coast. In *The Swahili World*, ed. S. Wynne-Jones and A. LaViolette, 487–499. New York: Routledge.

Horton, M. C., N. Boivin, and A. Crowther. 2021. Eastern Africa and the early Indian Ocean: Understanding mobility in a globalising world. *Journal of Egyptian History* 13 (1–2): 380–408.

Horton, M. C., and J. Middleton. 2000. *The Swahili: The social landscape of a mercantile society.* London: Blackwell.

Horton, M. C., and N. Mudida. 1993. Exploitation of maritime resources: Evidence for the origins of the Swahili communities of East Africa. In *The Archaeology of Africa: Food, metals and towns*, ed. T. Shaw, P. J. J. Sinclair, B. Andah, and A. Okpoko, 673–693. London: Routledge.

Horton, M. C., J. Olsen, J. Fleisher, and S. Wynne-Jones. 2022. The Chronology of Kilwa Kisiwani, AD 800–1500. *African Archaeological Review* 39 (2): 143–166.

Hoskins, J. 1998. *Biographical objects: How things tell the story of people's lives.* London: Routledge.

Huffman, T. N. 2007. *A Handbook to the Iron Age: The archaeology of pre-colonial societies of southern Africa.* Pietermaritzburg: University of KwaZulu-Natal Press.

Huffman, T. N. 2015a. Mapela, Mapungubwe and the origins of states in southern Africa. *South African Archaeological Bulletin* 70:15–27.

Huffman, T. N. 2015b. Settlements and culture: Cognitive models in African prehistory. In *Theory in Africa, Africa in Theory*, ed. S. Wynne-Jones and J. Fleisher, 111–136. London: Routledge.

Ichumbaki, E. B., and E. mitche. 2019. Valuing the Swahili cultural heritage: A maritime cultural ecosystem services study from Kilwa, Tanzania. *Conservation and Management of Archaeological Sites* 21 (4): 230–255.

Inskeep, R. R. 1961. The present state of archaeology in South Africa. *South African Museums Association Bulletin* 7:225–227.

Insoll, T. 1996. The archaeology of Islam in sub-Saharan Africa: A review. *Journal of World Prehistory* 10 (4): 439–504.

Jolly, P. 1996. Symbiotic interaction between black farmers and south-eastern San: Implications for southern African rock art studies, ethnographic analogy, and hunter-gatherer cultural identity. *Current Anthropology* 37 (2): 277–305.

Kaps, K., and A. Komlosy. 2013. Centers and peripheries revisited: Polycentric connections or entangled hierarchies? *Review (Fernand Braudel Center)* 36 (3–4): 237–264.

Karega-Munene, J. 2002. *Holocene foragers, fishers and herders of Western Kenya.* Oxford: British Archaeological Reports International Series.

Kelly, K. 1997. The archaeology of African-European interaction: Investigating the social roles of trade, traders and the use of space in the seventeenth and eighteenth century Huéda Kingdom, Republic of Bénin. *World Archaeology* 28:351–369.

Kent, S. 1992. The current forager controversy: Real versus ideal views of hunter-gatherers. *Man* 27:45–70.

Kessy, E. T. 1997. Archaeological site survey from Kisuji to Dar es Salaam. *Nyame Akuma* 48:57–69.

Killick, D. 2016. A global perspective on the pyrotechnologies of sub-Saharan Africa. *Azania: Archaeological Research in Africa* 51 (1): 62–87.

Killick, D. J. 2009. Cairo to Cape: The spread of metallurgy through eastern and southern Africa. *Journal of World Prehistory* 22:399–414.

Kirkman, J. S. 1966. *Ungwana on the Tana.* The Hague: Mouton.

Kleinitz, C., and C. Näser. 2011. The loss of innocence: Political and ethical dimensions of the Merowe Dam Archaeological Salvage Project at the Fourth Nile Cataract (Sudan). *Conservation and Management of Archaeological Sites* 13 (2–3): 253–280.

Kuper, A. 1992. Post-modernism, Cambridge and the great Kalahari debate. *Social Anthropology* 1 (1a): 57–71.

Kusimba, C. M. 1993. *The Archaeology and Ethnography of Iron Metallurgy on the Kenya coast.* PhD Thesis. Bryn Mawr College, Bryn Mawr.

Kusimba, C. M. 1999. *The rise and fall of Swahili States*. Walnut Creek: AltaMira Press.
Kusimba, C.M. and Kusimba, S.B., 2005. Mosaics and interactions: East Africa, 2000 BP to the present. African archaeology*:* A critical introduction, 392–419.
Kusimba, C. M., and Kusimba, S. B., 2017. Mosaics: Rethinking African connections in coastal and hinterland Kenya. In *The Swahili World*, ed. S. Wynne-Jones and A. LaViolette, 403–418. London: Routledge.
Laforgue, P. 1924. Une station préhistorique dans le secteur nomade de Tichitt. *Bulletin De La Société De Géographie Et D'archéologie D'oran* 44 (3–4): 267–279.
Laforgue, P., and R. Mauny. 1939. Contribution à la préhistoire de la région de Tichitt. *Bulletin de l'Institut Francais de l'Afrique Noire, série B* 1 (4): 691–696.
Lane, P. J. 2004. The 'moving frontier' and the transition to food production in Kenya. *Azania: Archaeological Research in Africa* 39 (1): 243–264.
Lane, P. J. 2011a. Trajectories to pastoralism in northern and central Kenya: An overview of the archaeological and environmental evidence. In *Pastoralism in Africa: Past, present and future*, ed. M. Bollig, M. Schnegg, and H.-P. Wotzka, 105–143. Oxford: Berghahn Books.
Lane, P. J. 2011b. Possibilities for a postcolonial archaeology in sub-Saharan Africa: Indigenous and usable pasts. *World Archaeology* 43 (1): 7–25.
Lane, P. J. 2021. Recent approaches to the archaeological investigation of slavery in Africa. In *The Archaeology of slavery in early medieval Northern Europe*, ed. F. Biermann and M. Jankowiak, 23–39. Cham: Springer International Publishing.
Lane, P. J., C. Ashley, O. Seitsonen, P. Harvey, S. Mire, and F. Odede. 2007. The transition to farming in eastern Africa: New faunal and dating evidence from Wadh Lang'o and Usenge, Kenya. *Antiquity* 81:62–81.
LaViolette, A., W. B. Fawcett, N. J. Karoma, and P. R. Schmidt. 1989. The coast and the hinterland: University of Dar es Salaam archaeological field schools, 1987–88. *Nyame Akuma* 32:38–46.
LaViolette, A., W. B. Fawcett, N. J. Karoma, and P. R. Schmidt. 1999. Survey and excavations between Dar es Salaam and Bagamoyo: University of Dar es Salaam archaeological field school 1988 (Part II). *Nyame Akuma* 52:74–78.
LaViolette, A., and J. Fleisher. 2005. The archaeology of sub-Saharan urbanism: Cities and their countrysides. In *African Archaeology: A critical introduction*, ed. A. B. Stahl, 327–353. Malden: Blackwell.
Leacock, E., and R. B. Lee. 1982. Introduction. In *Politics and history in band society*, ed. E. Leacock and R. B. Lee, 1–21. Cambridge: Cambridge University Press.
Leakey, M. D., W. E. Owen, and L. S. B. Leakey. 1948. *Dimple-based pottery from Central Kavirondo, Kenya Colony*. Nairobi: Coryndon Memorial Museum Nairobi.
Leclant, J., 1990. *Rapport sur une mission de l'UNESCO pour l'etude archeologique de la zone de la IVe cataracte du Nil*. Unpublished report to UNESCO.
Lee, R. B. 1979. *The! Kung San: Men, women and work in a foraging society*. Cambridge: Cambridge University Press.
Lee, R. B., and I. DeVore, eds. 1968. *Man the hunter: The first intensive survey of a single, crucial stage of human development - man's once universal hunting way of life*. Chicago: Aldine Publishing.
Lee, R. B., and M. G. Guenther. 1991. Oxen or onions? The search for trade (and truth) in the Kalahari. *Current Anthropology* 32:592–601.
Lee, R. B., and M. G. Guenther. 1995. Errors corrected or compounded? A reply to Wilmsen. *Current Anthropology* 36:298–235.
Lemos, R. 2020. Material culture and colonization in ancient Nubia: Evidence from the New Kingdom cemeteries. In *Encyclopedia of Global Archaeology*, ed. C. Smith, 6812–6836. Chame: Springer International Publishing.
Lemos, R. 2022. Can we decolonize the ancient past? Bridging postcolonial and decolonial theory in Sudanese and Nubian Archaeology. *Cambridge Archaeological Journal* 33 (1): 19–37.
Leroi-Gourhain, A. 1965. *Le Geste et la Parole*. Second. Paris: Albin Michel.

Lewis-Williams, J. D. 1993. Southern African Archaeology in the 1990s. *South African Archaeological Bulletin* 48:45–40.
Linares-Matás, G. J. 2022. Spatial organization and socio-economic differentiation at the Dhar Tichitt Center of Dakhlet el Atrouss I (southeastern Mauritania). *African Archaeological Review* 39 (2): 167–188.
Lombard, M., M. V. Caruana, J. van der Walt, and A. Högberg. 2020. The Keimoes 3 desert kite site, South Africa: An aerial lidar and micro-topographic exploration. *Antiquity* 94 (373): 197–211.
Luke, C., and L. Meskell. 2023. New deals for the past: The Cold War, American archaeology, and UNESCO in Egypt and Syria. *History and Anthropology* 34 (2): 194–214.
MacDonald, K. C. 1998. Before the Empire of Ghana: Pastoralism and the origins of cultural complexity in the Sahel. In *Transformations in Africa: Essays on Africa's later past*, ed. G. Connah, 71–103. London: Leicester University Press.
MacDonald, K. C. 2011a. A view from the South. In *Money, trade and trade routes in pre-Islamic North Africa*, ed. A. Dowler and E. R. Galvin, 72–82. London: British Museum Press.
MacDonald, K. C. 2011b. Betwixt Tichitt and the IND: The pottery of the Faita Facies, Tichitt Tradition. *Azania: Archaeological Research in Africa* 46:49–69.
MacDonald, K. C. 2015. The Tichitt tradition in the West African Sahel. In *The Cambridge World History: A world with agriculture (12000 BCE - 500 CE)*, ed. G. Barker and C. Goucher, 499–513. Cambridge: Cambridge University Press.
MacEachern, S., 1998. Scale, style, and cultural variation: Technological traditions in the northern Mandara Mountains. In: Stark, M. (ed.), *The Archaeology of Social Boundaries*. Washington, DC: Smithsonian Institution Press, pp.107–131.
Maddy-Weitzman, B. 2006. Ethno-politics and globalisation in North Africa: The Berber culture movement. *Journal of North African Studies* 11 (1): 71–84.
Maggs, T. 2000. African naissance: An introduction. *South African Archaeological Society Goodwin Series* 8:1–3.
Mapunda, B. B. 1991. The role of archaeology in development: The case of Tanzania. *TransAfrican Journal of History* 20:19–34.
Marean, C. 1992. Hunter to herder: Large mammal remains form the hunter-gatherer occupation at Enkapune ya Muto rockshelter. *African Archaeological Review* 10:65–127.
Marshall, F. 1991. Appendix II - Mammalian fauna from Gogo Falls. *Azania* 26:175–179.
Marshall, F. 1994. Archaeological perspectives on East African pastoralism. In *African pastoralist systems*, ed. E. Fratkin, K. A. Galvin, and E. A. Roth, 17–43. Lynne Reinner: Boulder.
Marshall, F., K. M. Grillo, and L. Arco. 2011. Prehistoric pastoralists and social responses to climatic risk in East Africa. In *Sustainable Lifeways: Cultural persistence in an ever-changing environment*, ed. N. F. Miller, K. M. Moore, and K. Ryan, 39–74. Philadelphia: University of Pennsylvania Press.
Martin, P. M. 1972. *The external trade of the Loango Coast, 1576–1870*. Oxford: Oxford University Press.
Mattingly, D. J. 1996. From one colonialism to another: Imperialism and the Maghreb. In *Roman imperialism: Post-colonial perspectives*, ed. J. Webster and N. Cooper, 49–69. Leicester: Leicester University Press.
Mauny, R. 1951. Du nouveau sur la préhistoire et l'archéologie de l'Aouker et du Hodh (Mauritanie). *Bulletin de la Société Préhistorique de France* 48 (1/2): 78–83.
Mazel, A.D., 1987. The archaeological past from the changing present: Towards a critical assessment of South African Later Stone Age studies from the early 1960s to the early 1980. *In*: J. Parkington and M. Hall, eds. Papers in the Prehistory of the Western Cape, South Africa. Oxford: British Archaeological Reports International Series, 504–529.
Mazel, A. D. 1989. People making history: The last ten thousand years of hunter-gatherer communities in the Thukela Basin. *Southern African Humanities* 1 (07): 1–168.
Mbeki, L., L. M. Kootker, H. Kars, and G. R. Davies. 2017. Sickly slaves, soldiers and sailors: Contextualising the Cape's 18th–19th century green point burials through isotope investigation. *Journal of Archaeological Science: Reports* 11:480–490.

McDonald, K., P. Bosshard, and N. Brewer. 2009. Exporting dams: China's hydropower industry goes global. *Journal of Environmental Management* 90:S294–S302.

McDougall, J. 2006. *History and the Culture of Nationalism in Algeria.* Cambridge: Cambridge University Press.

McGranaghan, M. 2017. Ethnographic analogy in archaeology: Methodological insights from southern Africa. In *Oxford research encyclopedia of African History*, ed. T. Spear. Oxford: Oxford University Press.

McIntosh, R. J. 1998. *The peoples of the Middle Niger*. Oxford: Blackwells.

McIntosh, R. J. 2015. Different cities: Jenne-jeno and African urbanism. In *The Cambridge World history*, ed. N. Yoffee, 364–380. Cambridge: Cambridge University Press.

McIntosh, R. J. 2021. Urbanization in the Middle Niger of Mali. In *Oxford research encyclopedia of Anthropology*, ed. T. Spear. Oxford: Oxford University Press.

McIntosh, S. K. 1994. Changing perceptions of West Africa's past: Archaeological research since 1988. *Journal of Archaeological Research* 2:165–198.

McIntosh, S. K. 1999. Modeling political organization in large-scale settlement clusters: A case study from the Inland Niger delta, Mali. In *Beyond chiefdoms: Pathways to complexity in Africa*, ed. S. K. McIntosh, 66–79. Cambridge: Cambridge University Press.

McIntosh, S. K. 2020. Long-distance exchange and urban trajectories in the first millennium AD: Case studies from the Middle Niger and Middle Senegal River valleys. In *Urbanisation and State formation in the ancient Sahara and Beyond*, ed. M. Sterry and D. Mattingly, 521–563. Cambridge: Cambridge University Press.

McIntosh, S. K. 2024. Africa, west: Villages, cities, and early states. In *Encyclopedia of Archaeology*, ed. E. Nikita and T. Rehren, 144–158. Oxford: Academic.

McIntosh, S. K., and R. J. McIntosh. 1981. West African prehistory. *American Scientist* 69:602–613.

McIntosh, S. K., and R. J. McIntosh. 1984. The early city in West Africa: Towards an understanding. *African Archaeological Review* 2 (1): 73–98.

McIntosh, S. K., and R. J. McIntosh. 1988. From stone to metal: New perspectives on the Later Prehistory of West Africa. *Journal of World Prehistory* 2:89–133.

McIntosh, S. K., and R. J. McIntosh. 1993. Cities without citadels: Understanding urban origins alng the middle Niger. In *The Archaeology of Africa: Food, metals and towns*, ed. T. Shaw, P. J. J. Sinclair, B. Andah, and A. Okpoko, 622–641. London: Routledge.

McIntosh, S. K., and R. J. McIntosh. 1995. Background to the 1981 research. In *Excavations at Jenne-Jeno, Hambarketolo and Kaniana: The 1981 season*, ed. S. K. McIntosh, 1–26. Berkley: University of California Press.

Miller, D. E., and N. J. Van Der Merwe. 1994. Early metal working in sub-Saharan Africa: A review of recent research. *Journal of African History* 35 (1): 1–36.

Mitchell, P. J. 2005a. *African Connections: An archaeological perspective on Africa and the wider world*. Oxford: AltaMira Press.

Mitchell, P., I. Plug, G. Bailey, and S. Woodborne. 2008. Bringing the Kalahari debate to the mountains: Late first millennium AD hunter-gatherer/farmer interaction in highland Lesotho. *Before Farming* 2008 (2): 1–22.

Mitchell, P. J. 2003. Anyone for hxaro? Thoughts on the theory and practice of exchange in Southern African Later Stone Age archaeology. In *Researching Africa's past: New perspectives from British Archaeology*, ed. P. J. Mitchell, A. Haour, and J. Hobart, 35–43. Oxford: Oxbow Books.

Mitchell, P. J. 2005b. Why hunter-gatherer archaeology matters: A personal perspective on renaissance and renewal in southern African Later Stone Age research. *South African Archaeological Bulletin* 60 (182): 64–71.

Mitchell, P. J., E. Loftus, and A. B. Babalola. 2024. Archaeological science in Africa: Twenty-one papers for the twenty-first century. *Journal of Archaeological Science* 163:105933.

Mitchell, P. J., and J. Seneši. 2023. Trends in Southern African archaeology 1980-2019: Changing publication patterns in the 'South African Archaeological Bulletin'. *South African Archaeological Bulletin* 77:127–139.

Mlambo, D. N., M. A. Mubecua, and V. H. Mlambo. 2023. Post-colonial independence and Africa's corruption conundrum: A succinct South African critique post-democratisation. *Insight on Africa* 15 (2): 184–202.

Monroe, J. C. 2013. Power and agency in precolonial African states. *Annual Review of Anthropology* 42:17–35.

Morgan, L. H. 1982. *Ancient society*. Calcutta: K. P. Bagchi & Company.

Munson, P. J. 1971. *The Tichitt Tradition: A late prehistoric occupation of the southwestern Sahara.* Champaign: University of Illinois at Urbana-Champaign.

Murdock, G. 1968. The current status of the world's hunting and gathering peoples. In *Man the Hunter: The first litensive survey of a single, crucial stage of human development— man's once universal hunting way of life*, ed. R. B. Lee and I. DeVore, 13–20. Chicago: Aldine Publishing.

Nelson, C. M. 1995. The work of the Koobi Fora Field School at the Jarigole Pillar site. *Kenya Past and Present* 27:49–63.

Nikis, N., and A. Livingstone Smith. 2017. Copper, trade and polities: Exchange networks in southern central Africa in the 2nd Millennium CE. *Journal of Southern African Studies* 43 (5): 895–911.

Nurse, D., and T. J. Hinnebusch. 1993. *Swahili and Sabaki: A linguistic history*. Berkley: University of California Press.

Nurse, D., and T. Spear. 1985. *The Swahili: Reconstructing the history and language of an African society AD 800–1500.* Philadelphia: University of Pennsylvania Press.

Padilla-Iglesias, C., L. M. Atmore, J. Olivero, K. Lupo, A. Manica, E. Arango Isaza, L. Vinicius, and A. B. Migliano. 2022. Population interconnectivity over the past 120,000 years explains distribution and diversity of Central African hunter-gatherers. *Proceedings of the National Academy of Sciences* 119 (21): e2113936119.

Parkington, J. E. 1984. Soaqua and Bushmen: Hunters and robbers. In *Past and Present in Hunter-Gatherer Studies*, ed. C. Schrire, 151–174. New York: Academic.

Pearce, D. G. 2012. Ethnography and history: the significance of social change in interpreting rock art. In *Working with Rock Art: Recording, presenting and understanding rock art using indigenous knowledge*, ed. B. W. Smith, Helskog, and D. Morris, 135–145. Johannesburg: Wits University Press.

Phillipson, D. W. 1989. Editorial: The ethnographic present is past. *African Archaeological Review* 7:1.

Pikirayi, I. 2015. The future of archaeology in Africa. *Antiquity* 89 (345): 531–541.

Pollard, E., R. Bates, J.-C. Comte, E. Graham, C. Lubao, N. Munisi, and E. B. Ichumbaki. 2025. Climate change, coastal heritage digitization, and local community engagement at the ruins of Kilwa Kisiwani World Heritage Site, Tanzania. *Journal of Field Archaeology* 50 (1): 6–21.

Pollard, E., J. Fleisher, and S. Wynne-Jones. 2012. Beyond the stone town: Maritime architecture at fourteenth–fifteenth century Songo Mnara, Tanzania. *Journal of Maritime Archaeology* 7 (1): 43–62.

Pollard, E. J. 2008a. The maritime landscape of Kilwa Kisiwani and its region, Tanzania, 11th to 15th century AD. *Journal of Anthropological Archaeology* 27 (3): 265–280.

Pollard, E. J. 2008b. The maritime landscape of Kilwa Kisiwani and its region, Tanzania, 11th to 15th century AD. *Journal of Anthropological Archaeology* 27:265–280.

Posnansky, M. 2017. Archaeology and the local community in Africa: A retrospective. *Journal of Community Archaeology & Heritage* 4 (2): 77–84.

Prendergast, M. E. 2010. Kansyore sher-foragers and transitions to food production in East Africa: The view from Wadh Lang'o, Nyanza Province, Western Kenya. *Azania: Archaeological Research in Africa* 45:83–111.

Prendergast, M. E. 2020. The history of Eastern African foragers. In *Oxford research encyclopedia of African history*, ed. T. Spear. Oxford: Oxford University Press.

Prendergast, M. E., K. Grillo, A. Z. Mabulla, and H. Wang. 2014. New dates for Kansyore and Pastoral Neolithic ceramics in the Eyasi Basin, Tanzania. *Journal of African Archaeology* 12:89–98.

Purdy, J. M. 2024. The Great Mosque of Kilwa: An architectural lodestone. In *The Routledge companion to global renaissance art*, ed. S. Campbell and S. Porras, 657–676. New York: Routledge.

Robbins, L. H., A. C. Campbell, M. L. Murphy, G. A. Brook, F. Liang, S. A. Skaggs, P. Srivastava, A. A. Mabuse, and S. Badenhorst. 2008. Recent archaeological research at Toteng, Botswana: Early domesticated livestock in the Kalahari. *Journal of African Archaeology* 6:131–149.

Robertshaw, P. 1990. A history of African Archaeology: An introduction. In *A history of African Archaeology*, ed. P. Robertshaw, 3–12. Oxford: James Currey Ltd.

Robertshaw, P. 2021. Archaeology of early pastoralism in East Africa. In *Oxford research encyclopedia of African history*, ed. T. Spear. Oxford: Oxford University Press.

Robertshaw, P. T. 1991. Gogo Falls: A complex site east of Lake Victoria. *Azania* 26:63–195.

Robins, S. 2001. NGOs, 'Bushmen' and double vision: The Khomani San land claim and the cultural politics of 'community' and 'development' in the Kalahari. *Journal of Southern African Studies* 27:833–853.

Rocheleau, C. M. 2008. *Amun Temples in Nubia: A typological study of New Kingdom, Napatan and Meroitic temples*. Oxford: Archaeopress.

Rüther, H., and G. Palumbo. 2012. 3D laser scanning for site monitoring and conservation in Lalibela World Heritage Site, Ethiopia. *International Journal of Heritage in the Digital Era* 1:217–232.

Sadr, K. 1997. Kalahari archaeology and the Bushman debate. *Current Anthropology* 38 (1): 104–112.

Sadr, K. 2003. The Neolithic of Southern Africa. *Journal of African History* 44 (2): 195–209.

Sadr, K. 2015. Livestock first reached Southern Africa in two separate events. *PLoS One* 10 (8): e0134215.

Sahlins, M. 1972. *Stone Age Economics*. Chicago: Aldine Publishing.

Samuels, K. L. 2009. Trajectories of development: International heritage management of archaeology in the Middle East and North Africa. *Archaeologies: Journal of World Archaeological Congress* 5:68–91.

Schmidt, P. R. 2009. *Postcolonial archaeologies in Africa*. Santa Fe: School for Advanced Research Press.

Schmidt, P. R., and K. W. Arthur. 2018. Community-based approaches to African history. In *Oxford research encyclopedia of African history*, ed. T. Spear. Oxford: Oxford University Press.

Schmidt, P. R., and B. B. Mapunda. 1997. Ideology and the archaeological record in Africa: Interpreting symbolism in iron smelting technology. *Journal of Anthropological Archaeology* 16 (1): 73–102.

Schrire, C. 1980. An inquiry into the evolutionary status and apparent identity of San hunter-gatherers. *Human Ecology* 8:9–32.

Schrire, C., ed. 1984a. *Past and present in hunter gatherer studies*. New York: Academic.

Schrire, C. 1984b. Wild surmises on savage thoughts. In *Past and present in hunter-gatherer studies*, ed. C. Schrire, 1–25. Orlando: Academic.

Schrire, C. 1990. Excavating archives at Oudepost 1. *Cape. Social Dynamics* 16 (1): 11–21.

Segobye, A. 2006. Divided commons: The political economy of southern Africa's cultural heritage landscapes observations of the Central Kalahari Game Reserve, Botswana. *Archaeologies* 2:52–72.

Segré, C. G. 1974. *Fourth shore: The Italian colonization of Libya*. Chicago: Chicago University Press.

Seitsonen, O. 2010. Lithics use at Kansyore sites in East Africa: Technological organisation at four recently excavated sites in Nyanza Province, Kenya. *Azania: Archaeological Research in Africa* 45:49–82.

Shaw, T. 1989. African Archaeology: Looking back and looking forward. *African Archaeological Review* 7 (1): 3–31.

Shennan, S. J. 1989. Introduction. In: Shennan, S. J. (ed.), Archaeological Approaches to Cultural Identity. London: Unwin Hyman, pp. 1-32.

Shepherd, N. 2002. The politics of archaeology in Africa. *Annual Review of Anthropology* 31:189–209.

Sietsonen, O. 2010. Lithics use at Kansyore sites in East Africa: Technological organisation at four recently excavated sites in Nyanza Province, Kenya. *Azania: Archaeological Research in Africa* 45:49–82.

Silberbauer, G. B. 1981. *Hunter and habitat in the Central Kalahari Desert*. Cambridge: Cambridge University Press.

Smith, S. T. 2003. *Wretched kush: Ethnic identities and boundaries in the Egyptian Nubian empire*. London: Routledge.

Solway, J. S., and R. B. Lee. 1990. Foragers, genuine or spurious? Situating the Kalahari San in history. *Current Anthropology* 31 (2): 109–146.

Stahl, A. B. 2009. The archaeology of African history. *International Journal of African Historical Studies* 42 (2): 241–255.

Stahl, A. B. 2014. Africa in the world: (Re)centering African history through archaeology. *Journal of Anthropological Research* 70 (1): 5–33.

Stein, G. 1999. *Rethinking World-Systems: Diasporas, colonies and interaction in Uruk Mesopotamia*. Tucson: University of Arizona Press.

Steindorff, G. 1937. *Aniba II*. Glückstadt: J.J. Augustin.

Stewart, K. A. 1993. Iron Age ceramic studies in Great Lakes eastern Africa: A critical and historiographical review. *African Archaeological Review* 11 (1): 21–37.

Stump, D. S. 2010. Ancient and backward or long-lived and sustainable: the role of the past in developmental debates in eastern Africa. *World Development* 38 (9): 1251–1262.

Sulas, F., and I. Pikirayi. 2020. From centre-periphery models to textured urban landscapes: Comparative perspectives from sub-Saharan Africa. *Journal of Urban Archaeology* 1:67–83.

Sutton, J. 2018. The East African coast: Researching its history and archaeology. In *The Swahili World*, ed. S. Wynne-Jones and A. LaViolette, 53–66. London: Routledge.

Swan, L. M. 2007. Economic and ideological roles of copper ingots in prehistoric Zimbabwe. *Antiquity* 81 (314): 999–1012.

Sylvain, R. 2015. Foragers and fictions in the Kalahari: Indigenous identities and the politics of deconstruction. *Anthropological Theory* 15 (2): 158–178.

Tanaka, J. 1980. *The San Hunter-Gatherers of the Kalahari*. Tokyo: University of Tokyo Press.

Thill, F. 2017. The 'pyramid' of Sai: State of research. In *Nubia in the New Kingdom: Lived experience, pharaonic control and indigenous traditions*, ed. N. Spencer, A. Stevens, and M. Binder, 193–211. Leuven: Peeters.

Thomas, D. S. G., and D. Sporton. 2002. Sustainable livelihoods in Kalahari environments: A contribution to global debates. In *Sustainable Livelihoods in Kalahari Environments: Contributions to global debates*, ed. D. Sporton and D. S. G. Thomas, 1–20. Oxford: Oxford University Press.

Thomas, E. M. 1959. *The Harmless People*. New York: Alfred Knopf.

Thondhlana, T. P., E. C. Lyaya, and E. Mtetwa. 2022. The politics of knowledge production: Training and practice of archaeological science in Africa. *African Archaeological Review* 39:461–477.

Tixier, J. 1967. Procédés d'analyse et questions de terminologie concernant l'étude des ensembles industriels du Paléolithique récent et de l'Epipaléolithique dans l'Afrique du Nord-Ouest. In *Background to Evolution in Africa*, ed. W. W. Bishop and J. D. Clark, 771–820. Chicago: Chicago University Press.

Togola, T. 1996. Iron Age occupation in the Méma Region, Mali. *African Archaeological Review* 13:91–110.

Trigger, B. G. 1990. The history of African Archaeology in world perspective. In *A history of African Archaeology*, ed. P. Robertshaw, 303–319. Oxford: James Currey Ltd.

Trigger, B. G. 2003. *Understanding early civilizations: A comparative study*. Cambridge: Cambridge University Press.

Ucko, P. J. 1990. *Academic freedom and apartheid: The story of the World Archaeological Congress*. London: Duckworth.

Van Doornum, B. L. 2005. *Changing places, spaces and identity in the Shashe Limpopo region of Limpopo Province, South Africa.* PhD Thesis. University of the Witwatersrand.
Van Grunderbeek, M.-C. 1992. Chronologie de l'age du fer ancient au Burundi, au Rwanda et dans la région des grandos lacs. *Azania* 27:53–80.
Van Pelt, W. P. 2013. Revising Egypto-Nubian relations in New Kingdom Lower Nubia: From Egyptianization to cultural entanglement. *Cambridge Archaeological Journal* 23:523–550.
Vansina, J. 1990. *Paths in the Rainforests: Toward a history of political tradition in Equatorial Africa.* London: James Currey Ltd.
Vansina, J. 2004. *How Societies are Born: Governance in West Central Africa before 1600.* Charlottesville: University of Virginia Press.
Verneau, R. 1920. Nouveaux documents sur l'ethnographie ancienne de la Mauritanie. *L'Anthropologie* 30 (3): 323–368.
Wadley, L. 1987. *Later Stone Age hunters and gatherers of the southern Transvaal.* Oxford: British Archaeological Reports.
Wallerstein, I. M. 2004. *World-Systems Analysis: An introduction.* Durham: Duke University Press.
Wandibba, S. 1980. The application of attribute analysis to the study of Later Stone Age/Neolithic pottery ceramics in Kenya (summary). In *Proceedings of the 8th Panafrican Congress of prehistory and quaternary studies, Nairobi, 5 to 10 September 1977*, ed. L. S. B. Leakey and B. Ogot, 283–285. International Louis Leakey Memorial Institute for African Prehistory: Nairobi.
Welsby, D. A. 2008. Dams on the Nile: From Aswan to the Fourth Cataract. *Sudan Studies* 37:5–18.
Widlok, T. 1994. Space and the 'other': Social experience and ethnography in the Kalahari debate. In *Social experience and Anthropological knowledge*, ed. K. Hastrup and P. Hervik, 135–149. London: Routledge.
Wilmsen, E. N. 1978. Prehistoric and historic antecedents of a contemporary Ngamiland community. *Botswana Notes and Records* 10:5–18.
Wilmsen, E. N. 1989a. *Land Filled with Flies: A political economy of the Kalahari.* Chicago: University of Chicago Press.
Wilmsen, E. N. 1989b. The antecedents of contemporary pastoralism in western Ngamiland. *Botswana Notes and Records* 20:29–39.
Wilmsen, E. N. 1997. Introduction. In *The Kalahari Ethnographies (1896–1898) of Siegfried Passarge: Nineteenth century Khoisan- and Bantu-speaking peoples*, ed. E. N. Wilmsen, 13–37. Cologne: Rüdiger Köppe Verlag.
Wilmsen, E. N. 2002. Mutable identities: Moving beyond ethnicity in Botswana. *Journal of Southern African Studies* 28 (4): 825–841.
Wilmsen, E. N. 2003. Further lessons in Kalahari ethnography and history. *History in Africa* 30:327–420.
Wilmsen, E. N., and J. R. Denbow. 1990. Paradigmatic history of San-Speaking peoples and current attempts at revision. *Current Anthropology* 31 (5): 489–524.
Wood, M., S. Panighello, E. F. Orsega, P. Robertshaw, J. T. Van Elteren, A. Crowther, M. C. Horton, and N. Boivin. 2017. Zanzibar and Indian Ocean trade in the first millennium CE: The glass bead evidence. *Archaeological and Anthropological Sciences* 9 (5): 879–901.
Wynne-Jones, S. 2005. *Urbanisation at Kilwa, Tanzania, AD800–1400.* PhD Thesis. Cambridge: University of Cambridge.
Wynne-Jones, S. 2007. Creating urban communities at Kilwa Kisiwani, Tanzania, AD 800-1300. *Antiquity* 81:368–380.
Wynne-Jones, S. 2018. Kilwa Kiswani and Songo Mnara. In *The Swahili World*, ed. S. Wynne-Jones and A. LaViolette, 253–259. London: Routledge.
Wynne-Jones, S., and A. J. LaViolette, eds. 2018. *The Swahili World.* London: Routledge.
Zeebroek, R. 2015. Perles et tissus: Les instruments monétaires au Katanga. *Afrique: Archéologie & Arts* 11:21–38.

Chapter 8
Why Archaeology in Africa matters

Abstract Pivoting from history to purpose, this chapter makes the case for archaeology's value today. It advocates integrating archaeology and history as mutually informing practices for reconstructing complex pasts and addressing present challenges. The discussion centres on the community as the ethical ground of research design and heritage care. It then confronts loss: war, looting, development pressures, climate change, and under-resourced institutions that imperil sites and collections. In response, the chapter surveys management frameworks, repatriation and restitution efforts, and participatory models that align conservation with livelihoods and education. It also reflects on cultural commodification, including tourism, branding, and popular media, warning against extractive logics while acknowledging opportunities for sustainable economies. The closing section returns to "the past matters" as a civic proposition: archaeology can enable reparative African futures when it is collaborative, reflexive, and oriented to public good.

> ...archaeology provides a new basis on which to write an account of Africa's precolonial past, one that pays due attention to the continent's dynamic interactions with the rest of the world. (Mitchell 2005, p. 7)

In northern South Africa, in what is now part of the Kruger National Park, two rivers converge: the Limpopo and Luvuvhu. This region is replete with a host of animals, birds, and large riverine trees that abound along the rivers' banks. Along the Luvuvhu is a narrow gorge, Lanner, that places the observer about 80 m above the river to survey up- and downstream as the river meanders, cutting through the sandstone bedrock. Below are hippos, crocodiles and fish, and along the banks herds of antelope graze and browse the river margins. It is a sight that shakes you with its beauty. East from Lanner by a short way the sandstone hills give way to a wide, floodplain that is largely flat other than the occasional small hillock. At the edge of this topographic change, on the final hill, is Thulamela.

Whispers of an immense archaeological site in the area had reached the ears of Tol Pienaar (1990), the park's warden between 1978 and 1987. He told his field rangers that while performing their daily duties they should keep an eye out for a site in the hope of rediscovering the mostly forgotten settlement. In 1983, Flip Nel, while patrolling the southern bank of the Luvuvhu River, climbed the hill to find the extensive walled citadel perched on its edge overlooking the floodplain. A team

T. Forssman, *Archaeology in Africa: Why the Past Matters*, Archaeology of Africa,
https://doi.org/10.1007/978-3-032-13365-6_8

was quickly assembled and dispatched to inspect the site a few days later, and they confirmed that it was indeed a site of high importance. Seven years after its identification, an archaeological team from the National Museum of South Africa visited Thulamela, along with two other sites known in the area, Makahane and Matjigwili (Eloff and De Vaal 1965), with the intention of mapping each and performing limited archaeological investigations (Küsel 1992). The team excavated test trenches and dated charcoal samples, but only at Thulamela did they report substantial archaeological remains from a large midden and the site's surface (Fig. 8.1). The assemblage included perforated shells, glass trade beads, a late seventeenth/early eighteenth century CE Chinese porcelain sherd, earthenware ceramic sherds and faunal remains, several gold beads, and two pottery crucibles with gold-bearing slag adhering to the surface suggesting local gold processing. These finds demonstrated the great archaeological and scientific potential of the site, and because of its monumentality, was considered a suitable tourist destination. As such, funds were raised and a largescale rehabilitation and excavation programme was initiated beginning in 1993 (Miller 1996b).

In charge of the work at Thulamela was Sidney Miller (Meskell 2007). He was not an archaeologist or formally trained in archaeology, but was in fact an engineer with a Masters degree in the conservation of architecture. Nonetheless, and despite there being many archaeologists in South Africa at the time, he was tasked with this crucially important goal of rebuilding and understanding this precolonial kingdom. Ten local men were appointed to assist him with the programme of work, and together they completed their activities in 1997, at which point work at the site ended. One of the most notable finds were human burials within walled enclosures. According to his published 'T. V. Bulpin-style', romanticised novel, *Thulamela: The lost gold of the VhaVenda* (2018, p. 19):

> After my friends left last Sunday afternoon leaving me glutted with food and liquid refreshment, I felt the need to go to the Mountain and clear my mind and body. When I got there I first wandered around a bit. Then I went to the equipment store, took out a trowel, brush and dustpan and walked to enclosure 5. I randomly chose a place in the enclosure and started excavating. Within ten minutes I opened up the edge of a human hip-bone.

Soon after Miller (2018) had uncovered human remains, he alerted the Thulamela Committee, comprised of community members, stakeholders, South African National Parks officials, and heritage specialists including an archaeologist (Nemaheni 2004, p. 256). After consultation, it was decided that the finds should be exhumed by specialists but examined on site. Work began on the human burial, named UP43, which was found to be a female buried 400 mm below a hut floor. During the course of the investigation, a male burial was identified (UP44) in a western enclosure. His remains were bundled together and not in the common foetal position, as was the case with UP44. Both burials contained a golden trove of items (Steyn et al. 1998).

A flurry of excitement followed (Miller 1996a). There had not been another archaeological site that had captured the public's interest so forcefully as Thulamela (Steyn et al. 1998). Partly driving its appeal was the country's political context at the time. When excavations began South Africa was heading towards the end of

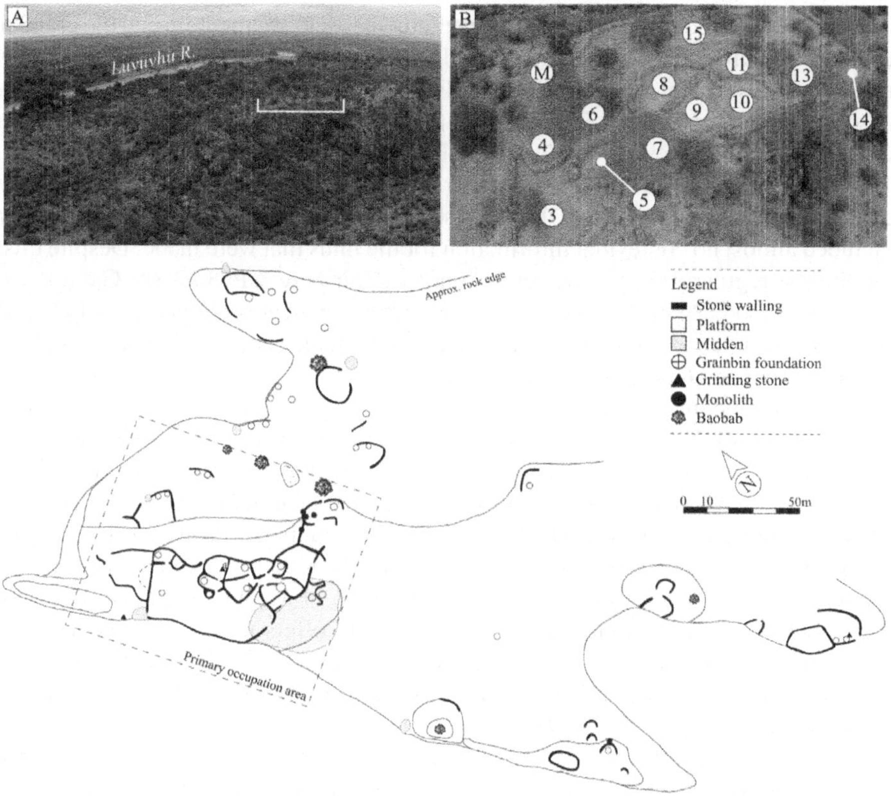

Fig. 8.1 (**A**) A view over Thulamela with the Luvuvhu river in the background, (**B**) An aerial image of the citadel areas with the enclosures indicated, and (**C**) A map of the archaeological site (photographs: Clive Morris Productions)

apartheid, and by the time the finds were made it had exited this era into a democratic dawn. Along with that, the sciences opened to become more inclusive and aware of African pasts with national and institutional hinderances removed. In light of these new possibilities and nation building imperatives, Thulamela became a site that the new government flagged as a message bearer – African precolonial prehistory was rich, and filled with opulence, advancement, and innovation. Pallo Jordan (1997, quoted in Meskell 2007, p. 387), a National Executive Committee member for the governing African National Congress, declared at the opening of Thulamela in 1996 in his speech titled *Thulamela excavation proves black heritage*: "Great Zimbabwe may be the most famous archaeological site in southern Africa. But Thulamela is the most magical". To Jordan, the site debunked the notion that history began when Europeans arrived in 1652 (Koch 1996; see also Delius et al. 2024). The Thulamela story was quickly co-opted by new nationalistic fervour and media hype (Miller 1996a).

With the work completed, the initial excitement lost its momentum and the grander challenges facing South Africa took hold. Thulamela fell from national narratives and eventually social memory. The finds, equally, were left alone in a museum basement and never studied. The only focussed work that was published pertained to the human burials (Steyn et al. 1998; Bodiba et al. 2019) and metals (Grigorova et al. 1998). The final report compiled by Miller (1997), which was never published in any considerable manner, was heavily criticised by Huffman (1998) and unfortunately included almost no contextual information for the finds that were made. Despite this, the site was regularly cited in academic sources (Chirikure & Pwiti 2008; Galla 1999; Nemaheni 2004; Pwiti & Ndoro 1999), but what was being said was largely based on assumptions made through comparisons with other, better studied sites such as Mapungubwe and Great Zimbabwe.

Work at Thulamela was shrouded in controversy. Lynn Meskell's (2012) *The Nature of Heritage* provides a pointed critique of the events that took place between 1993 and 1997, as well as into the time she was writing her book. She spoke to various informants that reported deeply concerning and unethical treatment of Thulamela's heritage. Accusations were made that students were taking artefacts for themselves, and even wore beaded bracelets they had found. Even worse, a plated golden item recovered from the site, similar to the golden rhino of Mapungubwe, disappeared, and auctioneers were phoning team members with offers to sell the golden finds. Whether this is true, Meskell 2012) is not sure, but in 2016 a collection of gold items was stolen from their display case from a museum in Skukuza, a tourist camp situated inside the national park (Wild 2017).

Thulamela's history and tragic mistreatment is a hurtful example of why the past matters, and what happens when it is treated as if it does not. The site evolved from a whisper to a national icon, and then to neglected heritage. It was shrouded in romanticism; the mystery of Thulamela and the lure of gold was hard to refuse and lulled archaeologists and the media into constructing their own narratives (Meskell 2007). However, egos, mischief, conflict, and fiasco bubbled to the surface as the project unfolded (Meskell 2012). The appointment of non-archaeologists to examine and restore the significant site is a clear demonstration of the kind of value that was placed on this important, precolonial settlement. Their focus on only the citadel, where the royalty or elite would have lived, and the attention given to finds of contemporary and western value displays a particular Eurocentric perspective and parochial approach towards understanding kingdoms and society. The focus never truly engaged descent communities but instead linked the site to a local family based on no evidence at all: no oral history, genetic work, memory, or archaeological relations. The site's interpretation then hinged not on evidence but analogy with other, similar sites, accepting unproblematically that these histories are homogenous across time, space, and politics. It was also intended to be a significant environmental education programme for local communities, which undermined the heritage: the value of heritage in this case was only emphasised if coupled with conservation efforts (Meskell 2007, p. 395). Finally, the neglect of Thulamela's artefacts is striking, in particular the theft of its gold in a democratic South Africa.

Thulamela's story demonstrates a general callousness towards history when it has the potential to play a significant transformative role in society (Meskell 2012). A senior official remarked to Meskell (2007, p. 396) during her study that the value of such a site would especially be to "black children, who might start to understand, and redefine themselves…it's not just economic. It's social. It's rebuilding the nation. It's actually giving you new vigour". The colonial context of South Africa with its apartheid history provides the past with greater impetus in addressing indigenous identities and histories. Instead, what we see is that archaeology's "governing paradigms and epistemologies often conflict with African historical needs, views of the past, and ways of structuring time and space" (Schmidt 1995, p. 119). It is not unusual that people "have a concept of their past, which is divergent from the past presented by archaeologists" (Eze-Uzomaka 2000, p. 153). Thulamela, like many of the examples in this book, demonstrate a larger issue of liberating knowledge of the past from the constraints of Eurocentric perspectives (Mudimbe 1988).

What these examples ultimately confront is the central theme of this chapter, why the past matters. From one perspective, learning about the past is a matter of pursuing knowledge and developing a robust understanding of the world that surrounds and surrounded us. However, this chapter considers why the past matters over and above our desire for knowing. To make this argument, it is suggested that the 'sibling' relationship between archaeologists and historians be revised (Robertshaw 2000; Vansina 1995b), and instead greater coherency between the two fostered. From this perspective, the role archaeology plays in making the past matter will be enhanced.

8.1 Archaeology as History, History as Archaeology

> Where writing is unknown, where the transmission of memory from one generation to the next fails, only archaeology—the exploration of the material traces left by those who came before us—can make up for the lack of any other sources (Schnapp 2014, p. 216)

Much of Africa was viewed as a space void of history. The accounts of the continent's past are unwritten and many historians, even in the mid-twenty-first century CE, denied it a substantive history, or at least one of significance, despite Africanist scholars' attempts at contesting these views. Africans were "the people without history" (in the title of Wolf 1982); Africa did not have a history as far as many in the global west were willing to admit. Peter Schmidt and Stephen Mrozowski (2013a) referred to this in the title of their book as the "death of prehistory". Early views provided the basis that still to this day influence perspectives of the continent's people and past via school curricula and stereotypes (Russell-Wood 1984; Fuglestad 1992; Lane 2005; King 2012). The past has influence on the present. On the one hand, this is through connections with contemporary groups (Ngaba-Waye 1996, p. 26), but on the other, it is in the way archaeology and history have shaped current socio-political faculties in modern nations (Delius et al. 2024). As such, African heritage and archaeology create opportunities to reinforce identity and self-understanding of individuals and communities. This has the potential to create a wider sense of belonging and social cohesion within the continent (Mitchell 2019, p. 11). Viewing archaeology as history, or history as archaeology in Africa, is vital to redressing archaeology's impact in the present.

The classic distinction between archaeology or prehistory and history is the advent of writing (Sauer 2004). The concept of prehistory, the time before writing, emerged in the mid-nineteenth century CE (Connah 2013, p. 17). It was co-opted in Africa and used largely only to refer to the Stone Age past. In this framework, history in Africa was construed as principally the domain of European activities. An example of this narrow view of history is Cornelis Muller's (1969) edited book *Five Hundred Years* in which a history of English and Afrikaans groups is presented in a "unilinear trend of "progress" and "development" brought by white men to southern Africa" (Legassick 1970, p. 491). A cursory examination of earlier texts demonstrates that Muller's (1969) attitude was not unique. Henriette Alimen's (1957) book *The Prehistory of Africa* committed 10 of its 428 pages to the Iron Age of Africa, whereas Desmond Clark's (1970) book by the same title grew this meagre number of pages substantially to 35 of 223. In this case, it constituted a single chapter that condensed farmer history and that of present communities into one. In the nine volumes in the *Cambridge History of Africa,* published between 1975 and 1986, archaeology was prevalent in the first two, had a single contribution in the third, and did not feature in volumes four to nine. Similarly, the *UNESCO General History of Africa* follows the same approach in which prehistoric pasts are subdued compared to the periods that followed (cf. Stahl 2009, p. 242). Archaeology was only considered important to historians in the appropriate contexts (Vansina et al. 1964), and for archaeologists the focus was keenly set on precolonial pasts in Africa (Swanepoel et al. 2008; Stahl 2009).

Some historians and archaeologists envisioned complimentary methods and interdisciplinary projects (Stahl 2009, p. 241); Robin Collingwood (1962, p. 199), for example, did not, and argued that an archaeologist can "arrange his relics in some kind of tidy order" but the result "is not history". Archaeology was to be history's *longue durée* and aid in establishing chronological sequences for Africa (Fagan 1961; Miller and Van der Merwe 1994; Mitchell and Whitelaw 2005). But, only using archaeology for the deeper past excluded the discipline from its contemporary counterpart: colonial and post-colonial histories (Stahl 2009). Initially, imprecision in radiocarbon dating undermined this hope for archaeology, alongside the cost of obtaining dates, with calendric years and error margins causing consternation. Making matters worse was the lack of refined chronologies archaeologists were capable of gaining with radiocarbon dating after about 1750 CE as a result of the Suess effect caused by human activities, particularly the Industrial Revolution and burning of fossil fuels (Tans et al. 1979). Jan Vansina (1995b), however, was further disillusioned and felt that the disparate theoretical positions of archaeological and historical thought would limit their intersectionality. As a result of these differences, their goals varied, sources were incompatible, and temporalities problematic. This view, which was held by others too, contributed to the marginalisation of Africa's precolonial history (Reid

2011). Vansina's (1995b) critique was largely influenced by processual archaeological approaches and did not account for the shifts that post-processual archaeology was driving in the discipline (Robertshaw 2000).

Scholars interested in Africa's past, in its politics, economics, ideologies, indigenous knowledge systems, and societies often have only but the archaeological record to call upon (Miller 1985). These pasts are not stored in texts as they are elsewhere, and even when they are those written sources are often highly selective and problematic (Pikirayi 1999, 2001, 2009a; Reid and Lane 2004, p. 7). As such, archaeology is the single most useful outlet to understanding the past (Lightfoot 1995a; Schmidt and Pikirayi 2018, p. 449) – it is not the only discipline though, with anthropology, genetics and linguistics also contributing significantly. Archaeology is, however, the only way of challenging the notion of a timeless African history. Obtaining a historical narrative for Africa, in most contexts, an interdisciplinary approach is necessary. The Kalahari Debate, for example, captures in many ways the frameworks adopted to understand African pasts, with its intersectionality between contemporary societies and their development, and the role archaeology can play in challenging archetypal conceptions of prehistory.

Archaeology is not problem free. The notion provided up until now might be that it is a magical pill to soothe the unsettled grumbles of history. Far from this. Archaeology's major limitations are significant. The tangibility of archaeological traces is paramount – not all humans used, ate, produced, or collected leave physical remains. Even when they do, it is usually only the durable materials that last, such as glass, stone, or tooth enamel. Others, despite being rigid, gradually disappear, like bone and metal. Moreover, their preservation hinges not only on the parent material's durability, but post-depositional change, soil acidity levels, animal interferences, and other issues such as leaching of collagen or subsurface root charring (Rapp and Hill 2006). Not to mention the perpetual challenge of chronology (Lucas 2004). Compounding archaeologists problems are the total absence of intangible cultural heritage in buried sequences or painted panels. While the finds are indicators of meaning and semiotics, recalling these is impossible without additional aids, such as ethnography (Pearce 2012), which as is readily acknowledged has its own problems (see Barham 1992; Lane 1994; Mitchell 2003; Denbow 2016; McGranaghan 2017). Although briefly summarised, it is clear that archaeology is not without its own inherent biases and epistemological gaps.

Studies integrating archaeological and historical datasets are infrequent. It is rare to find papers with both archaeologists and historians listed as authors (Stahl 2009, p. 242) and not until more recently were archaeological and historical sequences separated between chapters even when in the same book (cf. Mitchell 2024). A recent attempt at bringing these fields together more intrinsically was the *Five Hundred Year Initiative* in South Africa (Swanepoel et al. 2008). In 2006, archaeologists, historians and social anthropologists from universities and museums met to address a gap in research focussing on the last five-hundred years. Participants from a workshop held in the following year submitted papers to begin the processes of rooting out these knowledge gaps and filling them. These topics ranged from the establishment of local urban landscapes to translating missionary documents. Other studies that integrated archaeology and history was on the Bokoni sequence (Delius and Schoeman 2008; Wright 2010; Delius et al. 2012) and more recently the Indian Ocean trading network's footprint across southern Africa (Delius et al. 2024). Such collaborations cross the divide between archaeology and history and have generated longer, more integrated narratives of regional sequences.

The term 'historical archaeology' is intended to draw together history and archaeology (Stahl 2009, p. 246). While it entwines these disciplines, it has not passed seamlessly into the archaeological or historical lexicons (e.g., Reid and Lane 2004; Pikirayi 2006a; Orser 2012; Schmidt and Pikirayi 2018). The term emerged in North America in studies examining literate post-Columbian colonial society that were aided by texts (Little 1992). An early example in Africa of a historical archaeological study was by Carmel Schrire (1988, 1990) at Oudepost in Cape Town. Oudepost is a seventeenth/eighteenth century CE Dutch East India Company outpost. Her work integrated archaeological evidence with written accounts to extract from history far greater detail that she argued neither one approach would be capable of doing alone. Her work with Janette Deacon (1989), for example, was able to identify traces of indigenous people at Oudepost who were under-represented in historical texts. Schrire's historical approach was not met without criticism (e.g., Penn 1991; see Schrire 1991 for a response), but despite these the approach has emerged as an important field within the discipline (Schmidt 2006; Stahl 2010). However, historical archaeology still grapples with framing Africa's past beyond a colonial lens, where it sits in "the orbit of colonial influence" (Schmidt and Walz 2005, p. 319), as well as placing emphasis on ethnic categories and groups (Lightfoot 1995b).

Separating archaeology and history in Africa is flimsy at best (Pikirayi 2014). Issues involving the arrival and spread of writing is one aspect, but another is the disciplines' inter-related topics. Both the archaeologist and historian are interested in people, they are focussed on the past but acknowledge precedence in, and interference from, the present, and each uses human-produced correlates to understand past people, occurrences, and beliefs, among other things. The form of the correlates varies, from tools and food waste to architecture and texts. However, ultimately the disciplines ask the same questions (Sauer 2004). The distance between the archaeologist and historian is from a methodological and less theoretical view (e.g., Vansina 1995a), but this is entirely a matter of perspective. The terms 'archaeology' and 'history' are both disciplinary headings, within which a great variety of praxis exists. The tasks deployed by a Stone Age archaeologist, for example, as opposed to one interested in the Iron Age may vary but at times overlap. And yet, despite their differences, both practitioners are archaeologists. More discordant are those approaches used by an Earlier Stone Age specialist and a rock art researcher – the former relies on preferably stratified sites containing well-preserved items of material culture, whereas the other typically draws interpretations of painted panels on a rock wall from oral history, indigenous knowledge, or historic texts. Once again, both are archaeologists even though the latter is conceptually far more like a historian than the former. From one archaeologist to the other the difference in their research may at times be greater than those between another archaeologist and a historian.

Despite the apparent similarities between archaeology and history, from an archaeological perspective, archaeologists have struggled to build interpretive narratives over the years and have instead provided descriptive accounts that sometimes fall midway (Miller 1985, p. 293). Oliver Fage and Roland Oliver's (1975) *Cambridge History of Africa*, according to Joseph Miller (1985), falls within the latter style in that much of it attempts to be interpretive but it still presents history in archaeological discourse. To a historian, this may be a discomfort, such as the pains an archaeologist would take to present morphology, long sequences, or technological change, but to an archaeologist these variables are crucial to understand material culture. Without these data, archaeological arguments would lack the appropriate evidential detail the discourse demands to support any claims that are made. Troubling anyone writing from cultural material to historical narratives are the mute artefacts. They do not themselves layout interpretive histories, but rather lean more towards descriptive approaches given their technical complexities. In this sense, anthropological approaches bring additional meaning to the finds (Laudan 1996) but are themselves laden with problems despite claims overriding these issues (e.g., Pearce 2012).

In the context of arguing why the past matters, why does the difference between archaeology and history matter? For one, the distinguishing premise between the two is a European construct. The arrival of European writing also ebbed across the African region and did not appear rapidly, homogenously, or everywhere; its reach was limited for the first centuries after it appeared (Pikirayi 2009a). This results in the 'historic period' being chronologically disparate across the continent. Additionally, it generally includes only the last five centuries outside of North Africa, a short epilogue in humanity's continent-wide sequence. Separating the one from the other distinguishes Africa's past into before and after Europeans arrived, as if Africa's past needs to be defined by whether Europeans were present or not. Additionally, very few societies globally developed writing and it represents a tiny part of the human lived experience (Stahl 2023, pp. 2–3). It presents a reductionist perspective on a lengthy, significant, and diverse past, placing emphasis on an external influence as tantamount to justifying the partitioning of prehistory/history. It was the division setup by these two faculties that led a Tanzanian community informant to ask Schmidt (2013, p. 92): "Why do you whites call our history 'prehistory'?". These divisions are questionable at best, as demonstrated by some (Mitchell 2005; Robertshaw 2005), and on other's standards, useless (Schmidt and Pikirayi 2018, p. 444).

Keeping archaeology and history apart limits the usability and impact of archaeology in the present. David Cohen (2007,p. 1) argued that the historical project on the continent is to "bring Africa into history". What is striking about this, he continued, is that "Africa unwritten was already a part of, and long deeply engaged in, the wider world" (cf. Stahl 2014, p. 9). With this in mind, dividing archaeology and history not only contributes to separating Africa from the world but further separates archaeology from the present, when it absolutely has contemporary precedence. Moreover, it separates people from their past in cases where it is not stored in written texts but oral histories, ancestral knowledge, and buried deposits. The division, therefore, plays a deleterious role (Schmidt and Mrozowski 2013b, p. 1) and detracts from the longer-term continuity of socio-cultural, political and economic change (Lightfoot 1995a). Past sequences, especially those in the Holocene for much of Africa and certainly from the mid-Holocene, echo into the present in terms of settlement histories, social relations, the emergence of kingdoms and dynasties, and global trade relations. These phases are only conventionally disconnected by our own imposed divisions, not by anything in reality. By reconnecting them, other forms of knowledge can be considered, a single entity or pathway to knowledge is not privileged, and the influence of oppressive histories on contemporary societies can be addressed (Schmidt and Mrozowski 2013a, p. 8). In Africa, making archaeology history, and history archaeology, connects more meaningfully the present with the past, and accepts the challenge of threading deeper time into historical sequences.

8.2 The Past Matters

> Unquestionably, archaeology provides a powerful tool to recapture histories erased, excluded, and ignored over time. (Schmidt and Pikirayi 2018, p. 449)

> Archaeology has a lot to gain if it accepts the opportunity to learn from local people, but it also has a lot to contribute to the decolonisation of knowledge. Its local commitment, its bodily (and not merely intellectual) intervention, its easiness for crossing over different languages/writings/textures/texts and its usual bridging of realms severed by modern colonial knowledge (such as past and present, alive and dead, and so on), makes archaeology a potential art of decolonially relinking the world formerly severed by coloniality. (Haber 2014: 235)

The past matters because it is a narrative that defines us (Fagan 2018, p. 6); at least as much an image of us in the past as in the present. The past is because we were, then, and because we are, now; it reflects both. It matters because of the power it holds in how it reflects human society from history to the present day. In this regard, it has been used axiomatically, us and them, thereby constructing the 'other'. History is not just a record of events, or an ordering of relics, but a tool in the present. The way the past is framed is usually organised along power dynamics, which typically leads to the loss of indigenous heritage (Meskell 2007; Gosden 2012; Konishi 2019) and personhood (Wolfe 2006). Historical narratives are shaped by those in power, whether that is in terms of institutional, intellectual or access capitals. Memory and power work in tandem. Today there is pressure to amend historical injustices through archaeological and historical faculties, among others. The drive to return looted items such as the Benin Bronzes is one such example (Fig. 8.2) (Hicks 2020), but more abound (Shelton 2003; Little 2009; Stump 2013; Batt 2021). Recently, France's President Emmanuel Macron after commissioning a report stated that retaining objects constituted cultural colonialism (Hassett 2024). This sentiment has been around at least since the 1970s when Mobutu Sese Seko of then Zaire, now the Democratic Republic of the Congo, instituted *Authenticité*, a state ideology demanding the return of indigenous cultural objects and the rejection of colonial influence (Henriet 2022). Archaeology mobilises the ability to rebuild and reclaim history and to combat colonial narratives (Nkrumah 1963). Shadreck Chirikure's

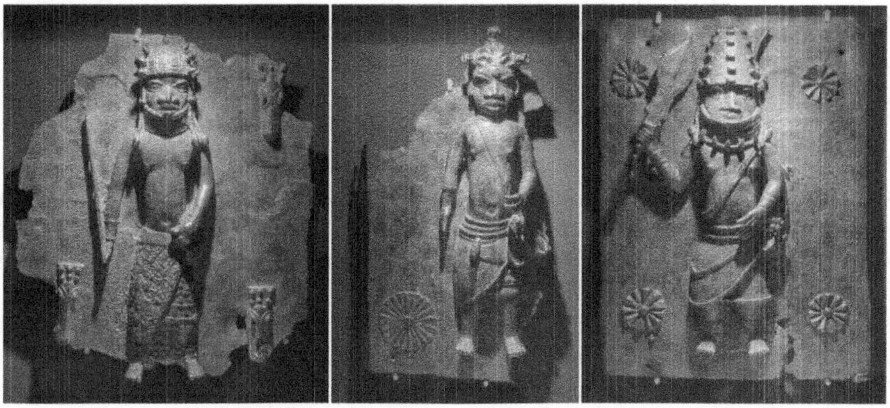

Fig. 8.2 Three Benin Bronzes from the Horniman museum and gardens, London (photographs: Mike Peel). *Sources* (left to right): https://commons.wikimedia.org/wiki/File:Benin_Bronzes,_Horniman_Museum_7.jpg; https://commons.wikimedia.org/wiki/File:Benin_Bronzes,_Horniman_Museum_5.jpg; and https://commons.wikimedia.org/wiki/File:Benin_Bronzes,_Horniman_Museum_3.jpg)

(2020) approach to Great Zimbabwe demonstrates the importance of reclaiming a 'confiscated' past, but in so doing highlights the complexity in doing so (Fontein 2021). Archaeology has a powerful role to play in Africa if the past can be made to intersect "with contemporary social problems" (Dawdy 2009, p. 142). Africa's past lives on vividly in the social fabric – in knowledge systems, collective memories, and the bonds (or fractures) within communities.

Archaeology is being forced to reckon with developments in real-time and confront present-day challenges (Rosenzweig 2020, p. 285). It is often further pressed towards activism and future-building narratives (this might not be distinctly different to its use in the early- and mid-twentieth century CE, in some respects). Whether archaeology is prepared to confront the present, "the present confronts archaeology". Very much as this book opened, the issue of the present emerges here once again. Archaeology has for its history in Africa reflected the present variably over its own historical trajectory. In some cases, this was as a tool for colonialism, in pursuit of objective science, or to reject narratives and focus on indigenous histories and ways of living. It also had a post-independence nationalist agenda, which Mahmood Mamdani (2019) observed of the 1960s and 1970s in Tanzania where scholars such as Al Mazrui argued academic work should be "socially relevant", effectively referring to its alignment with political ideology. This view continues the long tradition in archaeology of referencing itself in its contemporary context. Considering the grand challenges Africa faces, how is archaeology to confront these?

8.2.1 Community Matters

A problem faced in many parts of the world is how archaeology relates to indigenous communities (Pikirayi 2009b, p. 125; Schoeman and Pikirayi 2011; Posnansky 2017). For much of Africa archaeologists have not articulated archaeology's relevance to society beyond knowledge production (Evans 1975). It tends to call on a positivist framework that distances itself from social contexts (Shepherd 2007, p. 16). In this sense, politics does not intrude archaeological thought, which is aimed at uncovering information from the ground. This is a deep-seated attitude with a long history. However, hopefully it has been made clear by now that this understanding further entrenches bias and hides a priori assumptions inherent in archaeological approaches. Nick Shepherd (2007, p. 24) called these the "necessary entanglements" of post-colony life. There is a growing shift in creating emancipatory futures for archaeology based on the intersection of the past and its shaping of the present. In doing so, a cause for change is conducive (Harrison 2016) towards archaeology that is "transformative, politically engaged, and aspirational" (Reilly 2019, p. 3).

Engaging in epistemic justice is an important goal for archaeology. Tsim Schneider (2019) defined the concept of "heritage in-between", which refers to the missing heritage in the present because of extirpation in the past. These layers of heritage often survive in spite of near-extinction events and can be revived, as is the case in the United States of America (Vizenor 1999). Sonja Atalay (2019, p. 519) was positive about the emancipatory role of archaeology but argued that this required collaborative archaeologies involving indigenous members, inter-disciplinary studies, transepistemic approaches, and spheres of public discourses. She termed this "braided knowledge". Shepherd (2007, p. 15) also criticised knowledge construction and called the trend of ignoring other ways of knowing and doing "archaeologizing", stating the archaeologists need to move beyond this trap in their pursuit of impact and influence in the contemporary world.

Making the past matter links to the need for decolonisation since colonial legacies are still enmeshed within the cultural sphere. Archaeology is uniquely situated in that it has the ability to peer beyond the veil (Lane 2011), and archaeological studies are in many cases examples of shifting the gaze. The goal is to dismantle colonial biases and power imbalances that pervade Africa's past through scientific disciplines. Bethwell Ogot (2009, p. 1), for example, argued that archaeology can challenge the "false image of cultural isolation and temporal stagnation" that has been assigned to Africa, which represents intellectual assumption and prejudices. Before her, David Cohen (1985) argued that the external voices that shaped Africa is illustrative of the need to reconstruct the continent's history. It is worth being explicit, at this point, that the fact that external voices have contributed to building the continent's past is not inherently a problem and the drive to decolonise is not a project only from within that can be achieved by African scholars alone. Rather, it should be considered as a deeply collaborative process that seeks to redress past reconstructions with a collective approach.

An impassioned example is the *Rhodes Must Fall* movement that began at the University of Cape Town (Fig. 8.3), South Africa, but spread to many other campuses within and outside of the country. The movement was born out of the sense of alienation many students felt (Nyamnjoh 2017), symbolically represented in the Cecil Rhodes centre-piece statue at the top of the university's main staircase (Ndlovu-Gatsheni 2018 see Chapter 9: Rhodes Must Fall). The transformative movement shifted dialogue around pedagogy in higher education, questioning, for example, whose history is taught and how (Heleta 2016; Ntloedibe 2019). The movement ultimately found its thematic purchase in the past and the injustices that had not adequately been dealt with in contemporary society. Studies have shown that heritage is capable of reinforcing civil society (Pikirayi 2009b, p. 126), and the *Rhodes Must Fall* movement demonstrates how. The importance of decolonising the past may provide a constructivist framework to help address social contexts.

Communities, however, have increasingly asked what heritage conservation and use does for them (Ndoro and Chirikure 2017a, 2017b; Taruvinga 2020; Ndoro 2021). Chirikure and Gilbert Pwiti (2008, p. 467) argued that community archaeology leads to "empowering previously powerless peoples, particularly the indigenous and local communities that have lost rights to their heritage through colonialism". Chapurukha Kusimba (2017) navigated this complex process along Kenya's coast where he worked with communities in unravelling the Swahili past while training youths in archaeological method. Studies at Kuumbi Cave, Zanzibar, were carried-out with engaged community participation, and as a result the Hadimu community assisted the archaeological group with avoiding desecrating sacred areas and working towards shared and common goals (Chami 2019). Similarly, the University of Cambridge's

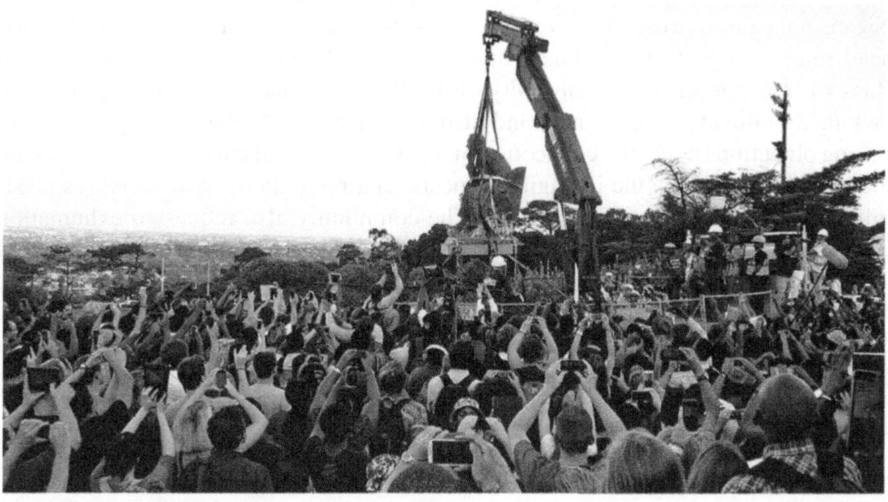

Fig. 8.3 The statue of Cecil Rhodes at the University of Cape Town is removed in front of students and onlookers in 2015 (photograph: Desmond Bowles). *Source* https://commons.wikimedia.org/wiki/File:-RMF_Statue_Removal_32_Desmond_Bowles.jpg)

collaboration with the Ministry of Culture on the Cape Verde islands has dealt with fragile heritage and examined early life in island towns while involving local communities (Sørensen and Evans 2011). Community engaged work is not a smooth process. It often involves the difficult task of defining communities, determining who is indigenous, and negotiating multiple and competing interests (Chirikure and Pwiti 2008), as well as confronting the often-held perception that archaeology is a tool that desecrates the past (Pikirayi 2009b, p. 125). Although in many contexts the stated goal of archaeology is to repopulate history unwritten with history lived, and give history back to people, its praxis fails to account for indigenous ways of knowing and desires to know. This is important because communities use pasts and archaeology deals in them (e.g., Pikirayi 2006b). It also allows archaeologists to address inequalities and upend the destructiveness of development.

The Prestwich Street example in Cape Town neatly illustrates various Afro-specific entanglements with archaeology. During excavations for the development of a luxury apartment building in Green Point, where Prestwich Street is located, in mid-May of 2003 human remains were discovered. The developer reported the finds to the South African Heritage Resources Authority and a company to exhume the remains was contracted. By August, over 500 individuals had been exhumed in a 1200 square metre area, although estimates place the total at likely double that. This work was carried out under a permit designed for preliminary investigation to establish the site's parameters. Most of the remains were retrieved from shallow graves without evidence of coffins or markers. As part of the process, the graves were left exposed for public viewing from behind a fence. Sixty days were allowed for the retrieval of the remains, and beyond this, which the project headed, it would be at the discretion of the developer.

Community engagement began seven weeks after the finds were made. When it began, opposition arose from various quarters: community and religious leaders, academics at a historically black university, and NGOs (Shepherd 2007). Ciraj Rassool, a historian at the University of the Western Cape, accused the process of lacking a political consciousness and displaying naivety (Malan 2003, p. 3). Those raising objections noted the connection many descendants of enslave people had with the buried individuals, the intangible aspects relating to their lives, social responsibilities, and community cohesiveness. The community also requested exhumation activities be halted, requesting a lengthier and detailed consultation period (Shepherd 2007, pp. 10–11). The community's views were widely dismissed by the CEO of the heritage authority as being emotional and without strong reasoning (Kassiem 2003, p. 1). The Hands off Prestwich Street Ad Hoc Committee (HOC 2003, p. 3) stated that the:

> needs of archaeology as a science seem to have been given precedence over other needs: the needs of community socio-cultural history, of collective remembering and of acknowledging the pain and trauma related to the site and this history that gave rise to its existence.

The committee further stated that the removals of the remains erases "the apartheid regime's forced removals from the same area" (HOC 2003, p. 8). Exhumations continued. Additional burials were found and disinterred from their final resting grounds and sent to the Woodstock Day Hospital mortuary across town with a city-centre parade. Construction activity was permitted to continue and appeals by the ad hoc committee, and its later reformation as the Prestwich Place Project Committee, were all unsuccessful. The case highlights the issue of culture, citizenship, identity, memory, politics, and the past (Shepherd 2007, p. 14). It demonstrates the intersectionality of archaeology and social well-being in South Africa, and serves as an informative model for elsewhere (another well-known example of this is Kennewick Man from the Unites States of America; Zimmerman 2005). It also highlights archaeologists' role within a racially and ethnically divided context (Fontein 2006; Schoeman and Pikirayi 2011).

As Prestwich Street shows, the weight of history is acutely felt in African societies that have endured traumatic pasts. Confronting those histories openly has been essential for healing and building social cohesion. Africa has been a global pioneer in using truth-telling and memory as tools of reconciliation, the prime example being the Truth and Reconciliation Commission in South Africa after the end of apartheid in 1994 (Androff 2010). South Africa is not alone in using truth commissions to deal with legacies of conflict and oppression. Other countries following a similar approach include Liberia, Kenya, Morrocco, Rwanda, Sierra Leone, and Tunisia. In Rwanda, a traditional court was established called *Gacaca* in which the community would gather to hear confessions. These courts blended pre-colonial conflict resolution practices with the need for contemporary accountability for actions. While *Gacaca* courts faced criticism, they positioned themselves between the past and present, conceptually at least, and drew on indigenous knowledge and customs to ease social and national healing (Chakravarty 2006; Doughty 2015). In all instances, the notion is that ultimately the truth heals (Buckley-Zistel 2005). What does archaeology have to do with any of these contemporary social issues? Archaeology and history reach into the *longue durée* and grapple with the roots of society that shaped its modern counterparts. Understanding these histories, their complexities, and the mechanisms at play contributes to examining the causes and patterns of violence (Bakiner 2016). Additionally, archaeology and history provide information grounded in disciplinary methods that include indigenous knowledge, collective memory, forensic evidence, and human rights violations. The war in Argentina, for example, introduced the notion of *los desaparecidos,* the disappeared, referring to the victims of the military dictatorship, in which archaeological and forensic work could tangibly track crimes, corroborate testimonies, and even name the victims (Crossland 2000). Archaeology and history serve to reconstruct memory and the past in these traumatic histories that are poorly represented in relevant texts (Suárez 2009).

One feature of archaeology that scholars have argued is profitable in post-colony states is the culturally rich, precolonial past that presents Africa before domination (Pikirayi 2009b). The colonial-era categorising of African communities was as primordial and conquered, but this did not reflect the reality of pre-European contact social groupings (Earle 2018). Stelios Michalopoulos and Elias Papaioannou's (2020) meta-analysis led to the conclusion that ethnic malleability was crystallised through the colonial process, which contributed to reshaping the cultural landscape of Africa and its future. To contest these characterisations, local voices emerged along with international scholarship to counter colonial essentialism (Boahen 1987). In the context of archaeology, these perspectives stem from the things (cultural material or artefacts) from the past that have preserved into the present. These provide first-hand experiences and personal histories of daily, lived precolonial life, illuminating pre-domination ways of being. Terence Ranger (1999) did just this in Zimbabwe's Matopo Hills. He weaved together a transepistemic narrative that populated the historical account with oral history and African spirituality (Mlambo 2001). This type of approach enters humanistic traits more intrinsically into research and does not negate descendant's rights to their own understandings of the past and its use in the present (Pikirayi 2015, p. 535).

Many post-independent states specifically invoked precolonial histories to inspire nationhood (Coker 2019). After independence in French Sudan, for example, the President Modibo Keïta renamed the country Mali after the medieval Mali Empire, signalling a revival of the golden age as part of national identity (Foltz 1965). In Ethiopia, although not colonised, Emperor Menelik II used archaeology and legend to solidify national unity while portraying his regime as heir to the Solomonic Dynasty. He reportedly commissioned excavations to legitimise these claims (Zena 2018). Seko's *Authenicité* applies similarly (Henriet 2022). In 2021, as part of "a manifestation of the new Egyptian ideological discourse", the 'Golden Parade of the Pharaohs' was held in the streets of Cairo. Twenty-two mummies were moved by the government from the Egyptian Museum to the new National Museum of Egyptian Civilisation. The elaborate parade adopted Egyptian statehood, religious and moral traditions as a statement of nationhood and identity (Tüske 2024). Cheik Anta Diop's (1960) revalorising of African pasts was aimed to demonstrate the contributions from the continent to global history and invoke racial pride and assert black humanity (Dunstan 2023). Ranger (2004) referred to this use of the past in Zimbabwe, where Great Zimbabwe was appropriated by Robert Mugabe, as "patriotic history".

However, in this guise, the use of the past in post-colonies has to grapple with creating inclusive histories without effacing the richness of local memories, pasts, and spirituality. Being often composed of a variety of ethnic groups or language speakers complicates this process, creating anxiety around plurality. In Nigeria there has been debate over history representations in the school curriculum, such as how the Nigerian-Biafran War (1967–1970), the only civil war in Africa during the independent era, is presented (Onuoha 2016). State history in Ethiopia has also had to face hegemonic representations of Christian history from the highland region in an Amhara-Tigray narrative. This approach marginalised other histories, such as Oromo and Somali, growing tensions within the country. As part of forging national cohesion in Ethiopia, the histories and heroes of other groups have now been celebrated (Adamu 2009, 2013; Finneran 2013). The interplay between colonial/postcolonial, indigenous/settler, but also languages groups stimulates visions of the past that suit agendas but not always everyone involved (Kaarsholm 1990).

8.2.2 *Losing the Past*

Newly formed precolonial pasts were undermined by the rise of fringe or pseudoarchaeology, which germinates readily in non-European contexts. Its appearance in Africa attacks the foundation of African heritage and reassigns it to other, often outer worldly or science fiction protagonists. Such narratives "are routinely used in the service of white supremacy, racialized nationalism, colonialism, and the dispossession and oppression of indigenous peoples" (Hoopes 2019, p. 9). It constitutes cultural violence, defined as the advancement of harmful traits in society such as racism, oppression, or elitism (Galtung 1969, 1990). These theories, and many others, often wrest agency and legitimacy from local communities to present esoteric narratives. Many of the seeds of pseudoarchaeology are grounded in racialised perspectives that shape the past and indigenous cultural denialism (Seitz 2012; Colavito 2019). Rather than exploring the interlinkages and developments in the past that societies underwent, they seek disruptive devices that disarticulate contemporary, typically indigenous, people from their own historical sequences. There is probably also a component of anti-intellectualism where professionals are viewed with disdain and mistrust, and the lack of transparency and access to archaeological knowledge may foster some of this (Anderson 2019). Addressing fringe theories may require finesse and humanising strategies. Confronting these matters is not a process of gatekeeping but promoting responsible science through engaging with contemporary controversies (Hoopes 2019) and not using the past to subvert the present (Shanks and Tilley 1992).

Africa has had many imagined pasts (Derricourt 2011). Mentioned several times already is Leo Frobenius' (1911) African Atlantis and, from a different perspective, Diop's (1960) Egyptian origins argument. A theory yet to be discussed are the claims made by Cyril Hromnik (1981) that innovations in southern Africa are linked to Indian influences. He argued that dry-packed stone walled settlements in Mpumalanga Province, South Africa, are Indian/Hindu temples. The Indian settlers occupied nearby caves or shelters where they interacted with the local San, resulting in the appearance of the Quena (Khoekhoe herders). He further suggested that the BaPedi, an eastern Bantu-language speaking group that still lives in Mpumalanga, only arrived when Indian communities came to the province in search of gold (Hromnik 1999). Unfortunately, Indian settlers left few traces, making their presence difficult to confirm. This is at odds with an abundance of Iron Age remains found in the same stone structures that unequivocally support a local origin, referred to as Bokoni (Delius and Schoeman 2010). Despite this, new theories have emerged. Richard Wade (2009) argued that the Bokoni structures predate Mapungubwe, despite the well-dated mid-second millennium AD chronology for the investigated settlement structures, and that both settlements were astronomical observatories. On a different tangent, Johan Heine and Michael Tellinger (2008) interpreted the same stone structures as portals used by off-worldy beings.

Dealing with alternate archaeologies is tricky from a post-processual perspective. Ian Hodder (1984, pp. 30–31) argued that "different pasts will be constructed within different but limited sets of social interests", which Michael Shanks and Chris Tilley (1987, p. 195) suggested should be judged on political grounds or moral and practical consequences. Bruce Trigger (2006, pp. 467–468) felt that an argument's logic should be the discerning factor. This is an important question to consider because depending how archaeologists decide to exclude pseudoarchaeology, other knowledges might also be undermined. These may include oral histories, ancestral traditions, and memory, and more broadly indigenous knowledge when archaeological data contradicts or cannot support the claims. Robin Derricourt (2012) asked if all contested histories need to be accepted, or if being a critical archaeologist means making a commitment to one despite its political positioning? However, we could equally ask that if archaeologists do not take a position, is that in of itself a political stance? If left unopposed, pseudoarchaeological theories successfully strip local communities of their histories, and commit historical colonisation.

The intellectual violence pseudoarchaeology inflicts on the past is a different form of destruction to the rampant looting, demolishment, vandalism, and neglect African heritage contends. This is often linked to conflict, terrorism, agricultural expansion, and urban development (e.g., Amineddoleh 2015). Underscoring this is an inadequate response from most quarters (Brodie and Renfrew 2005) and a lack of interest in preserving Africa's past outside of tourist areas (Abungu and Ndoro 2023). Some archaeologists have proposed heritage crime as a crucial task for archaeologists to engage, either as it takes place outside of the academy (Grove 2013; Vollgraaff 2014) or through archaeology's collusion (Hutchings and La Salle 2019, p. 1655). Both are pertinent on the African continent which has higher rates of internal conflict than most other global regions (Colton 2015; Abungu and Ndoro 2023, p. 1; Beldados et al. 2023). During European expansionism and the subsequent colonisation of Africa, cultural heritage was plundered wantonly with little regard for human life in some instances (McGuire 1990). Time Magazine authors Aisha Labi and Simon Robinson (2001) wrote "Africa, its people already plundered by slavers, its animals by poachers and its mineral wealth by miners, is now yielding up its cultural heritage. Across the continent, artifacts are looted from museums, from universities and straight from the ground". The loss of African antiquities is enormous (Shaw 1997; Brodie and Renfrew 2005) and it is part of a global crime network surpassed only by drug trade and arms trafficking (Calvani 2009,p. 29; this list excludes human trafficking). The trafficking of illegal African antiquities has resulted in some scholars referring to the trade as 'cultural genocide' due to its prevalence (Bedaux and Rowlands 2001). Sadly, it has been described as one of the continent's greatest unfolding cultural disasters (Schmidt and McIntosh 1996).

West Africa faces considerable challenges in overcoming illicit trafficking of cultural heritage. Archaeologists in the 1980s noted the theft of Dogon-region terracotta statuettes in southern Mali (Kouroupas 1995). This has intensified, and with it the plundering for archaeological treasures has posed an increased threat to the preservation and protection of antiquities and their enquiry (Bedaux et al. 2001). The problem has been ongoing since the 1970s and has not abated (Colton 2015), but in the 1990s it worsened considerably (Brodie and Renfrew 2005, p. 346). An article by Mamadou Dembélé and Jacques van der Waals (1991) about looting in

Mali, written in 1991, begins with the announcement: "Here is more news, from the ground, of the catastrophe which is killing the archaeological sites of Mali". By that stage, 45% of a sample of 830 sites had been damaged, and five years later this had increased by 20% (Brodie and Renfrew 2005, p. 346). It is estimated that 80–90% of the Jenné-Jeno sites in the Niger River Valley have been looted (Barker 2018), with higher estimates for Niger (Gado 2001). Nigeria also faces rampant plundering of Ife sites, among others, with a specific incident taking place in 1995 that involved over 2000 people digging in Kawu for bronze heads (Labi and Robinson 2001). That same year, Igbo-Ukwu cultural items were stolen from the University of Ibadan, and in 1999 three of the Nok and Sokoto terracotta items appeared in France. In 1996, 24 Nigerian museum and community repositories were looted (Eluyemi 2002), with much of the crime being organised by syndicates (Filani 2003). Ghana, however, was able to stave off illicit trade through Museums and Monuments Board interventions, but development here now poses significant threats to heritage (Kankpeyeng and DeCorse 2004). In Egypt it differs because of a depressed economy and prevalence of conflict, but estimates predict that in 25 years' time most of the country's cultural heritage will be destroyed or looted (Vergano 2014). The theft of Thulamela's gold has already been mentioned but applies here. These examples, from a constrained region in Africa with intense interest, reflect what is happening in other parts of the continent (Schmidt and McIntosh 1996), and hinge on a growing international market for high-valued items and criminal networks (Elia 1997; Shaw 1997; Campbell 2013). These factors contribute to incongruent valuations of the past that layer heritage crime (Barker 2018).

Further adding to the destruction of Africa's antiquities and heritage, and enabling trafficking of cultural items (Gearon 2013), is conflict and war (Brodie 2003; Kila 2013; Colton 2015). Statistical analysis in Egyptian cases of looting from 1997 to 2014, during which various conflicts played out, showed that theft in these contexts is not opportunistic but strategic (Fabiani 2018). This worsened after 2011 when the Egyptian revolution came to an end and heritage policing and management declined, leaving many sites at greater risk. Ensuing attacks resulted in the damage and destruction of churches, museums, and various historic buildings (Tassie et al. 2015). It was initially estimated that 2% of artefacts held in 65 locations around the country were looted in the first 16 months after the revolution, amounting to 50,000 items (Joseph 2012), but later revised to 4000 (Brederova 2014); this reflects an unfortunate database management crisis (cf. Tassie et al. 2015). It has also been found that at least in some instances antiquity looting also provides a source of funding for armed forces (Baker and Anjar 2012; Robins-Early 2015). Conflict obviously leads to destruction, sometimes as a casualty of war but in other cases the destruction is intentional. Conflict in the Tigray Region between Ethiopia and Eritrea between 1998 and 2000 resulted in the toppling of the Stella of Matara, a 2500-year-old sculpture. It included the shelling and looting of heritage sites, including churches, monasteries, and mosques, with the intention of dominating local histories and narratives, suppressing communities, and exploiting resources for personal gain (Mulubrhan et al. 2024). Mali's Timbuktu was widely vandalised in 2012 when rebel groups entered the city and destroyed mosques, mausoleums, and tombs. Similarly, sacred sites were destroyed in Senegal when civilians took refuge in them between 1990 and 2011 as combatants hid from government forces. Oran Kepi figurines were used as firewood in Nigeria by troops who did not realise the items' value (Adewumi 2022a, 2022b). The Merowe Dam development in Sudan is a further example of how conflict can manifest into a destructive agent regarding local heritage when incongruent values interact (Kleinitz and Näser 2013). These are some of the many cases that exist, a list that presumably excludes a large number never recorded. Ultimately, the impact of the various destructive forces on heritage is wide ranging and includes the loss of heritage, lives, tourism potential, and scientific value. As non-renewable resources, its loss is irreversible (Elia 1997), and therefore it is imperative that it is confronted.

Another key driver of heritage loss is environmental degradation. Africa's disproportionate vulnerability to climate change is often linked to historical injustices. Climate change and vulnerable communities should chiefly be considered, Innocent Pikirayi (2019) suggested, to identify the best practices for future prosperity. Joy McCorriston and Julie Field's (2019, p. 6) *World Prehistory and the Anthropocene* contended that learning about the past helps make better decisions in the present and with the future in mind (Adeleye et al. 2021), but it also assists in generating useful baselines to which human adaptations and change can be related (e.g., Davies 2012; Thomas and Burrough 2012; Gowlett 2019; Thompson et al. 2021; Patalano et al. 2023). Despite some reservations (Lane 2015; Shaw 2016), the potential that archaeology can contribute to future-proofing is certainly present and its contributions may be dynamic (Mitchell 2008; Hudson et al. 2012). For example, food sustainability can be examined by studying past practices and contrasting these with contemporary challenges, climatic contexts, and indigenous agricultural approaches (Reed and Ryan 2019; Fisher 2020). Examining past land use patterns has also demonstrated the cross-section of food-producing regions, which in some cases were not thought of as such, including the areas of the Sahara (Lancelotti et al. 2019). There have also been claims that early states invited disaster and over-domestication, degradation, war, and inequality (Scott 2017). Stephanie Wynne-Jones (2019), for example, noted the exclusion of African states in James Scott's (2017) oversimplification of historical regimes and their reliance on grains (see comments by Campbell 2019). She draws on Jenné-Jeno and the yam cultivation in West Africa to demonstrate where states have emerged and persisted in regions without a reliance on grain-based agriculture. Furthermore, Wynne-Jones (2019) argued that African state formations should be understood through their entanglement with global systems, particularly European expansionism and capitalism, in order to better comprehend contemporary geopolitics. In a related critique, Atalay (2019) calls for the inclusion of multiple epistemologies to challenge the inherently capitalist framework of archaeology and to support its potential for social justice. These examples relate to the useable past model, developed in Africa (Andah 1995; Lane 2011), to advocate for local, historical strategies as they relate to contemporary problems (Logan et al. 2019). Archaeology cannot solve these problems or provide every answer, but the dataset with which it deals will aid in "developing appropriate, workable, and durable" adaptation and mitigation attempts (Rockman 2011, p. 194).

Several scholars have argued that archaeological and historical ecology in Africa has the potential to examine human responses and resilience to environmental or climatic challenges (Mitchell 2008; Douglass and Cooper 2020), and relate these to contemporary context in a transformative fashion (Van de Noort 2011). This is especially pertinent as it relates to agricultural sustainability, a field marked by contested definitions and no consensus on its key dimensions (Hayati et al. 2010). Augustin Holl (2020) examined the end of the African Humid Episode (9000–6000 BP) in the Sahara where pastoralist communities adapted their ways of living to suit ecological changes (shifts in grazing), and engaging with the cognitive anxieties that it caused (ritual appearance). For example, communities developed cattle burials that may have come after consumption or may have included whole carcasses. Selective burials during the wet season are suggested as a possible indication that it was linked to crisis management, health issues, or other forms of rituality. In all instances, this practice may have been linked to social healing. In Ethiopia, the Konso established innovative stone terraces to cope with semi-arid conditions (Fig. 8.4). Their strategy assists with soil and water conservation and has sociocultural values, labour partitions, and indigenous institutions (Gashure and Wana 2023). Also facing severe water constraints were the Garamantes in Libya's Fezzan region. Desertification in the area drove local change in land use and settlement patterns. It led to a shift from oases exploitation in the mid-first millennium CE to irrigation via *foggaras* (underground water conduits drawing from springs and distributing water to the surface) and long-distance trade (Liverani 2000). Albeit only three examples, they illustrate the human adaptations, whether innovative or migratory, intended to mitigate ecological pressure. However, studies into African pasts can also demonstrate how environmental change has altered societies and civilisations irreparably. The decline of the Aksumite Empire in Ethiopia corresponds with environmental change linked to reduced rainfall in the sixth and seventh centuries CE, in concert with conflict and shifting trade (Phillipson 2009), and the early nineteenth century CE Mfecane (scattering) period in South Africa, when the Zulu Kingdom raided large regions to sustain their own society, was partly linked to environmental and economic interactions (Eldredge 1992).

An important shift to consider is the local impact colonialism had on Africa's environmental context. European expansionism and later colonialism considerably altered the continent's ecological and geological history through mining, plantation agriculture, deforestation, draining wetlands, and damming, as well as moving and congregating people in small areas, and introducing new diseases. These initiatives and industries were often at odds with traditional management or extractive processes. The terms environmental colonialism (Bedarff et al. 1989) or climate colonialism (Bhambra and Newell 2023) describes these contexts. Similarly, Nnimmo Bassey (2016) described it as climate apartheid with reference to Africa's role as a dumping ground for carbon offsets rather than real reparations. The Intergovernmental Panel on Climate Change (2022) listed colonialism as a driver of climate change and noted that it continues to exacerbate vulnerabilities in certain communities (Douglass and Cooper 2020). Indigenous communities have argued that colonialism is at the centre of the climate crisis and engaging this is crucial in dealing with historic injustices

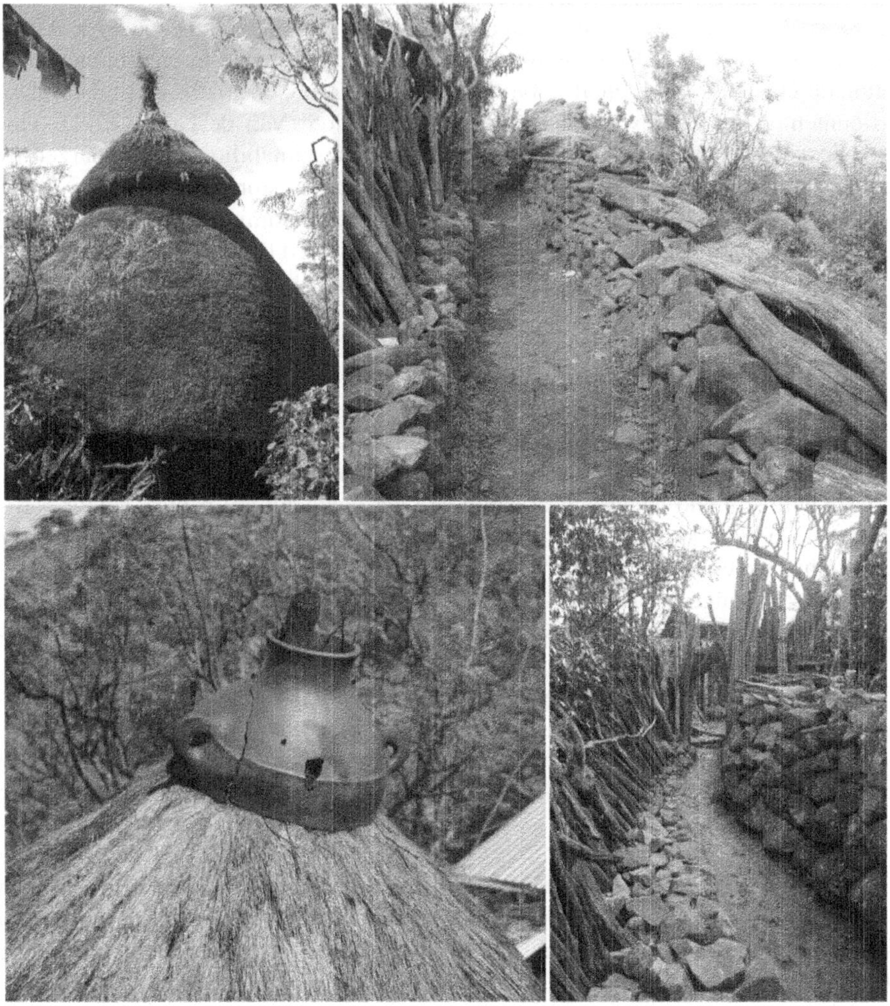

Fig. 8.4 Konso residences and stone-wall-lined village pathways (photographs: Tim Forssman)

(Whyte 2016) through approaches such as environmental self-determinism (Tsosie 2007). As with the examples above, archaeological and historical entanglements offer deeper understanding of social issues and sequences as they relate to climate colonialism, or the climate crisis more generally (Shaw 2016). Archaeological and historical studies can play a role in environmental activism and engage one of society's most pressing global challenges.

The climate crisis also poses significant risks on the conservation of cultural heritage, made worse by a lack of baseline evidence (Westley et al. 2023). Rising sea-levels, for example, pose serious risk to maritime archaeology. In a recent assessment, Michalis Vousdoukas et al. (2022) found that of 213 cultural heritage sites with 'outstanding universal value', 71 face damage and destruction due to coastal flooding. By 2050, if projections are accurate, this number will more than triple, and 20% of the UNESCO World Heritage sites along the coast will be impacted by erosion or flooding (18–34% according to Westley et al. 2023). Mozambique Island faces considerable threat (Fig. 8.5). The island was an early seat of Portuguese colonial government in eastern Africa, where their largest fort was constructed, São Sebastião (Newitt 2004). Severe weather events, particularly tropical cyclones, have increased in recent decades, along with the threat of flooding and sea-level rise (Mavume et al. 2021). According to a World Bank (2023) report, Mozambique is the country most affected by climate change on the continent. These changes threaten the preservation of the island's stone town heritage. For example, in March 2022, over 5500 buildings were damaged on the island by Cyclone Gombe, which brought with it 190 km/h winds and 200 mm of rainfall within a 24-hour period, resulting in widespread flooding. Gombe followed two cyclones in the months before that also unusually tipped the severity scale, Ana and Dumako (Milão et al. 2025). However, much more of the Swahili world is under threat, such as Kilwa and Songo Mnara where dynamic interventions involving digitisation, community engagement, and research initiatives have been deployed to promote conservation and sustainable living (Pollard et al. 2025). Preserving these forms of cultural heritage can be considered from a futurist perspective – the need to look after them for the next generations – but there are many other reasons for taking care of them. Dirk Spennemann (2011, p. 18) argued that it is crucial to also consider "community pride, identity, and social cohesiveness" offered by these cultural resources, making it important to disentangle the economic benefits they may or may not possess from their social importance.

8.2.3 Managing Heritage

How do archaeologists confront the loss of heritage? They have been trying in various ways, as evinced by the citations above and the many that have not been included here, but it is a complicated process. Dealing with conflict, looting, and war are not easily handled and archaeologists are largely not in a position to do so. Involving oneself in these matters invites risk, and potentially for collaborators and teams as well, as it might involve dealing with criminals, terrorists, soldiers, or law enforcement. The consequences can be severe. The Syrian archaeologist Khaled al-Asaad was reported beheaded in 2015 for refusing to provide his captors with the location of valuable antiquities (Barker 2018, p. 457). However, archaeologists can place systems of governance and institutions under pressure to advocate for change. Such activism has happened. Community pressure in Zimbabwe has led to more effective conservation approaches (Chirikure and Pwiti 2008). In South Africa, the Mapungubwe World Heritage Site was at risk of mining-linked damage and the loss of its world heritage status due to nearby coal mining, but pressure from stakeholders, local communities, and NGOs was able to permanently halt development (Chirikure 2013). Other remote sensing approaches have also helped track the destruction of

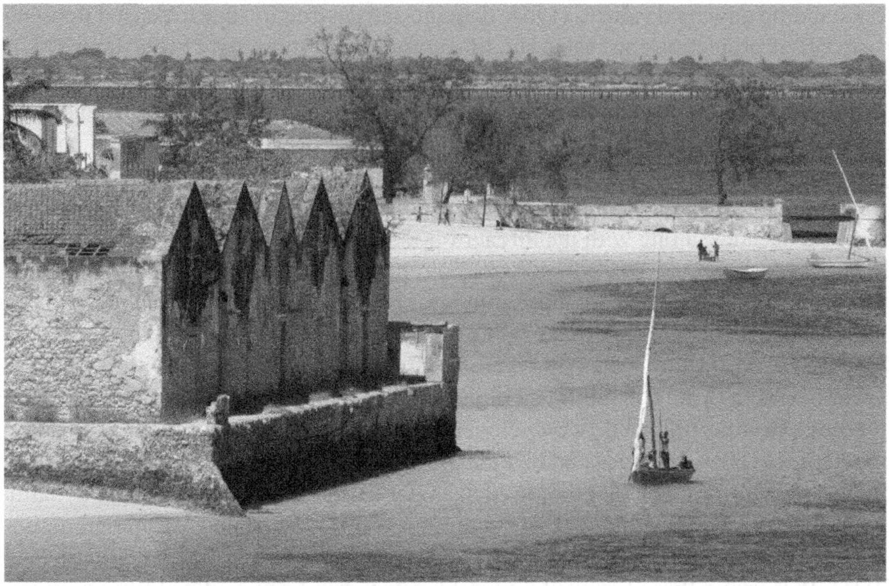

Fig. 8.5 Part of the Fort São Sebastião on Mozambique Island (photograph: Stig Nygaard; *source* https://commons.wikimedia.org/wiki/File:Ilha_de_Mocambique.jpg)

archaeological heritage, including identifying looting from space (Parcak et al. 2016; Tapete and Cigna 2019). The Endangered Archaeology in the Middle East and North Africa programme uses satellite imagery to rapidly record and produce data relating to archaeological landscapes. The project records actual and potential threats, and trains custodians on the ground to help establish historic environmental records. Their aim is to produce a heritage inventory of threatened landscapes and sites, and mitigate potential damage (Bewley et al. 2016; Sheldrick and Zerbini 2017). The method they use combines satellite imagery with published data and field surveys to analyse the condition of sites (Rayne et al. 2017).

Adding to the complexity of preserving heritage are the links between bodies charged with taking care of this resource and their own social histories with industry and governments. Their efficacy in swaying national decision-making and inserting themselves into political scenarios has resulted in a lack of outcomes (e.g., Tassie et al. 2015: 16). In this framework an axiom that has polarised views is the need to preserve and protect versus the local need to spiritually engage (Jopela and Fredriksen 2015: 262). The hegemonic approach has been to conserve heritage through preservation strategies that essentially disconnect heritage and people (Meskell 2018) – excluding participants engaging with heritage, placing it behind glass, or fencing it off. This has erased the past and ignored what heritage means to local communities (Aouchal 2023). Additionally, exotic objects received the greatest interest rather than those with local value (Nhamo and Katsamudanga 2022; Manetsi 2023) and political and economic interests often dictate historical or cultural significance and preservation approaches (Meskell 2018). Meskell (2018) unpacked this with a specific focus on UNESCO sites, but her arguments can be applied more widely. She discussed the influence of colonial and post-colonial power networks and their interplay in the decision to protect, conserve, preserve and present heritage. Heritage, in her assessment, is a tool for international politics, and is not neutral. An example of this is Colin Breen's (2007) report that noted 65 of the 851 UNESCO World Heritage Sites are in sub-Saharan Africa, of which 31 are cultural sites. The past is actively shaped by ideologies and institutions and this in turn shapes false universalities. Archaeologists are capable of contesting these views and redressing narratives, placing African pasts into developmental and protection frameworks that advocate for sustainable development goals (Allen et al. 2022).

Heritage management also finds itself occasionally at odds with indigenous methods of conservation that tend to consider sites as ancestral resting places and spaces to be avoided or left alone. Western principles of heritage management, which are well intended and give primacy to cleaning, restoring, conserving, and protecting, interfere with local ways of engaging sites (Ndlovu 2011; Chirikure et al. 2015). Chirikure et al. (2015) used the example of the Khami World Heritage site (Fig. 8.6) where interventions to maintain the site, which included restoration, brought about positive local benefits, but they equally undermined indigenous ways of relating to the site, notably as an ancestral resting place that should be left alone even in the event of decay. Similarly, at Zimbabwe's Domboshava rock art site, rain making rituals were banned once the site became a National Monument in 1938. In 1988, a tourist gift shop was established but in 1995 angry locals burnt it down. Following this, in 1998, paint was smeared over the rock art, destroying between 60 and 70% of the painted area. The vandalism was widely thought to be retaliation against the management strategy opted for Domboshava, under the premise that without the rock art the site's listing would be removed and rituals could resume (Taruvinga and Ndoro 2003). At sites like Domboshava and Khami, but also elsewhere in Africa, local communities were marginalised in the process of commodifying African heritage.

Heritage management across the continent has been a point of discussion for the past five decades (e.g. Alexander, 2011, p. 94; Arazi, 2009, p. 96; see also Breen and Rhodes, 2010; Kankpeyeng and DeCorse, 2004; MacEachern, 2001; 2010). Limiting heritage management is legislation dating to the 1960s and 1970s (Munjeri 2008); only Botswana (2001), Kenya (2006), Namibia (2004) and South Africa (1999) have overhauled their heritage legislation post-independence (Arazi 2011, p. 28). The Environmental Impact Assessment process is also not present in all countries – it is strong in Ghana and Tunisia, and robust in Algeria, Benin, Botswana, Egypt, South Africa and Uganda – but in the absence of local legislation it is driven by international legislation around development requirements (Arazi 2011, p. 31). However, only Botswana, Namibia and South Africa enforce heritage assessments through legislation (Ndoro and Kiriama 2008). The use of generic, foreign-based legislation or approaches are not always effective. The Chad-Cameroon oil pipeline led to clashes between outside cultural resource managers and local archaeologists desperate to use the opportunity to excavate sites to learn more of the region's past; non-local managers preferred to preserve and avoid any form of destruction (MacEachern

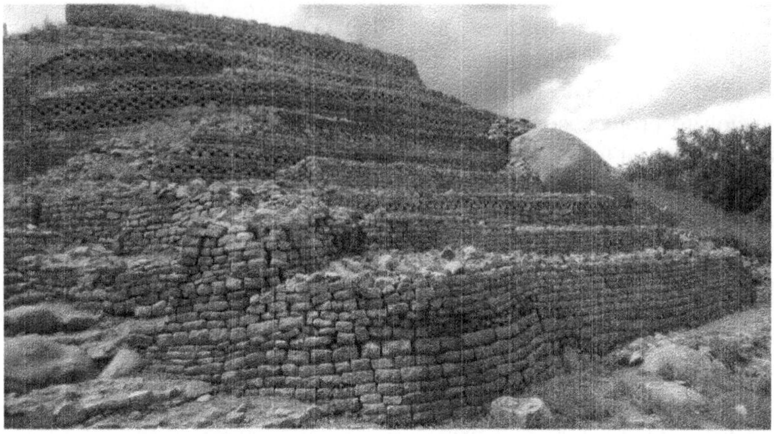

Fig. 8.6 A section of the Khami world heritage site after restoration showing decorative architectural features (photograph: Todinirunganga; *source* https://commons.wikimedia.org/wiki/File:Khami_Monuments.jpg)

2010). Despite legislation and attention to heritage management, there is, however, a persistent lack of compliance in all levels (Ashley and Bouakaze-Khan 2011, p. 98). Noemie Arazi (2011, p. 32), for example, noted that World Bank committed to enforcing cultural resource management in only 24% of its developments in sub-Saharan Africa since 1996. Heritage management is a challenge facing archaeologists as the continent moves into the future. It is difficult to strike a balance between the need for development, the deleterious impact it may have on heritage, and the up-rooting of peoples' lives that sometimes accompany growth (Brandt and Hassan 2000). However, if these challenges are not navigated carefully, the risks are disastrous for African heritage and the sustainability, both tangible and intangible, that it undermines. Preserving the past in a manner that blends value systems and ensures local communities are not marginalised in the process is critical.

Consequently, the views on heritage management across Africa is divisive with state and community presenting contrasting views (Aouchal et al. 2022). Ghana's and Nigeria's 'nothing about us, without us' approach was a direct response to the emergence of divergent views (Apoh and Osuagwu 2023). Wazi Apoh and Victoria Osuagwu (2023) presented the 'nothing about us, without us' approach taken in Ghana and Nigeria. In Ghana, a participatory community identification and management approach was established to examine and preserve slave heritage in the Volta Region. The approach disrupts the 'us/them' dichotomy that characterises much of African preservation approaches. Alternatively, Algeria experienced the reconstruction of cultural identities in the post-colonial period that ignored diverse local heritage and perspectives (Aouchal et al. 2022). French colonisation included the destruction of Muslim architecture and Islamic emblems and prioritised Roman archaeology. In the post-colonial state, a more diverse approach is being taken but in producing a national narrative a new version of exclusivism has emerged that requires local remedies. It is apparent that heritage management across Africa, while intending to enact positive good, results more commonly in negative outcomes (Jopela 2023). Systems of participation to heritage management, whether community-based (Smith 2006; Taruvinga 2007; Lupuwana 2024), engaged archaeological (Jopela and Fredriksen 2015; Ndoro and Chirikure 2017a, 2017b) or traditional custodianship (Jopela 2011), might help address some of the negative results (the contributions in Abungu 2016 discuss a range of management strategies across Africa).

8.2.4 Cultural Commodification

The commodification of heritage plays out in various sectors with variable impacts (Atalay 2019). In Africa, this is patently obvious in heritage tourism. The continent's rich historical attractions range from ancient monuments (e.g. the pyramids of Giza, the rock-hewn churches of Lalibela, the ruins of Carthage and Leptis Magna in North Africa) to sites relate to the Atlantic slave trade (such as Gorée Island in Senegal and Elmina Castle in Ghana) and modern historical landmarks (like Robben Island in South Africa). These places draw both local and international tourists, offering educational and often emotive encounters with the past (Gravari-Barbas and Jacquot 2014). However, this presents many issues, including financial constraints, negative impacts on sustainability, shifts caused by climatic change, crime, and land use change, and often the exclusion of local stakeholders (Mutanga et al. 2024). Tourism, unfortunately, is often thought to bring in significant jobs into regions, but heritage-based tourism has not met that hope (World Tourism Organization 2021). At South Africa's Mapungubwe National Park the perception that tourism would lead to upliftment and jobs was present in the local community, but it has not materialised to the extent that people had envisioned. Moreover, the site as a tourist attraction supersedes its cultural solemness and represents a painful exclusion of the region for some (Shabalala 2024). This example illustrates the negative impact tourism may have on community health and well-being (Brooks et al. 2023), although contemporary approaches to heritage are growing more aware of intangible cultural heritage and its impact (Ahmad 2006). Ghana's 2019 *Year of Return* appealed especially to African diaspora visitors to visit the former Gold Coast and Elmina as pilgrimage sites (Mensah 2022). Such roots campaigns are fraught with anxieties and concerns but represent an intangible homecoming-type approach to tourism that fosters identity construction (Aryee 2024). The *Year of Return* injected approximately $1.9 billion into Ghana's economy. Tours to Senegal's Maison des Esclaves on Gorée Island, a former slave house now museum, is similarly a powerful memorialisation. These examples show the double impact of tourism: confronting historical injustice can both educate and reconcile and simultaneously drive economic gains.

Cultural events and festivals also interface history with commerce and the representation of local and national identities. Across Africa, many communities have annual festivals with historical or ritual significance – for example, the Umhlanga reed dance in Eswatini, the Gerewol courtship festival in Niger, or the Fes Festival of sacred music in Morocco. Ikechukwu Ezeuduji (2012) examined event-based rural tourism in sub-Saharan Africa and found that it established authentic and unique tourist experiences. It contributed to preserving indigenous knowledge and cultural values (Mearns et al. 2006), while generating tourism branding. Over the past few decades, this form of cultural tourism has blossomed and led to not only the production of cultural practices and items but its consumption (Jovic 2016). It has transformed from niche to mass market, appealing to a range of people (Richards 2018). Cultural tourism also promotes cross-cultural learning and appreciation (Raymond and Hall 2008; Mokoena 2019). There are recognised risks with this model. Performers may alter their performances to suit tourist desires and in so doing dilute meaning and genuine cultural experience (Saarinen 2007). Archaeological and historical knowledge of the past works in tandem with tourism initiatives. They provide a depth of history that furnishes cultural experiences with additional knowledge, evidence of longevity, and they can enrich the experience. Naturally, this information should take into consideration voice and representation, and it should be incorporated by the performers as they see fit and appropriate.

Exposing people further to Africa's rich history are film productions, many of which include long sequences. Historical epics like Nigeria's film *Invasion 1897* (about the Benin Kingdom's fall) or South Africa's *Shaka iLembe* miniseries (detailing Shaka's family history and his origins) not only entertain but also shape public perception of the past, all while generating profit in the cultural marketplace. These productions can popularize history for broader audiences, though they sometimes sacrifice accuracy for drama (Graham Hancock's *Ancient Apocalypse,* for example, which is unashamedly pseudoscientific and intellectually destructive), or the complexity of the passed is pushed to the background. Still, they indicate the appetite for historical content and the power of media to disseminate Africa's past globally, contributing to cultural tourism. The commodification of history inevitably brings up the question: if heritage sites become commercialized through tourism, do local communities receive a fair share, or are they displaced and marginalized? There have been instances where authorities removed residents from around tourist sites (for example, around the pyramids of Giza or near wildlife parks with historical significance) to cater to visitors, leading to social conflict. Additionally, how do such movies reinforce stereotypes and commodify the 'other'? It has been argued that productions are intended to generate profit and cater to their own assumptions and bias in their economic pursuit (Reeves 2008). Once again, the need to strike balance emerges, and archaeology can aid in this process.

8.3 A Brief, Final Thought

John Fritz and Ted Plog (1970, p. 412) warned that if archaeologists cannot demonstrate the relevance of their discipline to the world, it will move on, leaving the past behind. Yet the world needs the past, and it needs archaeologists and other scholars to reveal its meanings, contradictions, and possibilities. The examples presented here show that the past is not singular or static; it is layered, contested, and deeply entangled with the present. To make this visible, archaeology must be activated in the world – not only as a scholarly pursuit, but as a socially engaged practice. Its role in community lives, social injustice, conservation strategies, heritage management, public engagement, and of course better understanding the many facets of the human past, from its earliest stone traces to contemporary histories, is pivotal. Moving beyond its roots in Eurocentric academia, archaeology must find traction in new footholds: in communities, classrooms, legislation, political spaces, and everyday life. Only then can it contribute meaningfully to the urgent conversations of our time and contribute to progress, growth, and redress.

References

Abungu, G. O. 2016. *Traditional management Systems at heritage sites in Africa.* Midrand: African World Heritage Fund.

Abungu, G. O., and W. Ndoro. 2023. Introduction: The heritage of the colonised. In *Cultural heritage management in Africa: The heritage of the colonized*, ed. G. O. Abungu and W. Ndoro, 1–10. Oxford: Routledge.

Adamu, A. Y. 2013. Diversity in Ethiopia: A historical overview of political challenges. *International Journal of Community Diversity* 12:17–27.

Adamu, M. M. 2009. The legend of Queen Sheba, the Solomonic Dynasty and Ethiopian history: An analysis. *African Research Review* 3 (1): 468–482.

Adeleye, M. A., S. E. Connor, and S. G. Haberle. 2021. A quantitative synthesis of Holocene vegetation change in Nigeria (Western Africa). *The Holocene* 31 (11–12): 1681–1689.

Adewumi, A.A. 2022a. *Africa's wars are hurting its rich heritage: how the law can help [online].* The Conversation. Available from http://theconversation.com/africas-wars-are-hurting-its-rich-heritage-how-the-law-can-help-180041 Accessed on 15 Mar 2025.

Adewumi, A. A. 2022b. The protection of cultural property in Africa: An analysis of policies and practices. *Policy Brief* 16:1–7.

Ahmad, Y. 2006. The scope and definitions of heritage: From tangible to intangible. *International Journal of Heritage Studies* 12:292–300.

Alimen, H. 1957. *The prehistory of Africa.* London: Hutchinson.

Alexander, J. 2011. Saving the African heritage is a global priority: How can a new subdiscipline of rescue archaeology aid it? *African Archaeological Review* 28: 93–96.

Allen, K. J., F. Reide, C. Gouramanis, B. Keenan, M. Stoffel, A. Hu, and M. Ionita. 2022. Coupled insights from the palaeoenvironmental, historical and archaeological archives to support social-ecological resilience and the sustainable development goals. *Environmental Research* 17:055011.

Amineddoleh, L. A. 2015. Cultural heritage vandalism and looting: The role of terrorist organizations, public institutions and private collectors. *Santander Art and Culture Law Review* 1:27–62.

Andah, B. 1995. European encumbrances to the development of relevant theory in African archaeology. In *Theory in archaeology: A world perspective*, ed. P. J. Ucko, 96–108. London: Routledge.

Anderson, D. S. 2019. 'I don't believe, I know': The faith of modern pseudoarchaeology. *SAA Archaeological Record* 19:31–34.

Androff, D. K. 2010. Truth and reconciliation commissions (TRCs): An international human rights intervention and its connection to social work. *British Journal of Social Work* 40:1960–1977.

Aouchal, H. 2023. Cultural heritage management in Africa: The heritage of the colonized. In *Built Heritage*, ed. G. O. Abungu and W. Ndoro, vol. 19.

Aouchal, H., K. Boufenara, and G. Verdini. 2022. Heritage exclusivism in postcolonial Algeria: Assessing local heritageness in Annaba, towards a holistic and participatory approach to urban heritage management. *Historic Environment: Policy & Practice* 13:399–425.

Apoh, W., and V. N. Osuagwu. 2023. 'Nothing about us, without us': Heritage, development and communities in West Africa. In *Cultural heritage management in Africa: The heritage of the colonized*, ed. G. O. Abungu and W. Ndoro, 105–119. Oxford: Routledge.

Arazi, N. 2009. Cultural research management in Africa: Challenges, dangers and opportunities. *Azania: Archaeological Research in Africa* 44: 95–106.

Arazi, N. 2011. Safeguarding archaeological cultural resources in Africa—Policies, methods and issues of (non) compliance. *African Archaeological Review* 28:27–38.

Aryee, R. 2024. Roots tourism experiences, identity construction, social equity and social justice: A mixed methods approach. *Journal of Heritage Tourism* 20:1–30.

Ashley, C., and D. Bouakaze-Khan. 2011. Conservation and management of archaeological sites in Sub-Saharan Africa. *Conservation and Management of Archaeological Sites* 13:95–102.

Atalay, S. 2019. Can archaeology help decolonize the way institutions think? How community-based research is transforming the archaeology training toolbox and helping to transform institutions. *Archaeologies* 15:514–535.

Baker, A., and M. Anjar. 2012. Syria's looted past: How ancient artifacts are being traded for guns. *Time* 12. Available from https://world.time.com/2012/09/12/syrias-looted-past-how-ancient-artifacts-are-being-traded-for-guns/. 15 March 2025.

Bakiner, O. 2016. *Truth commissions: Memory, power, and legitimacy*. Philadelphia: University of Pennsylvania Press.

Barham, L. 1992. Let's walk before we run: An appraisal of historical materialist approaches to the Later Stone Age. *South African Archaeological Bulletin* 47:44–51.

Barker, A. W. 2018. Looting, the antiquities trade, and competing valuations of the past. *Annual Review of Anthropology* 47:455–474.

Bassey, N. 2016. *Oil Politics: Echoes of ecological wars*. Wakefield: Daraja Press.

Batt, F. 2021. The repatriation of African heritage: Shutting the door on the imperialist narrative. *African Human Rights Yearbook* 5:328–350.

Bedarff, H., B. Holznagel, and C. Jakobeit. 1989. Debt-for-nature swaps: Environmental colonialism or a way out from the debt crisis that makes sense? *VRÜ Verfassung und Recht in Übersee* 22:445–459.

Bedaux, R. M., K. C. MacDonald, A. Person, J. Polet, K. Sanogo, A. Schmidt, and S. Sidibé. 2001. The Dia archaeological project: Rescuing cultural heritage in the Inland Niger Delta (Mali). *Antiquity* 75:837–848.

Bedaux, R. M. A., and M. Rowlands. 2001. The future of Mali's past. *Antiquity* 75 (290): 872–876.

Beldados, A., T. Tribe, C. Tribe, M. G. Wondim, D. Mamo, L. Bekele, and E. Abey. 2023. Effect of the 2020–2022 War in Northern Ethiopia on Archaeological and Historical Heritage and the Environmental Context in Amhara National Regional State. *Journal of Ethiopian Studies 56* (1): 69–96.

Bewley, R., A. Wilson, D. Kennedy, D. Mattingly, R. Banks, M. Bishop, J. Bradbury, E. Cunliffe, M. Fradley, and R. Jennings. 2016. Endangered archaeology in the Middle East and North Africa: Introducing the EAMENA project. In *CAA2015. Keep the Revolution Going: Proceedings of the 43rd annual conference on computer applications and quantitative methods in archaeology*, ed. S. Campana, R. Scopigno, G. Carpentiero, and M. Cirillo, 919–932. Oxford: Archaeopress.

Bhambra, G. K., and P. Newell. 2023. More than a metaphor: 'Climate colonialism' in perspective. *Global Social Challenges Journal* 2 (2): 179–187.

Boahen, A. A. 1987. *African perspectives on colonialism*. Baltimore: John Hopkins University Press.

Bodiba, M., M. Steyn, P. Bloomer, M. N. Mosothwane, F. Rühli, and A. Bouwman. 2019. Ancient DNA analysis of the thulamela remains: Deciphering the migratory patterns of a Southern African population. *Journal of African Archaeology* 17 (2): 161–172.

Brandt, S., and F. Hassan. 2000. *Dams and cultural heritage management*. Cape Town: World Commission on Dams.

Brederova, B. 2014. *The looting and deliberate destruction of cultural heritage during social and political unrest of the 21st century: The search for solution*. MA Dissertation. Reading: Reading University.

Breen, C. 2007. Advocacy, international development and world heritage sites in Sub-Saharan Africa. *World Archaeology* 39 (3): 355–370.

Brodie, N. 2003. Stolen history: Looting and illicit trade. *Museum International* 55:10–22.

Brodie, N., and C. Renfrew. 2005. Looting and the world's archaeological heritage: The inadequate response. *Annual Review of Anthropology* 34:343–361.

Brooks, C., E. Waterton, H. Saul, and A. Renzaho. 2023. Exploring the relationships between heritage tourism, sustainable community development and host communities' health and wellbeing: A systematic review. *PLoS One* 18 (3): e0282319.

Buckley-Zistel, S. 2005. "The truth heals"? Gacaca jurisdictions and the consolidation of peace in Rwanda. *Die Friedens-Warte* 80 (1/2): 113–129.

Calvani, S. 2009. Frequency and figures of organized crime in art and antiquities. In *Organized crime in art and antiquities*, ed. S. Manacorda, 28–38. New York: Springer.

Campbell, P. B. 2013. The illicit antiquities trade as a transnational criminal network: Characterizing and anticipating trafficking of cultural heritage. *International Journal of Cultural Property* 20:113–153.

Campbell, R. 2019. Scott, domestication and the end of history. *Cambridge Antiquary Society* 29:692–694.

Chakravarty, A. 2006. Gacaca courts in Rwanda: Explaining divisions within the human rights community. *Yale Journal of International Affairs* 1:132–145.

Chami, F. 2019. *"Sacred Limestone Caves": Management and the use of sacred heritage places in limestone cave areas along the Swahili Coast of Indian Ocean in Tanzania*. PhD Thesis. Brandenburg: Brandenburg University of Technology Cottbus–Senftenberg.

Chirikure, S. 2013. Heritage conservation in Africa: The good, the bad, and the challenges. *South African Journal of Science* 109 (1/2): 1–3.

Chirikure, S. 2020. *Great Zimbabwe: Reclaiming a 'confiscated' past*. London: Routledge.

Chirikure, S., T. Mukwende, and P. Taruvinga. 2015. Post-colonial heritage conservation in Africa: Perspectives from drystone wall restorations at Khami world heritage site, Zimbabwe. *International Journal of Heritage Studies* 22:165–178.

Chirikure, S., and G. Pwiti. 2008. Community involvement in archaeology and cultural heritage management: An assessment from case studies in southern Africa and elsewhere. *Current Anthropology* 49 (3): 467–485.

Clark, J. D. 1970. *The Prehistory of Africa*. London: Thames & Hudson.

Cohen, D. W. 1985. Doing social history from Pim's doorway. In *Reliving the past: The worlds of social history*, ed. O. Zunz, 191–235. Chapel Hill: University of North Carolina Press.

Cohen, D. W. 2007. One or many Africas? A few things bearing on 'Africa 2020'. In *Presented at the 2020 African Studies Conference*. Michigan: University of Michigan.

Coker, C. 2019. *The rise of the civilizational state*. Cambridge: Polity.

Colavito, J. 2019. Whitewashing American prehistory. *SAA Archaeological Record* 19:17–20.

Collingwood, R. G. 1962. *The idea of history*. Oxford: Clarendon Press.

Colton, F. 2015. The destruction of Mali's cultural heritage: Unveiling 'shadow powers' in the analysis of looting during modern warfare. *Potentia: Journal of International Affaris* 6:3–15.

Connah, G. 2013. In *Archaeological practice in Africa: a historical perspective*, ed. P. J. Mitchell and P. J. Lane, 15–36. Oxford: Oxford University Press.

Crossland, Z. 2000. Buried lives: Forensic archaeology and the disappeared in Argentina. *Archaeological Dialogues* 7 (2): 146–159.

Davies, M. I. J. 2012. Some thoughts on a 'useable' African archaeology: Settlement, population and intensive farming among the Pokot of northwest Kenya. *African Archaeological Review* 29:319–353.

Dawdy, S. L. 2009. Millennial archaeology. Locating the discipline in the age of insecurity. *Archaeological Dialogues* 16:131–142.

de Villiers Pienaar, Uys. 1990. *Neem uit die Verlede*. Pretoria: National Parks Board.

Delius, P., L. Chewins, and T. Forssman. 2024. Turning South African history upside down: Ivory and gold production, the Indian Ocean trading system and the shaping of southern African society, 600–1900 AD. *Journal of Southern African Studies* 50 (3): 499–520.

Delius, P., T. Maggs, and M. H. Schoeman. 2012. Bokoni: Old structures, new paradigms? Rethinking pre-colonial society from the perspective of the stone-walled sites in Mpumalanga. *Journal of Southern African Studies* 38 (2): 399–414.

Delius, P., and M. H. Schoeman. 2008. Revisiting Bokoni: Populating the stone ruins of the Mpumalanga Escarpment. In *Five hundred years rediscovered: Southern African precedents and prospects*, ed. N. Swanepoel, A. Esterhuysen, and P. Bonner, 135–167. Johannesburg: Wits University Press.

Delius, P., and M. H. Schoeman. 2010. Reading the rocks and reviewing red herrings. *African Studies* 69:235–254.

Dembélé, M., and J. D. van der Waals. 1991. Looting the antiquities of Mali. *Antiquity* 65 (249): 904–905.

Denbow, J. 2016. Analogy and the danger of over-simplifying the past. *Antiquity* 90 (352): 1086–1086.

Derricourt, R. M. 2011. *Inventing Africa: History, archaeology and ideas*. New York: Pluto Press.

Derricourt, R. M. 2012. Pseudoarchaeology: The concept and its limitations. *Antiquity* 86:524–531.

Diop, C. A. 1960. *L'Afrique Noire Précoloniale: Étude comparée des systèmes politiques et sociaux de l'Europe et de l'Afrique eoire, de l'antiquité à la formation des états modernes*. Paris: Présence Africaine.

Doughty, K. 2015. Law and the architecture of social repair: Gacaca days in post-genocide Rwanda. *Journal of the Royal Anthropological Institute* 21 (2): 419–437.

Douglass, K., and J. Cooper. 2020. Archaeology, environmental justice, and climate change on islands of the Caribbean and southwestern Indian Ocean. *Proceedings of the National Academy of Sciences* 117 (15): 8254–8262.

Dunstan, S. C. 2023. Cheikh Anta Diop's recovery of Egypt: African history as anticolonial practice. In *The anticolonial transnational: Imaginaries, mobilities, and networks in the struggle against empire*, ed. E. Manela and H. Streets-Salter, 135–161. Cambridge: Cambridge University Press.

Earle, J. L. 2018. African intellectual history and historiography. In *Oxford research encyclopedia of African History*, ed. T. Spear. Oxford: Oxford University Press.

Eldredge, E. A. 1992. Sources of conflict in southern Africa, c. 1800–30: The 'Mfecane' reconsidered. *Journal of African History* 33:1–35.

Elia, R. J. 1997. Looting, collecting, and the destruction of archaeological resources. *Nonrenewable Resources* 6:85–98.

Eloff, J. F., and J. B. De Vaal. 1965. Makahane. *Koedoe* 8:74–78.

Eluyemi, O. 2002. *The preservation of Nigeria cultural heritage: Challenges and prospects*. Nigeria: National Commission for Museums and Monuments.

Evans, J. 1975. *Archaeology as education and profession*. London: Institute of Archaeology.

Ezeuduji, I. O. 2012. Strategic event-based rural tourism development for Sub-Saharan Africa. *Current Issues in Tourism* 18:212–228.

Eze-Uzomaka, P. I. 2000. *Museums, archaeologists and Indigenous people: Archaeology and the public in Nigeria*. Oxford: British Archaeological Reports.

Fabiani, M. D. 2018. Disentangling strategic and opportunistic looting: The relationship between antiquities Looting and armed conflict in Egypt. *Arts* 7:22.

Fagan, B. 2018. *A little history of archaeology*. New Haven: Yale University Press.

Fagan, B. M. 1961. Radiocarbon dates for sub-Saharan Africa: From c. 1000 BC. *Journal of African History* 2:137–139.

Fage, J. D., and R. Oliver. 1975. *Cambridge history of Africa.* New York: Cambridge University Press.

Filani, K. 2003. *Museums in Nigeria: Historical antecedents and current practice.* Dakar: Aica Press.

Finneran, N. 2013. Lucy to Lalibela: Heritage and identity in Ethiopia in the twenty-first century. *International Journal of Heritage Studies* 19:41–61.

Fisher, C. 2020. Archaeology for sustainable agriculture. *Journal of Archaeological Research* 28:393–441.

Foltz, W. J. 1965. *From French West Africa to the Mali federation.* New Haven: Yale University Press.

Fontein, J. 2006. *The silence of Great Zimbabwe: Contested landscapes and the power of heritage.* London: Routledge.

Fontein, J. 2021. Reclaiming Great Zimbabwe: Progressive or regressive decoloniality? Great Zimbabwe: Reclaiming a 'confiscated' past, by Shadreck Chirikure. *Azania: Archaeological Research in Africa* 56 (3): 400–414.

Fritz, J. M., and F. Plog. 1970. The nature of archaeological explanation. *American Antiquity* 35:405–412.

Frobenius, L. 1911. *Auf dem Wege nach Atlantis.* Berlin: Vita.

Fuglestad, F. 1992. The Trevor-Roper trap or the imperialism of history: An essay. *History in Africa* 19:309–326.

Gado, B. 2001. The Republic of Niger. In *Trade in Illicit Antiquities: The destruction of the world's archaeological heritage*, ed. N. Brodie, J. Doole, and C. Renfrew, 57–72. Cambridge: McDonald Centre for Archaeological Research.

Galla, A. 1999. Transformation in South Africa: A legacy challenged. *Museum International* 51 (2): 38–43.

Galtung, J. 1969. Violence, peace, and peace research. *Journal of Peace Research* 6:167–191.

Galtung, J. 1990. Cultural violence. *Journal of Peace Research* 27:291–305.

Gashure, S., and D. Wana. 2023. Sustainability of the long-term indigenous soil and water conservation practices in the UNESCO designated cultural landscapes of Konso, Ethiopia. *Current Research in Environmental Sustainability* 5:100221.

Gearon, E. 2013. Mali and the Middle East: Viable solutions. *Middle East Policy* 20:134–144.

Gosden, C. 2012. Postcolonial archaeology. In *Archaeological theory today*, ed. I. Hodder, 251–266. Cambridge: Polity Press.

Gowlett, J. A. J. 2019. Human adaptation and long-term climatic change in Northeast Africa: An archaeological perspective. In *The ecology of survival: Cases from northeast African history*, ed. D. H. Johnson and D. M. Anderson, 27–45. Oxford: Routledge.

Gravari-Barbas, M., and S. Jacquot. 2014. World Heritage, tourism and sustainable development in Africa: Discourses, approaches and challenges. *Tourism Review* 4:4–5.

Grigorova, B., W. Smith, K. Stülpner, J. A. Tumily, and D. Miller. 1998. Fingerprinting of gold artefacts from Mapungubwe, Bostuswe and Thulamela. *Gold Bulletin* 31:99–102.

Grove, L. 2013. Heritocide? Defining and exploring heritage crime. *Public Archaeology* 12 (4): 242–254.

Haber, A. 2014. Commentary: On the debate on ethics in African archaeology. *Azania: Archaeological Research in Africa* 49 (2): 232–236.

Harrison, R. 2016. Archaeologies of emergent presents and futures. *Historical Archaeology* 50:165–180.

Hassett, D. 2024. Rupture and reconciliation: The neoliberal logics of Emmanuel Macron's colonial memory policies. *Modern & Contemporary France* 32 (1): 31–53.

Hayati, D., Z. Ranjbar, and E. Karami. 2010. Measuring agricultural sustainability. In *Biodiversity, Biofuels, Agroforestry and Conservation Agriculture*, ed. E. Lichtfouse, 73–98. Dordrecht: Springer Netherlands.

Heine, J., and M. Tellinger. 2008. *Adam's calendar: Discovering the oldest man-made structure on Earth*. Johannesburg: Zulu Planet.
Heleta, S. 2016. Decolonisation of higher education: Dismantling epistemic violence and Eurocentrism in South Africa. *Transformation in Higher Education* 1 (1): 1–8.
Henriet, B. 2022. Decolonizing African history: Authenticité, cosmopolitanism and knowledge production in Zaire, 1971–1975. *Journal of Eastern African Studies* 16 (2): 335–354.
Hicks, D. 2020. *The Brutish Museums: The Benin bronzes, colonial violence and cultural restitution*. London: Pluto Press.
HOC. 2003. *Substantiation of appeal submitted by the hands off Prestwich street Ad HOC Committee*. Cape Town: Hands Off Prestwich Street Ad Hoc Committee.
Hodder, I. 1984. Archaeology in 1984. *Antiquity* 58:25–32.
Holl, A. F. C. 2020. Dark side archaeology: Climate change and mid-Holocene Saharan pastoral adaptation. *African Archaeological Review* 37 (3): 491–495.
Hoopes, J. 2019. Introduction. *SAA Archaeological Record* 19:8–9.
Hromnik, C. 1981. *Indo-Africa: Towards an understanding of the history of sub-Saharan Africa*. Cape Town: Juta and co.
Hromnik, C. 1999. Gitlane: Where the moon sickle strikes—on the edge of time at Elandsdoorn. *Nordic Journal of African Studies* 8:1–17.
Hudson, M. J., M. Aoyama, K. C. Hoover, and J. Uchiyama. 2012. Prospects and challenges for an archaeology of global climate change. *WIREs Climate Change* 3 (4): 313–328.
Huffman, T. N. 1998. *The Goldfields Thulamela project*. Johannesburg: University of the Witwatersrand, Prepared for the South African National Parks.
Hutchings, R. M., and M. La Salle. 2019. Sustainable archaeology: Soothing rhetoric for an anxious institution. *Antiquity* 93:1653–1660.
Intergovernmental Panel on Climate Change. 2022. *Climate change 2022: Impacts, adaptation and vulnerability*. Cambridge: Cambridge University Press.
Jopela, A. 2011. Traditional custodianship: A useful framework for heritage management in southern Africa? *Conservation and Management of Archaeological Sites* 13 (2–3): 103–122.
Jopela, A. 2023. The trouble with participation: Heritage places, politics and communities in Africa. In *Cultural heritage management in Africa: The heritage of the colonized*, ed. G. O. Abungu and W. Ndoro, 88–104. Oxford: Routledge.
Jopela, A., and P. D. Fredriksen. 2015. Public archaeology, knowledge meetings and heritage ethics in southern Africa: An approach from Mozambique. *World Archaeology* 47 (2): 261–284.
Jordan, P. 1997. *Thulamela excavation proves black heritage*. Johannesburg: Mail & Guardian.
Joseph, M. 2012. *Minister: 2% of artifacts stolen during security vacuum*. Cairo: Egypt Independent.
Jovic, D. 2016. Cultural tourism in the context of relations between mass and alternative tourism. *Current Issues in Tourism* 19:605–612.
Kaarsholm, P. 1990. Mental colonisation or catharsis? Theatre, democracy and cultural struggle from Rhodesia to Zimbabwe. *Journal of Southern African Studies* 16:246–275.
Kankpeyeng, B. W., and C. R. DeCorse. 2004. Ghana's vanishing past: Development, antiquities, and the destruction of the archaeological Record. *African Archaeological Review* 21:89–128.
Kassiem, A. 2003. Public given time to appeal against moving graves, *Cape Times*, 6.
Kila, J. D. 2013. Inactive, reactive, or pro-active? Cultural property crimes in the context of contemporary armed conflicts. *Journal of Eastern Mediterranean Archaeology & Heritage Studies* 1:319–342.
King, R. 2012. Teaching archaeological pasts in South Africa: Historical and contemporary considerations of archaeological education. *Archaeologies* 8 (2): 85–115.
Kleinitz, C., and C. Näser. 2013. Archaeology, development and conflict: A case study from the African continent. *Archaeologies: Journal of World Archaeological Congress* 9:162–191.
Koch, E. 1996. *Unearthing a find of a different kind*. Johannesburg: Mail & Guardian.
Konishi, S. 2019. First nations scholars, settler colonial studies, and indigenous history. *Australian Historical Studies* 50 (3): 285–304.

Kouroupas, M. P. 1995. US efforts to protect cultural property: Implementation of the 1970 UNESCO convention. *African Arts* 28 (4): 32–41.

Küsel, M. 1992. A preliminary report on settlement layout and gold melting at Thula Mela, a Late Iron Age site in the Kruger National Park. *Koedoe* 35 (1): 55–64.

Kusimba, C. M. 2017. Community archaeology and heritage in coastal and western Kenya. *Journal of Community Archaeology and Heritage* 4:218–228.

Labi, A. and S. Robinson. 2001. *Looting Africa [online]*. Time. Available from: https://time.com/archive/6664439/looting-africa/ Accessed 15 Mar 2025.

Lancelotti, C., S. Biagetti, A. Zerboni, D. Usai, and M. Madella. 2019. The archaeology and ethnoarchaeology of rain-fed cultivation in arid and hyper-arid North Africa. *Antiquity* 93:1026–1039.

Lane, P. 1994. The use and abuse of ethnography in the study of the southern African iron age. *Azania: Archaeological Research in Africa* 29 (1): 51–64.

Lane, P. J. 2005. Barbarous tribes and unrewarding gyrations? The changing role of ethnographic imagination in African archaeology. In *African archaeology: A critical introduction*, ed. A. B. Stahl, 24–54. Oxford: Blackwell Publishing.

Lane, P. J. 2011. Possibilities for a postcolonial archaeology in sub-Saharan Africa: Indigenous and usable pasts. *World Archaeology* 43 (1): 7–25.

Lane, P. J. 2015. Archaeology in the age of the Anthropocene: A critical assessment of its scope and societal contributions. *Journal of Field Archaeology* 40 (5): 485–498.

Laudan, L. 1996. *Beyond Positivism and Relativism: Theory, method and evidence*. Boulder: Westview Press.

Legassick, M. 1970. Review of five hundred years: A history of South Africa. *African Historical Studies* 3 (2): 491–496.

Lightfoot, K. G. 1995. Culture contact studies: Redefining the relationship between prehistoric and historical archaeology. *American Antiquity* 60 (2): 199–217.

Little, B. J., ed. 1992. *Text-aided archaeologies*. Boca Raton: CRC Press.

Little, B. J. 2009. What can archaeology do for justice, peace, community, and the earth? *Historical Archaeology* 43 (4): 115–119.

Liverani, M. 2000. The Garamantes: A fresh approach. *Libyan Studies* 31:17–28.

Logan, A. L., D. S. Stump, S. T. Goldstein, E. A. Orijemie, and M. H. Schoeman. 2019. Usable pasts forum: Critically engaging food security. *African Archaeological Review* 36:419–438.

Lucas, G. 2004. *The archaeology of time*. London: Routledge.

Lupuwana, V. 2024. Heritage and social justice in southern Africa: Rethinking spaces of community involvement in heritage Management. In *Routledge handbook of critical african heritage studies*, ed. A. Sinamai, J. Giblin, S. Chirikure, and I. Odiaua, 88–100. Oxford: Routledge.

MacEachern, S. 2001. Cultural resource management and Africanist archaeology. *Antiquity* 75 (290): 866–871.

MacEachern, S. 2010. Seeing like an oil company's cultural heritage management programme: Exxon and archaeology on the Chad export project. *Journal of Social Archaeology* 10:347–366.

Malan, A., 2003. *Prestwich Place. Exhumation of accidentally discovered burial ground in Green Point, Cape Town [Permit no. 80/03/06/001/51]: Public consultation process 9 June to 18 August 2003*. Cape Town: Cultural Sites and Resources Forum, Prepared by Dr Antonia Malan, Cultural Sites and Resources Forum for the South African Heritage Resources Agency and the Developer.

Mamdani, M. 2019. Decolonising universities. In *Sharing knowledge, transforming societies: The norhed programme 2013–2020*, ed. T. Halvorsen, S. Orgeret, and R. Krøvel, 48–67. Cape Town: African Minds.

Manetsi, T. 2023. Heritage governance in post-colonial Africa. In *Cultural heritage management in Africa: The heritage of the colonized*, ed. G. O. Abungu and W. Ndoro, 57–69. Oxford: Routledge.

Mavume, A. F., B. E. Banze, O. A. Macie, and A. J. Queface. 2021. Analysis of climate change projections for Mozambique under the representative concentration pathways. *Atmosphere* 12:588.

McCorriston, J., and J. Fields. 2019. *World prehistory and the anthropocene: An introduction to human history*. London: Thames & Hudson.
McGranaghan, M. 2017. Ethnographic analogy in archaeology: Methodological insights from southern Africa. In *Oxford Research Encyclopedia of African History*, ed. T. Spear. Oxford: Oxford University Press.
McGuire, T. 1990. African antiquities removed during colonialism: Restoring a stolen cultural legacy. *Detroit College of Law Review* 1990:31–69.
Mearns, M. A., A. S. A. Du Toit, and G. Mukuka. 2006. Conservation of indigenous knowledge at cultural villages: An exploratory study. *Mousaion* 24:23–50.
Mensah, I. 2022. Homecoming events and diaspora tourism promotion in emerging economies: The case of the Year of Return 2019 campaign in Ghana. In *Marketing tourist destinations in emerging economies*, ed. I. Mensah, K. Balasubramanian, M. R. Jamaluddin, G. Alcoriza, V. Gaffar, and S. M. Rasoolimanesh, 211–229. Cham: Springer International Publishing.
Meskell, L. 2007. Falling walls and mending fences: Archaeological ethnography in the Limpopo. *Journal of Southern African Studies* 33 (2): 383–400.
Meskell, L. 2012. *The nature of heritage: The new South Africa*. Malden: Wiley-Backwell.
Meskell, L. 2018. *A future in ruins: UNESCO, world heritage, and the dream of peace*. Oxford: Oxford University Press.
Michalopoulos, S., and E. Papaioannou. 2020. Historical legacies and African development. *Journal of Economic Literature* 58:53–128.
Milão, S., T. Ribeiro, M. Correia, I. C. Neves, J. Flores, and O. Alvarez. 2025. Contributions to architectural and urban resilience through vulnerability assessment: The case of Mozambique Island's World Heritage. *Heritage* 8 (1): 25.
Miller, D. E. 1996a. Letter from Thulamela. *Southern African Review of Books* 45:19–20.
Miller, D. E., and N. J. Van der Merwe. 1994. Early metal working in Sub-Saharan Africa: A review of recent research. *Journal of African History* 35:1–36.
Miller, J. C. 1985. History and archaeology in Africa. *Journal of Interdisciplinary History* 16 (2): 291–303.
Miller, S. M. 1996b. Rebuilding the walls of 16th-century Thulamela. In *Aspects of African archaeology: Papers from the 10th Congress of the Pan-African association for prehistory and related studies*, ed. G. Pwiti and R. Soper, 837–839. Harare: University of Zimbabwe Publications.
Miller, S. M. 1997. *The archaeological investigation, the rebuilding of the walls and the public presentation of the Thulamela site in the northern Kruger National Park*. Pretoria: South African National Parks.
Miller, S. M. 2018. *Thulamela: The lost gold of the Vha Venda*. Pretoria: Aluwen.
Mitchell, P. 2008. Practising archaeology at a time of climatic catastrophe. *Antiquity* 82:1093–1103.
Mitchell, P. J. 2003. Anyone for hxaro? Thoughts on the theory and practice of exchange in southern African Later Stone Age archaeology. In *Researching Africa's past: New perspectives from British archaeology*, ed. P. J. Mitchell, A. Haour, and J. Hobart, 35–43. Oxford: Oxbow Books.
Mitchell, P. J. 2005. *African connections: An archaeological perspective on Africa and the wider world*. Oxford: AltaMira Press.
Mitchell, P. J. 2019. Carpe diem: Building African archaeology in the twenty-first century. In *Archaeology in Africa: Potential and perspectives on laboratory and fieldwork research*, ed. S. de Lernia and M. Gallinaro, 7–15. Sesto Florentino: All'Insegna del Giglio.
Mitchell, P. J. 2024. *The Archaeology of Southern Africa*. Cambridge: Cambridge University Press.
Mitchell, P. J., and G. Whitelaw. 2005. The archaeology of southernmost Africa from c. 2000 BP to the early 1800s: A review of recent research. *Journal of African History* 46 (2): 209–241.
Mlambo, A. S. 2001. Review of voices from the rocks: Nature, culture and historyin the Matopos Hills of Zimbabwe. By Terence Ranger. *Journal of African History* 42:158–159.
Mokoena, L. G. 2019. Cultural tourism: Cultural presentation at the Basotho cultural village, free state, South Africa. *Journal of Tourism and Cultural Change* 18:470–490.
Mudimbe, V. Y. 1988. *The invention of Africa: Gnosis, philosophy, and the order of knowledge*. Bloomington: Indiana University Press.

Muller, C. F. J. 1969. *Five hundred years: A history of South Africa*. Pretoria: Academica.

Mulubrhan, G., Tekulu, F. B. Gebre, H. T. Hailu, H. G. Asgedom, D. B. and Hadgu, T. B. 2024. The War in Tigray and Its Immediate Impact on Cultural Heritage in Eastern Tigray. Journal of African Archaeology, 22 (1–2), 1–11.

Munjeri, D. 2008. Introduction to international conventions and charters on immovable cultural heritage. In *Cultural Heritage and the law: Protecting immovable heritage in Sub-Saharan Africa*, ed. W. Ndoro, A. Mumma, and G. Abungu, 13–23. Rome: ICCROM Conservation Studies.

Mutanga, C. N., O. D. Kolawole, R. Gondo, and J. E. Mbaiwa. 2024. A review and SWOC analysis of natural heritage tourism in Sub-Saharan Africa. *Journal of Heritage Tourism* 19:49–67.

Ndlovu, N. 2011. Management versus preservation: Archaeological heritage management in a transforming South Africa. *Conservation and Management of Archaeological Sites* 13 (2–3): 123–133.

Ndlovu-Gatsheni, S. J. 2018. *Epistemic freedom in Africa: Deprovincialization and decolonization*. London: Taylor & Francis.

Ndoro, W. 2021. Cultural heritage and conflict in Africa. In *Oxford research encyclopedia of anthropology*, ed. M. S. Aldenderfer. Oxford: Oxford University Press.

Ndoro, W., and S. Chirikure. 2017a. Caring matters: The future of managing heritage in Africa. In *Managing Heritage in Africa*, ed. W. Ndoro and S. Chirikure, 237–250. London: Routledge.

Ndoro, W., and S. Chirikure. 2017b. Caring matters: The future of managing heritage in Africa. In *Managing heritage in Africa*, ed. W. Ndoro, S. Chirikure, and J. Deacon, 237–250. Oxford: Routledge.

Ndoro, W., and H. Kiriama. 2008. Management mechanisms in heritage legislation. In *Cultural heritage and the law: Protecting immovable heritage in Sub-Saharan Africa*, ed. W. Ndoro, A. Mumma, and G. Abungu, 53–62. Rome: ICCROM Conservation Studies.

Nemaheni, T. I. 2004. The reburial of human remains at Thulamela, Kruger National Park, South Africa. In *The dead and their possessions: Repatriation in principle, policy and practice*, ed. C. Fforde, J. Hubert, and P. Turnball, 256–261. London: Routledge.

Newitt, M. 2004. Mozambique Island: The rise and decline of an East African coastal city, 1500-1700. *Portuguese Studies* 20 (1): 21–37.

Ngaba-Waye, A. 1996. The future of African archaeology: Cultural continuity and the future. *African Archaeological Review* 13:5–34.

Nhamo, A., and S. Katsamudanga. 2022. Legal protection of African cultural heritage in the 21st century and beyond: A prognosis and futures perspective. In *Cultural heritage management in Africa: The heritage of the colonized*, ed. G. O. Abungu and W. Ndoro, 70–87. Oxford: Routledge.

Nkrumah, K. 1963. *Africa must unite*. New York: Frederick A. Praeger.

Ntloedibe, F. N. 2019. Where are our heroes and ancestors? The spectre of Steve Biko's ideas in Rhodes must fall and the transformation of South African universities. *African Identities* 17 (1): 64–79.

Nyamnjoh, A. 2017. The phenomenology of Rhodes Must Fall: Student activism and the experience of alienation at the University of Cape Town. *Strategic Review for Southern Africa* 39:256–277.

Ogot, B. A. 2009. Rereading the history and historiography of epistemic domination and resistance in Africa. *African Studies Review* 52 (1): 1–22.

Onuoha, G. 2016. Shared histories, divided memories: Mediating and navigating the tensions in Nigeria–Biafra War discourses. *Africa Today* 63 (1): 3–21.

Orser, C. E. 2012. An archaeology of eurocentrism. *American Antiquity* 77:737–755.

Parcak, S., D. Gathings, C. Childs, G. Mumford, and E. Cline. 2016. Satellite evidence of archaeological site looting in Egypt: 2002–2013. *Antiquity* 90 (349): 188–205.

Patalano, R., C. Arthur, W. C. Carleton, S. Challis, G. Dewar, K. Gayantha, G. Gleixner, J. Ilgner, M. Lucas, S. Marzo, R. Mokhachane, K. Pazan, D. Spurite, M. W. Morley, A. Parker, P. Mitchell, B. A. Stewart, and P. Roberts. 2023. Ecological stability of late Pleistocene-to-Holocene Lesotho, southern Africa, facilitated human upland habitation. *Communications Earth & Environment* 4 (1): 129.

Pearce, D. G. 2012. Ethnography and history: the significance of social change in interpreting rock art. In *Working with rock art: Recording, presenting and understanding rock art using indigenous knowledge*, ed. B. W. Smith, Helskog, and D. Morris, 135–145. Johannesburg: Wits University Press.

Penn, N. 1991. "Excavating archives at Oudepost": A riposte. *Social Dynamics* 17:101–105.

Phillipson, D. W. 2009. Aksumite civilization, its connections and descendants. *Der Antike Sudan. Mitteilungen der Sudanarchäologischen Gesellschaft zu Berlin e.* 20:75–92.

Pikirayi, I. 1999. Research trends in the historical archaeology of Zimbabwe. In *Historical archaeology: Back from the edge*, ed. P. Funari, M. Hall, and S. Jones, 67–84. London: Routledge.

Pikirayi, I. 2001. *The Zimbabwe culture: Origins and decline in Southern Zimbabwean states*. Walnut Creek: Alta Mira.

Pikirayi, I. 2006a. Gold, black ivory and houses of stone. In *Historical archaeology*, ed. M. Hall and S. W. Silliman, 230–250. Oxford: Blackwell.

Pikirayi, I. 2006b. The kingdom, the power and forevermore: Zimbabwe culture in contemporary art and architecture. *Journal of Southern African Studies* 32:755–770.

Pikirayi, I. 2009a. Palaces, feiras and prazos: An historical archaeological perspective of African Portuguese contact in northern Zimbabwe. *African Archaeological Review* 26:163–185.

Pikirayi, I. 2009b. What can archaeology do for society in southern Africa? *Historical Archaeology* 43 (4): 125–127.

Pikirayi, I. 2014. Sharing the past: Archaeology and community engagement in southern Africa. In *Sharing archaeology*, ed. P. Stone and Z. Hui, 150–166. London: Routledge.

Pikirayi, I. 2015. The future of archaeology in Africa. *Antiquity* 89 (345): 531–541.

Pikirayi, I. 2019. Sustainability and an archaeology of the future. *Antiquity* 93:1669–1671.

Pollard, E., R. Bates, J.-C. Comte, E. Graham, C. Lubao, N. Munisi, and E. B. Ichumbaki. 2025. Climate change, coastal heritage digitization, and local community engagement at the ruins of Kilwa Kisiwani world heritage site, Tanzania. *Journal of Field Archaeology* 50 (1): 6–21.

Posnansky, M. 2017. Archaeology and the local community in Africa: A retrospective. *Journal of Community Archaeology & Heritage* 4 (2): 77–84.

Pwiti, G. and W. Ndoro. 1999. The legacy of colonialism: Perceptions of the cultural heritage in southern Africa, with special reference to Zimbabwe. *African Archaeological Review* 16: 143–153.

Ranger, T. 1999. *Voices from the rocks: Nature, culture and history in the Matopos Hills of Zimbabwe*. Oxford: James Currey Ltd.

Ranger, T. 2004. Nationalist historiography, patriotic history and the history of the nation: The struggle over the past in Zimbabwe. *Journal of Southern African Studies* 30 (2): 215–234.

Rapp, G. R., and C. L. Hill. 2006. *Geoarchaeology: The earth-science approach to archaeological interpretation*. New Haven: Yale University Press.

Raymond, E. M., and C. M. Hall. 2008. The development of cross-cultural (mis)understanding through volunteer tourism. *Journal of Sustainable Tourism* 16:530–543.

Rayne, L., J. Bradbury, D. Mattingly, G. Philip, R. Bewley, and A. Wilson. 2017. From above and on the ground: Geospatial methods for recording endangered archaeology in the Middle East and North Africa. *Geosciences* 7 (4): 100.

Reed, K., and P. Ryan. 2019. Lessons from the past and the future of food. *World Archaeology* 51:1–16.

Reeves, H. L. 2008. Commodifying Africa on US network reality television. *Communication, Culture & Critique* 1:416–446.

Reid, A., and P. J. Lane. 2004. African historical archaeologies: An introductory consideration of scope and potential. In *African historical archaeologies*, ed. A. Reid and P. J. Lane, 1–32. New York: Kluwer.

Reid, R. 2011. Past and presentism: The 'precolonial' and the foreshortening of African history. *Journal of African History* 52 (2): 135–155.

Reilly, M. C. 2019. Futurity, time, and archaeology. *Journal of Contemporary Archaeology* 6:1–15.

Richards, G. 2018. Cultural tourism: A review of recent research and trends. *Journal of Hospitality and Tourism Management* 36:12–21.

Robertshaw, P. 2000. Sibling rivalry? The intersection of archaeology and history. *History in Africa* 27:261–286.

Robertshaw, P. 2005. African connections: Archaeological perspectives on Africa and the wider world. By Peter Mitchell. *Journal of African Archaeology* 3 (2): 301–303.

Robins-Early, N. 2015. Syria's historical artifacts aren't just being destroyed by ISIS, they're being looted. *The Huffington Post*, March 3.

Rockman, M. 2011. The necessary roles of archaeology in climate change mitigation and adaptation. In *Archaeology in society*, ed. M. Rockman and J. Flatman, 193–215. New York: Springer.

Rosenzweig, M. S. 2020. Confronting the present: Archaeology in 2019. *American Anthropologist* 122 (2): 284–305.

Russell-Wood, A. J. R. 1984. African history: Unrewarding gyrations or new perspectives on the historian's craft. *The History Teacher* 17 (2): 247–266.

Saarinen, J. 2007. Cultural tourism, local communities and representations of authenticity: The case of Lesedi and Swazi cultural villages in southern Africa. In *Culture and community: Tourism studies in eastern and southern Africa*, ed. B. Wishitemi, A. Spenceley, and H. Wels, 139–154. Amsterdam: Rozenburg.

Sauer, E. W. 2004. The disunited subject: Human history's split into 'history' and 'archaeology'. In *Archaeology and ancient history*, ed. E. W. Sauer, 29–58. London: Routledge.

Schmidt, P. R. 1995. Using archaeology to remake history. In *Making alternative histories: The practice of archaeology and history in non-western settings*, ed. P. R. Schmidt and T. C. Patterson, 119–147. Santa Fe: School for Advanced Research Press.

Schmidt, P. R. 2006. *Historical archaeology in Africa: Representation, social memory, and oral traditions*. Walnut Creek: AltaMira Press.

Schmidt, P. R. 2013. Historical archaeology, colonial entanglements, and recuperating 'timeless' histories through structuralism. In *The death of prehistory*, ed. P. R. Schmidt and S. A. Mrozowski, 92–116. Oxford: Oxford University Press.

Schmidt, P. R., and R. J. McIntosh. 1996. *Plundering Africa's past*. Oxford: James Currey Ltd.

Schmidt, P. R., and S. A. Mrozowski. 2013a. *The death of prehistory*. Oxford: Oxford University Press.

Schmidt, P. R., and S. A. Mrozowski. 2013b. The death of prehistory: Reforming the past, looking to the future. In *The death of prehistory*, ed. P. R. Schmidt and S. A. Mrozowski, 1–28. Oxford: Oxford University Press.

Schmidt, P. R., and I. Pikirayi. 2018. Will historical archaeology escape its Western prejudices to become relevant to Africa? *Archaeologies* 14:443–471.

Schmidt, P. R., and J. R. Walz. 2005. Historical archaeology in Africa: Noble claims, revisionist perspectives and African voices? *Journal of African History* 46 (2): 315–319.

Schnapp, A. 2014. The birth of the archaeological vision: From antiquaries to archaeologists. *West 86th: A Journal of Decorative Arts, Design History, and Material Culture* 21 (2): 216–229.

Schneider, T. D. 2019. Heritage in-between: Seeing native histories in colonial California. *Public Historian* 41:51–63.

Schoeman, M. H., and I. Pikirayi. 2011. Repatriating more than Mapungubwe human remains: Archaeological material culture, a shared future and an artificially divided past. *Journal of Contemporary African Studies* 29 (4): 389–403.

Schrire, C. 1988. The historical archaeology of the impact of colonialism in 17th-century South Africa. *Antiquity* 62 (235): 214–225.

Schrire, C. 1990. Excavating archives at Oudepost 1, Cape. *Social Dynamics* 16 (1): 11–21.

Schrire, C. 1991. Is the Penn mightier than the shovel? A sally to a riposte. *Social Dynamics* 17:106–109.

Schrire, C., and J. Deacon. 1989. The indigenous artefacts from Oudepost I, a colonial outpost of the VOC at Saldanha Bay, Cape. *South African Archaeological Bulletin* 44:105–113.

Scott, J. C. 2017. *Against the grain: A deep history of the earliest states*. New Haven: Yale University Press.

Seitz, P. 2012. No more white history. *Curator* 55:279–285.

Shabalala, L. P. 2024. Heritage sites as tourism attractions: Spiritual, psychological and emotional toll on communities. *Koedoe* 66 (2): a1800.

Shanks, M., and C. Tilley. 1987. *Social theory and archaeology*. Cambridge: Polity Press.

Shanks, M., and C. Tilley. 1992. *Reconstructing archaeology: Theory and practice*. London: Routledge.

Shaw, J. 2016. Archaeology, climate change and environmental ethics: Diachronic perspectives on human:non-human:environment worldviews, activism and care. *World Archaeology* 48 (4): 449–465.

Shaw, T. 1997. The contemporary plundering of Africa's past. *African Archaeological Review* 14 (1): 1–7.

Sheldrick, E., and A. Zerbini. 2017. A heritage inventory for documenting endangered archaeology in the Middle East and North Africa. *ISPRS Annals of the Photogrammetry, Remote Sensing and Spatial Information Sciences* IV-2/W2:237–241.

Shelton, D. 2003. The world of atonement: Reparations for historical injustices. *Netherlands International Law Review* 50:289–325.

Shepherd, N. 2007. Archaeology dreaming: Post-apartheid urban imaginaries and the bones of the Prestwich street dead. *Journal of Social Archaeology* 7:3–28.

Smith, B. W. 2006. Rock art tourism in southern Africa: Problems, possibilities and poverty relief. In *Of the past to the future: Integrating archaeology and conservation*. Proceedings of the conservation theme of the 5th World Archaeological Congress, Washington D.C., 22–26 June 2003, ed. N. Agnew and J. Bridgland, 322–330. The Getty Conservation Institute: Los Angeles.

Sorensen, M. L., C. Evans, and K. Richter. 2011. A place of history: Archaeology and heritage at Cidade Velha, Cape Verde. In *Slavery in Africa: Archaeology and memory* eds. P. J. Lane and K. C. MacDonald, 421–442. Oxford: British Academy.

Spennemann, D. 2011. Beyond 'preserving the past for the future': Contemporary relevance and historic preservation. *CRM Journal* 8:7–22.

Stahl, A. B. 2009. The archaeology of African history. *International Journal of African Historical Studies* 42 (2): 241–255.

Stahl, A. B. 2010. 'Route work' through alternative archives: Reflections on cross-disciplinary practice. *South African Historical Journal* 62 (2): 252–267.

Stahl, A. B. 2014. Africa in the world: (Re)centering African history through archaeology. *Journal of Anthropological Research* 70 (1): 5–33.

Stahl, A. B. 2023. *Archaeology: Why it matters*. Cambridge: Polity Press.

Steyn, M., S. Miller, W. C. Nienaber, and M. Loots. 1998. Late iron age gold burials from Thulamela (Pafuri region, Kruger National Park). *South African Archaeological Bulletin* 53:73–85.

Stump, D. S. 2013. On applied archaeology, indigenous knowledge, and the usable past. *Current Anthropology* 54:268–298.

Suárez, R. R. 2009. The archaeology of a search: An archaeological search; the history of the finding of "Che" Guevara's remains. In *Memories from darkness: Archaeology of repression and resistance in Latin America*, ed. P. Funari, A. Zarankin, and M. Salerno, 129–144. New York: Springer New York.

Swanepoel, N., A. Esterhuysen, and P. Bonner, eds. 2008. *Five hundred years rediscovered: Southern African precedents and prospect*. Johannesburg: University of the Witwatersrand Press.

Tans, P. P., A. F. M. De Jong, and W. G. Mook. 1979. Natural atmospheric 14C variation and the Suess effect. *Nature* 280 (5725): 826–828.

Tapete, D., and F. Cigna. 2019. Detection of archaeological looting from space: Methods, achievements and challenges. *Remote Sensing* 11 (20): 2389.

Taruvinga, P. 2007. Community participation and rock art management in Zimbabwe. In *African Rock Art: The future of Africa's past. Proceedings of the 2004 International Rock Art Conference*, ed. J. Deacon, 39–48. Nairobi: TARA.

Taruvinga, P. 2020. World heritage, sustainable development, and Africa. In *Oxford research encyclopedia of anthropology*, ed. M. S. Aldenderfer. Oxford: Oxford University Press.

Taruvinga, P., and W. Ndoro. 2003. The vandalism of the Domboshava rock painting site, Zimbabwe: Some reflections on approaches to heritage management. *Conservation and Management of Archaeological Sites* 6 (1): 3–10.

Tassie, G., A. De Trafford, and J. van Wetering. 2015. Egypt's heritage in times of conflict and crisis. In *The management of Egypt's cultural heritage*, ed. F. A. Hassan, G. Tassie, L. Owens, A. De Trafford, J. van Wetering, and O. El Daly, 14–47. London: Golden House Publications.

Thomas, D. S. G., and S. L. Burrough. 2012. Interpreting geoproxies of late Quaternary climate change in African drylands: Implications for understanding environmental change and early human behaviour. *Quaternary International* 253:5–17.

Thompson, J. C., D. K. Wright, S. J. Ivory, J.-H. Choi, S. Nightingale, A. Mackay, F. Schilt, E. Otárola-Castillo, J. Mercader, S. L. Forman, T. Pietsch, A. S. Cohen, J. R. Arrowsmith, M. Welling, J. Davis, B. Schiery, P. Kaliba, O. Malijani, M. W. Blome, C. A. O'Driscoll, S. M. Mentzer, C. Miller, S. Heo, J. Choi, J. Tembo, F. Mapemba, D. Simengwa, and E. Gomani-Chindebvu. 2021. Early human impacts and ecosystem reorganization in southern-central Africa. *Science Advances* 7 (19): eabf9776.

Trigger, B. G. 2006. *A history of archaeological thought*. 2nd ed. Cambridge: Cambridge University Press.

Tsosie, R. 2007. Indigenous people and environmental justice: The impact of climate change. *University of Colorado Law Review* 78 (4): 1625–1678.

Tüske, L. 2024. Pharaonism and contemporary Egypt: A new 'civilizational state' in statu nascendi. *The Arabist: Budapest Studies in Arabic* 47:171–182.

Van de Noort, R. 2011. Conceptualising climate change archaeology. *Antiquity* 85 (329): 1039–1048.

Vansina, J. 1995a. Historians, are archeologists your siblings? *History in Africa* 22:369–408.

Vansina, J. 1995b. New linguistic evidence and 'The Bantu Expansion'. *Journal of African History* 36:173–195.

Vansina, J., R. Mauny, and L. V. Thomas. 1964. The techniques of the historian in Africa. In *The historian in tropical Africa*, ed. J. Vansina, R. Mauny, and L. V. Thomas, 59–76. London: Oxford University Press.

Vergano, D. 2014. *Archaeologists warn of pillaged Egypt as U.S. weighs tougher antiquities laws*. Washington, D.C: National Geographic.

Vizenor, G. 1999. *Manifest manners: Narratives on post-Indian survivance*. Lincoln: University of Nebraska Press.

Vollgraaff, H. 2014. Developing policy on heritage crime in southern Africa. In *Heritage crime*, ed. L. Grove and S. Thomas, 169–187. London: Palgrave Macmillan UK.

Vousdoukas, M. I., J. Clarke, R. Ranasinghe, L. Reimann, N. Khalaf, T. M. Duong, B. Ouweneel, S. Sabour, C. E. Iles, C. H. Trisos, L. Feyen, L. Mentaschi, and N. P. Simpson. 2022. African heritage sites threatened as sea-level rise accelerates. *Nature Climate Change* 12 (3): 256–262.

Wade, R. 2009. *A systematics for interpreting past structures with possible cosmic references in Sub-Saharan Africa*. MA Dissertation. Pretoria: University of Pretoria.

Westley, K., G. Andreou, C. El Safadi, H. O. Huigens, J. Nikolaus, R. Ortiz-Vazquez, N. Ray, A. Smith, S. Tews, L. Blue, and C. Breen. 2023. Climate change and coastal archaeology in the Middle East and North Africa: Assessing past impacts and future threats. *Journal of Island and Coastal Archaeology* 18 (2): 251–283.

Whyte, K. 2016. Is it colonial déjà vu? Indigenous peoples and climate Iijustice. In *Humanities for the Environment: Integrating knowledge, forging new constellations of practice*, ed. J. Adamson and M. Davis, 88–104. Rochester: Social Science Research Network.

Wild, S. 2017. Theft of South African relics riles researchers. *Nature* 548:22479.

Wolf, E. 1982. *Europe and the people without history*. Berkley: University of California Press.

Wolfe, P. 2006. Settler colonialism and the elimination of the native. *Journal of Genocide Research* 8 (4): 387–409.

World Bank. 2023. *Mozambique country climate and development report*. Washington: World Bank.

World Tourism Organization. 2021. *International tourism highlights, 2020 edition*. Madrid: UNWTO.

Wright, J. 2010. Putting Bokoni on the historian's map. *African Studies* 69 (2): 229–233.

Wynne-Jones, S. 2019. On inclusions and exclusions. *Cambridge Archaeological Journal* 29:714–716.

Zena, A. 2018. Archaeology, politics and nationalism in nineteenth- and early twentieth-century Ethiopia: The use of archaeology to consolidate monarchical power. *Azania: Archaeological Research in Africa* 53:1–19.

Zimmerman, L. J. 2005. Public heritage, a desire for a "white" history for America, and some impacts of the Kennewick Man/ Ancient One decision. *International Journal of Cultural Property* 12 (2): 265–274.

Chapter 9
From Then, to Now, to Beyond: An Archaeological-Naissance

Abstract The concluding chapter looks forward. It sketches the "immediate beyond": practical steps that may strengthen training, archives, and legal regimes; deepen regional and transoceanic research; and open the way for multilingual, community-anchored scholarship. It then imagines "Africa reclaiming", considering African leadership within the field, funding priorities, publication venues, and curatorial decisions. Finally, it reflects on archaeology's public futures: how to tell fuller stories that dislodge lingering myths, link deep histories to contemporary justice, and invite broad participation. Rather than recap the volume, the chapter offers a horizon; an archaeological-naissance grounded in ethical partnerships, methodological plurality, and sustained attention to how pasts are made to matter in policy, classrooms, and everyday life.

> Archaeology defines us as human beings. (Fagan 2018, p. 6)

Understanding the past as archaeologists is about revealing human histories. But, archaeologists create the past in the present using contemporary agendas, politics, values, and disciplinary discourse (whether intentionally or unwittingly). These features, and others, influence how the past is interpreted, and therefore, how people in the past are understood. Returning to this book's opening page, archaeology is "perched on the present" (Bernbeck and Pollock 1996, p. 138, quoting Singh 1994). The tripartite of past people, present practitioners, and perceptions of the past coalesce in our academic pursuit of defining human beings; we are defined not only by archaeologists interpreting the past, but by the very framework those archaeologists use to do so. As this book has attempted to show, archaeology does not shape us as human beings, but rather, archaeology, and our understanding of the past, is shaped by us as human beings. From this perspective, archaeology and the past it constructs is a tool, which in Africa has been used in various ways as its function, positionality, and impact has changed.

The African past is not a distant, inert timeline of events. It shapes politics, economies, societies, and responses to local and global challenges. History and heritage are continually invoked and reinterpreted across the continent in nation-building, identity formation, economic development, and social cohesion. The uses of African archaeology and history are diverse and powerful. In contemporary Africa,

T. Forssman, *Archaeology in Africa: Why the Past Matters*, Archaeology of Africa,
https://doi.org/10.1007/978-3-032-13365-6_9

it is leveraged in multiple dimensions, illustrated by the case studies drawn on in this book, and has ongoing influence, from the past into the present and beyond. However, as a product of the present, its theoretical framework is part of that time and space (Said 1983, pp. 241–242). As this book has until now packaged archaeology with a wider historical context, the aim of this final chapter is to consider where to, from now, into the beyond?

Just as much as the discipline's history was shaped by contemporaneous contexts, like the discipline's current state, going forward it will likely continue to be a reflection of its new present. In light of this, envisioning a future of archaeology is contingent on the present, both here and now, and perspectives of it. As this changes, so will the endeavours of archaeology. In a world of uncertain political, social, and economic upheaval and ongoing crises, it might not be possible or even wise to think too far ahead. Therefore, beyond is considered the immediate next, rather than the distant future. Here, some ideas are charted and how they might draw from their historical roots, which penetrate the annals of archaeology in Africa. They are not conclusive and may very well not even represent more than a single voice, or a handful, but hopefully they add to the ensemble of archaeologists speaking out about Africa's past and where the discipline can profitably head.

9.1 The Immediate Beyond

> We need prehistoric archaeology to show what was happening before the coloniality of power entered the scene.... But we also need archaeology of the contemporary past to complete the story; a historical archaeology that stops short in the nineteenth century is insufficient. The archaeology of the present allows us to check whether the promise of the past, as creative and empowering was fulfilled. Or if it was actually a promise in the first place or a warning (González-Ruibal 2014, p. 20)

Graham Connah's (2004, p. 176) view that we know exceedingly little of Africa's past than we realise is probably not an exaggeration. Even with the time that has passed since he penned those words, while incredible progress has been made, it surely still holds true. Regions are better understood, and these tend to be those where universities are based, but vast blind spots persist. In regions such as the Congo River system, even though covering a massive area, very little is known (De Matos et al. 2021; Clist et al. 2023). The Marmatica region, which spans from the Libyan Sea to the southern desert and includes parts of northwest Egypt, has seen little focus, despite it being a crucial transit region connecting important and well-studied archaeological landscapes (Laguna-Palma et al. 2023). The Kalahari Desert has featured prominently in palaeoclimatic research and the contemporary past, but its earlier archaeological sequences have not been as well explored and current study programmes are revealing unexpected results regarding Pleistocene archaeology (Hatton et al. 2022; Stone et al. 2024). Research is also showing that West Africa played an important evolutionary role in human history, which at present represents a gap in our understanding (Cerasoni et al. 2022). The Swahili world has

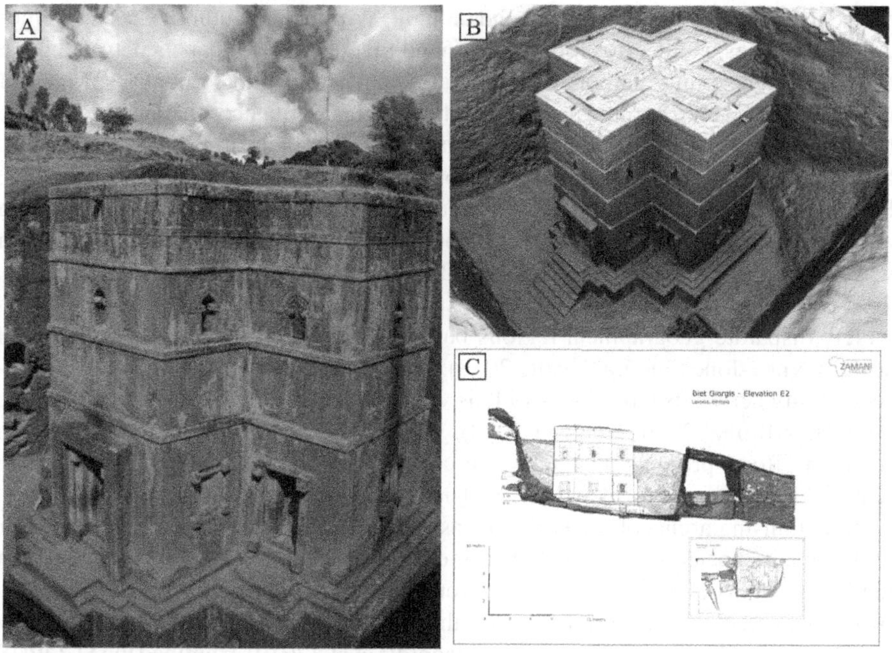

Fig. 9.1 The Biet Giorgis Church (Church of Saint George) at Lalibela: (**A**) photograph; (**B**) 3D scan; and (**C**) plan view. *Courtesy*: Zamani Project.

seen considerable research over the years (Wynne-Jones and LaViolette 2018), but gaps in the wider trading network exist, such as those between the east coast and southern Africa's interior (Chirikure 2014a), and much of Mozambique's archaeology outside of a few core areas remains understudied (Sinclair et al. 1993; Duarte 2012). Archaeological research is covering ground in many new areas and over time these gaps are expected to reduce and a far more detailed and expanded understanding developed.

Expanding into new areas and covering poorly visited frontiers will redress the colonial-shaped geopolitical landscape of archaeology. Most research was carried out in colonised nations and still is to this day. Coastal regions, for example, have seen considerably more researched than many interior zones, and Anglophone and Francophone countries have seen more investigations than Lusophone regions. Furthermore, where there are significant risks to safety or difficult access, regions have been avoided, such as large parts of Central Africa. Time will no doubt fill the many gaps, but it would be worth targeting areas for research to assess what exists in these spaces before they potentially become damaged or destroyed. Advances in remote sensing will likely make doing so far more possible, and coupled with machine learning the rate at which areas can be surveyed is increasing (Davis and Douglass 2020). A key challenge, despite this, will remain the imposed separation caused by national boundaries on archaeological work and thought. Within the Southern African Democratic Countries, Nelius Boshoff (2010) found that only 3% of papers between 2005 and 2008 were jointly authored by scholars from two or more countries. Many of these countries share borders and have archaeological sequences that paid these little heed, and yet those artificial, contemporary boundaries are treated as sacrosanct. Studies intentionally crossing national borders have returned with valuable results. For example, trade across the Mozambique landscape into the interior of southern Africa breaches contemporary national boundaries and demonstrates connectivity in ways severed by colonialism (Chirikure 2014a; Delius et al. 2024; Antonites et al. 2025). The entire Swahili world shows expansive interconnectedness from between widely disparate geographical regions but also transoceanic networks on a global scale (Wynne-Jones and LaViolette 2018). North Africa, too, shows incredible intersectionality across its territory as well as with the Middle East and southern Europe (González-Ruibal 2020; Hitchner 2022). The imposition of national boundaries on research efforts presents an immutable character to the past that would not have featured in its present form and likely changed periodically.

Decolonising archaeology is not an easy process. European influence existed for 500 years, if expansionism is included, and this impacted the fabric of science. What tends still to be found is that "[p]ersons from one part of the world study the problems of another part of the world and prescribe their solutions" (Brown 1988, p. 633). A few simple metrics illustrate this well. John Ioannidis et al. (2019) examined the SCOPUS database and generated a list of 100,000 scientists using standardised information, including citations, h-index, co-authorship and other fields. They found that only 10% of top-rated scientists are from global south nations, with less than 1% from South America and Africa. In another study on published geoscience papers, 182,996 articles were examined, 7162 on African topics, of which 2181 (30%) were written by African authors (North et al. 2020). This means that foreign authors have written more about Africa than African authors have. Moreover, African scholars tend to publish more on African topics than on regions beyond the continent. In effect, foreign authors write more easily and frequently about Africa than Africans do about other parts of the world – and even more than Africans write about Africa itself. Publication trends have displayed general stagnation in African-authored articles since the 1970s, with a slight increase from the 2000s (ibid). Scholars have considered various reasons for this, such as the 'brain drain' across Africa (King 2004; Capuano and Marfouk 2013) and wage deficits – in 1999, at Nigeria's Ahmadu Bello University, 75% of staff had a second job that contributed more to their monthly income than their university salary (Waast 2002). Publications also tend to come from a limited set of countries in Africa, such as Algeria, Egypt, Nigeria, South Africa and Tunisia, based on an analysis of papers from 2000–2015 in science disciplines (Sooryamoorthy 2018). Although these metrics are not directly related to historical research, it is symptomatic of a significant challenge to local capacity building, infrastructural growth, and access.

In recent years, the term helicopter or parachute science has been used to describe foreign researchers entering the global south to collect data with their team and student cohorts only to take the findings back to their home nations without establishing meaningful local partners (Odeny and Bosurgi 2022). Confronting parachute science has been directly linked to confronting the impact and legacy of colonialism within research fields (Culotta et al. 2025). Archaeology has the means to overcome parachute science, more than other disciplines. At a basic level, fieldwork requires assistance and it can be costly. The use of local students as aids in fieldwork is a brilliant way of training local scholars, exposing them to research and research teams, and having them participate in analysis. It is also the easiest and cheapest method of getting field help for foreign teams, who need the help regardless (Posnansky 2017). While this provides benefits for local students and institutions, these really are at a minimum effort on behalf of principle investigators and affect local change at only a surface level. For example, field experience will not get a student a job, the necessary funds for postgraduate degrees, or access to materials for postgraduate projects. Therefore, although probably the most common way foreign research teams are engaging locals, participating in fieldwork is the least impactful measure.

Meaningful change comes in other forms, and education ranks highly. In post-independence Africa, new training programmes emerged, which brought in new scholars, approaches and research interests (Posnansky 1982, p. 349; Schmidt 1995; Thondhlana et al. 2022). For example, in Nigeria the Benin and Yoruba Historical Research schemes emerged in the 1950s, whereas Uganda saw growing interest in the lacustrine states (Posnansky 1959). The value of oral histories also became more recognised as another source of historical data, as well as discovering and interpreting archaeological sites and helping to reconstruct past economies. In the years following independence, in Tanzania and Eritrea, archaeology at universities emerged with the aim of contesting Eurocentric narratives of the past, and each was met with mixed results largely predicated by local contexts (Schmidt 2005) Universities across Africa were epistemologically extremely colonial spaces. The *Rhodes Must Fall* movement, earlier described, is an example of related student experiences and their drive to create inclusive space in higher education systems. It is necessary to question the character of archaeological and historical studies in these contexts. How are the disciplines responding to massification in university spaces; are they perpetuating colonial epistemes; and how can they better respond to twenty-first century challenges facing contemporary students? Addressing this is not straightforward, but there is a great degree of scholarship on the matter that modern educators would likely find both informative and instructive (e.g., Luckett 2001, 2016; Northedge 2003; Boughey 2005, 2012; Schmidt 2005; Esterhuysen and Lane 2013; Boughey and McKenna 2016; Heleta 2016; Becker 2019; Luckett et al. 2019; Thondhlana et al. 2022; Govender and Naidoo 2023). Higher education has quite obviously much larger issues that it is grappling with, but archaeology and history are well suited to respond to many of them and chart epistemic reform going forward.

More deliberate collaborations are necessary at a partnership level. Nearly 80% of all scholarship from Central Africa has been undertaken in collaborative studies with partners from outside Africa (Boshoff 2010). In the same study by Boshoff (2010) it was found that 47% of southern African papers were co-authored with colleagues from high-income countries. Partnerships clearly play a significant role in advancing and supporting research in Africa. However, the author also concluded that there is a high degree of unequal partnerships and imbalances. The publication metrics that were presented earlier demonstrate this further. Scholars have complained that African scholars are used to facilitate access to collections and sites, rather than being integral stakeholders in project designs and research approaches (Fongwa 2018).

Infrastructural support is under-developed across Africa (Gabel 1985; Thondhlana et al. 2022), especially outside of countries such as Nigeria and South Africa. To an extent, this might be driving the need for foreign teams to return home with their finds. The lack of accessible laboratories also affects local archaeologists, and they often need to send samples to Europe or North America for testing at additional costs. Laboratories in the global north have not only facilities but budgets that dwarf most on the African continent (Chirikure 2017, p. 63). The impetus should be to change this axiom. There are no conditions in Africa that render laboratories impossible to establish, and enough fieldwork in a huge variety of fields takes place on the continent that requires laboratory science. As such, it would be profitable to all if such facilities existed on the continent: local skills training, enhancement of access and research, and support of local institutions and organisations by foreign teams who can also avoid the need for extraneous costs, permits, and risks in transporting their finds. There have been initiatives that have attempted and been successful with building infrastructure and capacity on the continent. The Swedish Agency for Research Collaborations/Swedish International Development Agency is a fine example of capacity building in southern Africa (Ogundiran 2016). Led primarily by Paul Sinclair since 1987 and later Anneli Ekblom (2024), the programme has resulted in a large number of graduates being trained through Uppsala University but also the University of Dar es Salaam, under the African Archaeology Network (Ichumbaki 2023), and more recently the University of Pretoria, and it has provided support for various initiatives and outputs (Chami et al. 2001, 2004; Sinclair and Bendegard 2004; Murimbika and Moyo 2008). Across the continent university offerings are growing with many new departments, whether archaeology or blended courses that involve archaeology (Esterhuysen and Lane 2013; Ichumbaki 2023), and at many of these institutions laboratories of various types are being established. While changes are afoot, it is not at the same pace as in higher income countries.

Since the 1980s, funding has crippled archaeological work (Posnansky 1982), and it continues to do so. Grants reflect national economic performance, and higher income nations tend to have more funding available for scholars (Coccia 2008). In these countries, approximately 1.7% of their GDP is spent on research, but in Africa it is 0.42% (Caelers and Okoth 2023). There are fewer grants presently available in Africa, of less value, than in higher income countries. In some cases this is linked to budget cuts, but in others to exclusion (ibid). Most African currencies are weak compared to the Dollar, Euro and Pound, which reinforces the local/foreign research divide. This disparity makes it difficult for African-funded projects to compete with those based in the global north. The consequence of not securing funding can restrict career progress and prospects (Powell 2016), as well as academic ratings, and have negative mental health impacts (Meirmans et al. 2019, p. 755).

Applying for grants takes time, and continued attempts or multiple applications to accrue the amount needed eats into other career tasks, including research time. A related issue is producing 'state-of-the-art' research when funds are limited, never mind pushing scholarly boundaries (Petersen 2021). Not being competitive worsens scholars' chances of being successful in international grants, and this further diminishes research efforts. Having access to grants not only facilitates fieldwork and other necessities, but it impacts the ability to publish in journals and pay for open access, where special agreements do not exist. This allows for those with larger grants to disseminate their work more widely and potentially receive greater citations. In such instances, researcher gaps in h-index scores grows and as a result what emerges are images as described above, where only 10% of the world top 100,000 scientists are found in the global south (Ioannidis et al. 2019). Increased publication rate is directly related to career growth, and while there are of course other milestones that are necessary, the old adage, *publish or perish*, is certainly still alive. The cycle of research poverty continues, and the ensuing funding dynamics reflect and entrench colonial histories. The academic gap between the north and south widens despite the south being the intellectual playground of the north.

A lack of resources not only influences higher education and research but also national capacity for managing heritage (Arthur et al. 2011, p. 234). Heritage management has risen in importance since the 1990s, accelerating into the 2000s (Arazi 2011). Challenges facing cultural resource management require serious consideration and, where possible, mitigation because of the global significance of Africa's heritage. Only Africa has a complete record of the human experience accompanied by cultural remains, genetic sequences, and ethnographic information (Alexander 2011). The development of dams, infrastructure, mines and agricultural growth put heritage items and places at risk (further to conflict, war and climate change as discussed in the previous chapter) (Arazi 2009; Chirikure 2014b). The realisation of this led to developer-funded archaeology that now contributes to the vast majority of jobs within the field (e.g., Darvill and Russell 2002). An excellent example of where industry, international relations, and financial support led to all-round benefits is the Metolong Dam project in Lesotho. The Metolong Dam was built to provide water to Maseru, Lesotho's capital, and ahead of construction the Lesotho Highlands Development Authority contracted Peter Mitchell and his team (Arthur et al. 2011, 2021; King and Eoin 2014; Dewar et al. 2018) to perform Phases 1 and 2 archaeological assessments. Their research integrated tangible and intangible studies, worked closely with local communities, trained members to be field technicians, and supported postgraduate studies. It was by most measures a great success. The widespread need for jobs and skills training that development brings complicates management processes. Africa is a developing continent and the preservation of heritage may obstruct pathways to growth (Chirikure 2014b). Preserving heritage is often in competition with social and well-being issues, and the need for job creation and skills development (Arazi 2011, p. 36). However, moving ahead, Africanist archaeologists and development strategies need to establish common ground to foster greater care for heritage resources and balance the need for job creation and skills transfer.

This brings me to the final point that I wish to discuss. The past is based on Eurocentric perceptions of history that originated from European enlightenment and colonialism (Fontein 2006, p. 131). Innocent Pikirayi (2015, p. 534) calls this the "colonial burden that archaeologists seek to rid themselves of". The broad aim is to counteract western views of indigenous communities, addressing the "systematic erasure of peoples, sites, and cultures from the land, from public memory, and the conventional writing of history" (Schneider and Hayes 2020, p. 127). Sonja Atalay (2006) called for a change that needs to come from within, although this may risk establishing an exclusionary approach and undermines the fine contributions and important collaborations from foreign scholars. In Africa, demographics and representation is still an issue (Pikirayi 2009, p. 125). In Mitchell and Jacob Seneši's (2023) review of the *South African Archaeological Bulletin* they found persistently low publications by black authors, despite an uptick in the 2010s. Similarly, Cameron Gokee and Akin Ogundiran's (2023) examination of the *African Archaeological Review* noted a majority of first-authored publications from Europe (38%), followed by Africa (30%) and North America (28%). African authors came from 28 countries, but Morocco, Nigeria, South Africa and Tanzania were dominant. An important part of decolonising is voice and representation (Spivak 1988). The under-representation of local voices in publications reflects the difficult and lengthy process involved in transforming the academy (for a South African example see Ndlovu and Smith 2019), which is likely further restricted by access to higher education and funding across the continent. Therefore, to address author demographics, and by extension professional demographics, it is important to look deeper at archaeological frameworks (Reilly 2022). The process of decolonising archaeology has, understandably, seen considered debate and discussion, but certain approaches do appear to be central or at least repeated. As discussed above, pedagogical approaches have been flagged as an important task for decolonising the field (Atalay 2019; Arday et al. 2021) and the need for transepistemes is evident in the alienation many students feel within university contexts (Heleta 2016; Nyamnjoh 2017). Engaging society more generally is necessary to improve archaeological and career prospect awareness before students arrive at their higher education institutions. Teaching archaeology at school is one method (Esterhuysen and Lane 2013) but presenting archaeology to community groups through museum initiatives, innovative travelling heritage displays, archaeological experiences, community-based research, public talks and online, multi-language articles are all viable and can be achieved with varying amounts of effort (Moser et al. 2002; Chirikure and Pwiti 2008; Abungu 2019; Atalay 2019; Lane 2021; Forssman and Van Heerden 2025). Some scholars have argued that the origins of archaeology and anthropology in white supremacy has not been reckoned and may be largely to blame (Reilly 2022; Beliso-De Jesús et al. 2023). This may require 'undisciplining' to change larger institutional structures (Schneider and Hayes 2020). Ultimately, the practice of archaeology and the discipline itself is tightly bound to Eurocentric value networks and histories that need to be reconciled as the field advances into the future.

Should the global north be co-opted to assist in addressing these issues? One may argue that it is not the problem of the west, and the current cohort of scholars are not those who laid the foundations of these issues. However, a reparative approach might rather acknowledge the longstanding colonial boot-print on Africa and its rippling shudders into the present. The influence that borders have and continue to have, the challenges of multi-ethnic, imagined societies being forced into Eurocentric, capitalist systems, the trauma and scarring that colonialism has had on peoples' livelihoods, and the permanently altered climatic trajectory that extractive endeavours of the global north in African populations and soils has had all push the continent towards a precipice not of its own making. Measures and approaches should be instilled in the fabric of archaeological endeavours that address these issues in effective ways that support disciplinary autochthony and independence.

9.2 Africa Reclaiming

Not hoping to end on a pessimistic note, after the many concerns in the preceding pages, it is worth recognising the tremendous growth archaeology has made – most notably the growing emphasis on Africa's past from imposed narratives, affirming its place within global history. From colonial-era expeditions to today's community-led and technologically sophisticated projects, the discipline's evolution in Africa reflects methodological advancements, theoretical shifts, and a drive to reclaim African history for Africans and by collaborative teams with a shared understanding of ethical archaeology.

African archaeology has witnessed revolutions in practice, method and theory. The basic field approaches from the mid-twentieth century CE have been replaced by cutting-edge scientific techniques that have propelled an understanding of the past in directions not imagined when the field was in its infancy. Advances in understanding chronology are critical to developing a complex history for Africa, but macro- and micro-analyses, isotope analysis, ancient DNA studies, x-ray fluorescence, geographic information systems, and mass-spectrometry analyses have all allowed archaeologists to understand local history in considerable depth. Accelerating since the 1990s, the result has been a scientific turn in African archaeology. A great example of how advanced technologies are revealing lost histories is the LiDAR (light detection and ranging) detection of Kweneng, a large, stone-walled settlement complex south of Johannesburg that had been lost from collective memory (Sadr 2019). Another is laser ablation analyses of glass beads found along the eastern coastline that have connected parts of Africa, like Zanzibar (Wood et al. 2017) and central southern African interior sites (Robertshaw et al. 2010), to south and south-eastern Asia, with local glass bead production recently being identified at Mkokotoni in the early second millennium CE (Rødland 2023). The science of archaeometallurgy had a particularly early start. In the 1970s, Nikolaas van der Merwe began training metallurgists and moved the department at the University of Cape Town into the science faculty, where they gained better resources to foster specialisations in archaeobotany, archaeozoology, and geoarchaeology (Thondhlana et al. 2022, p. 465). The Zamani Project based at the University of Cape Town is arguably the leading organisation digitally recording heritage sites mostly in Africa using advanced techniques (Rajan and Rüther 2007; Rüther et al. 2012a, 2012b). Their laser scanning of Lalibela, Ethiopia, produced 3D digital models of the churches that provide a conservation baseline that can be used for education and presentations (Fig. 9.1) (Rüther and Palumbo 2012). The Zamani Project demonstrates the incredible value in non-destructive, highly accurate recording methods for African heritage sites.

Another field that has held much promise for decades, but which has struggled to work neatly in tandem with archaeology, is ancient DNA (aDNA) (MacEachern 2013). New abilities to obtain aDNA have more recently led to an increase in studies, but African aDNA samples amount to only 3% of the global published genomic work (Prendergast 2023). In Mary Prendergast's (2023, p. 806) map of Africa it is also clear that most come from East Africa, followed by the north and very few studies in the southern and western regions. The growth of aDNA research is encouraging and has led to advances in understanding migrations, movements, and interactions across the continent, as well as faunal dynamics (Prendergast et al. 2017; Horsburgh 2020). However, they have been accompanied by concerns regarding ethics and communities, indigeneity, and global politics (see Prendergast and Sawchuck 2018; Gibbon 2020; MacEachern 2000). Research using aDNA has also been mostly conducted and led by non-African scholars (but see Bodiba et al. 2019), creating a research divide (Prendergast 2023), almost certainly reflecting a lack of access to local laboratories, specialist skills, and funding. It will still be some time before aDNA studies have continent-wide data to draw from and establish wider regional patterns, and for now it represents a frontier in African archaeological science.

Theoretical transitions have been met bravely in African archaeology, considering the apprehensiveness that they can cause. David Lewis-Williams made an early plea to shift archaeology to a historical-materialist approach after the significant advances he and Patricia Vinnicombe made in rock art studies (Mitchell 2005). This approach challenged Eurocentric perspectives from the time that emphasised scientific approaches based on quantification or other explanations that were not based in indigenous knowledge, such as art for the sake of art approach (Lewis-Williams 2006). Not only did rock art begin to challenge normative approaches, but continued work at Great Zimbabwe provided ample evidence dismissing the foreigner theories that dominated in the early twentieth century CE but which persisted after independence (Fontein 2006; Chirikure 2020). Bassey Andah (1995) by the 1990s was already urging scholars to decolonise archaeology by valuing African cultural contexts and rejecting western theory. Augustin Holl (1990) promoted 'Africanising' archaeology, and Thurston Shaw (1963, 1977) collaborated with elders in Nigeria to locate historical sites using oral traditions. He blended archaeology and ethnography to what today we know as ethnoarchaeology. These scholars appealed, essentially, to archaeologists that African communities were not only subject but knowledge holders. These shifts played out more generally in the processual to post-processual dichotomy, which caused considerable upheaval in archaeology globally, but was muted in Africa (see Wynne-Jones and Fleisher 2015). What strengthened instead was later frameworks such as cognitive archaeology, hybridised archaeological, historical, indigenous knowledge, and community-based archaeology (Huffman

2004). Peter Schmidt and Thomas Patterson's (1995) edited volume confronted this new disciplinary context and recognised the importance of addressing issues of power and 'othering', using archaeology to examine colonial practices, attitudes, and support reflexivity.

One of the most visible areas of change is in heritage management. Following decolonization in the 1960s, newly independent African states established antiquities departments, national museums, or legal frameworks to safeguard heritage. Countries like Ghana, Nigeria, Kenya, and Senegal passed laws to control the export of artefacts and designated national monuments (Pwiti 1996; Ndoro and Pwiti 2001; Deacon et al. 2004). These efforts have only grown; today, many more African country have heritage institutions tasked with conservation, often working with universities and local communities. Various initiatives at preserving, conserving and promoting African heritage have led to the protection of these irreplaceable resources. At Timbuktu, collaborations between UNESCO and the government of Mali rebuilt mausoleums that had been destroyed in conflict. Traditional knowledge and methods were used in the rehabilitation programme. The outcomes of this work are presented online for visitors to explore digitally (UNESCO 2012). At Jenné-jeno, Mali (Sacko 2021), and the Sukur Cultural Landscape, Nigeria (Day et al. 2022), communities actively maintain archaeological and heritage sites, often in cooperation with archaeologists. Heritage management, including contract archaeology and cultural resource management, has driven forward in many respects and is a global leader in the integration of tangible and intangible cultural heritage in management systems.

The rise of community and engaged archaeology is a significant advance that took hold in the independence era. It could be argued that this represents a grand shift in schools of thought in the practice of archaeology; a paradigm shift. When the discipline first left its tracks in Africa's soils it was for the gain of European settlers, imperialism, and the administration of colonies and people. Within this framework, it was practiced by the educated elite with local participation in the form of cheap labour, and whose names are often not known anymore (Shepherd 2002; Ndlovu 2009). It was typical at this time to not feed information back into communities, certainly before 1950, among whom archaeologists worked (Posnansky 2017). From the independence era, change began. Museums in countries like Somaliland and Uganda began to expand their focus with the aim to keep traditions alive and represent the locally diverse culture. In other countries, including Niger, Tanzania and Zambia, folk villages were established for visitors to experience local ways of living. The past ceased to be stones and bones and school children were now being exposed to a celebration of history (ibid). An integrated example is from Begho, Ghana, where Merrick Posnansky (2017) conducted work at a medieval, early modern market town. Between 1970 and 1975, annual field schools were organised and the University of Ghana built a research centre with housing, storage and other facilities, and from 1970 to 1998 longitudinal anthropological work in local villages began. Engaged archaeologies like the examples here are becoming more common. They allow archaeologists to recognise voice, acknowledge communities and stakeholders, include active participants in their research who have valuable knowledge, vested interest, and lived experience, and reconfigure the elitism that once characterised the discipline (Pikirayi 2014). This shift in paradigms – from us to them, expert to learner, on to with – is an important threshold that archaeology has passed through. Emphasis is now regularly placed on outreach initiatives, participatory work, shared interpretations, and benefit-sharing.

Although the process of decolonisation is on-going, intellectual space has been reclaimed. Archaeology has successfully challenged normative assumptions about local pasts and through the discipline dissolved many colonial perceptions. Sites such as Aksum, Great Zimbabwe, Jenné-Jeno, Thulamela, and the Nile Valley show complex societies flourishing before the arrival of Europeans. Archaeology highlights these accomplishments in both academic and public discourse. Academic colonialism is also being confronted and is now an occurrence that local and foreign researchers are acutely aware of and actively avoiding. A greater emphasis on local partnerships has emerged, even though it still requires greater thought and redress. Cultural items are also being returned to Africa as a reparative measure for the impact of colonial theft and looting (Colwell 2019). The repatriation of these items serves to repatriate history, and in cases where ancestral and spiritual links exist with those plundered artefacts, intangible cultural heritage (Simpson 2008; Ibanga 2020). Departments and institutions that were once mostly occupied by white archaeologists who were more often than not male has shifted, with more black and female academics taking up professional positions than before (Pikirayi 2015; Ndlovu and Smith 2019). These changes are happening, and while one might argue too slowly, they are complex matters that require scholars and educators to dismantle legacies of colonialism (Humphreys et al. 2020).

These developments, and many others not directly discussed here, have had a significant impact on African societies in their understanding of history and its wider context, and the enrichment of historical narratives. Archaeology in Africa is no longer esoteric or a tool divorced from every-day concerns; it is relevant to national identity, local economies, and cultural healing. Archaeology deepens historical knowledge, and the two disciplines work in tandem to fill the long, complex history of people and places on the continent with richer understandings; archaeology and history cannot be separated in Africa. Through the disciplines the *longue durée* of African societies is woven into a complex narrative. Part of this network is the rest of the world. When once Africa was considered to be a land apart, through archaeological and historical work it is now known that it was a land connected. Africa has a place in global history, through historic economic systems, the interests of community, kingdom or dynasty were pursued, power relations were renegotiated, and influence was meted out. Africa's history is not peripheral; it is paramount.

This book has traced archaeology through different 'presents', and examined the discipline's role within those contexts. As social and political agendas advanced, changed, or reformed, the role and purpose of archaeology shifted. On the African continent, with its unique contexts, this resulted in the construction of the past being dictated by others, and its character aligning with contemporary agendas and perspectives. The notion that archaeology can be apolitical is false. It is inextricably political. The past is constructed by looking back through a lens in the present. This has not changed. Contemporary archaeologists are as influenced by their present contexts as ever, and our revisions of the past, questions, methods, frameworks, and approaches, never mind uses, are focussed through a "vibrant coalesce of multiple temporalities" (Reilly 2019, p. 2). Within the contemporary context, Pikirayi (2015) and others envisioned a future of African archaeology with greater integration of scientific innovation and indigenous knowledge, more inclusive narratives, and sustained growth of local expertise – in short, a future where Africa's past belongs to its people and contributes to a global understanding of human heritage. Archaeology cannot "take place at a distance from society" (Shepherd 2007, p. 17); it must confront its present.

References

Abungu, G. O. 2019. Museums: Geopolitics, decolonisation, globalisation and migration. *Museum International* 71:62–71.

Alexander, J. 2011. Saving the African heritage is a global priority: How can a new subdiscipline of rescue archaeology aid it? *African Archaeological Review* 28:93–96.

Andah, B. 1995. European encumbrances to the development of relevant theory in African archaeology. In *Theory in archaeology: A world perspective*, ed. P. J. Ucko, 96–108. London: Routledge.

Antonites, A., A. R. Antonites, C. E. Peterson, T. Hopf, and N. Ndlovu. 2025. New evidence for early Indian Ocean trade routes into the South African interior. *Proceedings of the National Academy of Sciences* 122:e2419077122.

Arazi, N. 2009. Cultural research management in Africa: Challenges, dangers and opportunities. *Azania: Archaeological Research in Africa* 44:95–106.

Arazi, N. 2011. Safeguarding archaeological cultural resources in Africa—Policies, methods and issues of (non) compliance. *African Archaeological Review* 28:27–38.

Arday, J., D. Zoe Belluigi, and D. Thomas. 2021. Attempting to break the chain: Reimaging inclusive pedagogy and decolonising the curriculum within the academy. *Educational Philosophy and Theory* 53:298–313.

Arthur, C., P. J. Mitchell, L. Mallen, D. Pearce, A. Bonneau, F. Prinsloo, R. Mokachane, P. Nthunya, S. Mothopeng, and R. King. 2021. Record-making, research, and removal: Mitigating impacts on rock art in a CRM context in southern Africa—The case of the Metolong Dam, Lesotho. *African Archaeological Review* 38:675–694.

Arthur, C., M. Mohapi, and P. Mitchell. 2011. Archaeology and dam projects in Lesotho. *Conservation and Management of Archaeological Sites* 13:231–252.

Atalay, S. 2006. Guest editor's remarks: Decolonising archaeology. *American Indian Quarterly* 30:269–279.

Atalay, S. 2019. Can archaeology help decolonize the way institutions think? How community-based research is transforming the archaeology training toolbox and helping to transform institutions. *Archaeologies* 15:514–535.

Becker, H. 2019. Postcolonial African anthropologies. *Anthropology Southern Africa* 42:186–188.

Beliso-De Jesús, A. M., J. Pierre, and J. Rana. 2023. White supremacy and the making of anthropology. *Annual Review of Anthropology* 52 (1): 417–435.

Bernbeck, R., and S. Pollock. 1996. Ayodhya, archaeology, and identity. *Current Anthropology* 37:138–142.

Bodiba, M., M. Steyn, P. Bloomer, M. N. Mosothwane, F. Rühli, and A. Bouwman, 2019. Ancient DNA analysis of the Thulamela remains: deciphering the migratory patterns of a Southern African population. *Journal of African Archaeology*17 (2): 161–172.

Boshoff, N. 2010. South–South research collaboration of countries in the Southern African Development Community (SADC). *Scientometrics* 84:481–503.
Boughey, C. 2005. Epistemological access to the university: An alternative perspective. *South African Journal of Higher Education* 19 (3): 638–650.
Boughey, C. 2012. Social inclusion and exclusion in a changing higher education environment. *Multidisciplinary Journal of Educational Research* 2 (2): 133–151.
Boughey, C., and S. McKenna. 2016. Academic literacy and the decontextualised learner. *Critical Studies in Teaching and Learning (CriSTaL)* 4 (2): 1–9.
Brown, D.E. 1988. *Hierarchy, History, and Human Nature*. Tucson: University of Arizona Press.
Caelers, D., and D. Okoth. 2023. Research funding in Africa: Navigating sustainability and shifting perspectives. *Nature Africa*, December. Available from https://www.nature.com/articles/d44148-023-00360-4. 18 March 2025.
Capuano, S., and A. Marfouk. 2013. African brain drain and its impact on source countries: What do we know and what do we need to know? *Journal of Comparative Policy Analysis and Practice* 15:297–314.
Cerasoni, J. N., E. Y. Hallett, E. B. Arous, R. M. Beyer, M. Krapp, A. Manica, and E. Scerri. 2022. Archaeological sites and palaeoenvironments of Pleistocene West Africa. *Journal of Maps* 18:630–637.
Chami, F., G. Pwiti, and C. Radimilahy. 2001. *People, contacts and the environment in the African past*. Dar es Salaam: Dar es Salaam University Press.
Chami, F., G. Pwiti, and C. Radimilahy. 2004. *The African archaeology network: Reports and a review*. Dar es Salaam: Dar es Salaam University Press.
Chirikure, S. 2014a. Land and sea links: 1500 years of connectivity between southern Africa and the Indian Ocean rim regions, AD 700 to 1700. *African Archaeological Review* 31 (4): 705–724.
Chirikure, S. 2014b. 'Where angels fear to tread': Ethics, commercial archaeology, and extractive industries in southern Africa. *Azania: Archaeological Research in Africa* 49 (2): 218–231.
Chirikure, S. 2017. The metalworker, the potter, and pre-European African 'laboratory'. In *What do science, technology, and innovation mean from Africa?* ed. C. C. Mavhunga, 63–77. Cambridge, MS: MIT Press.
Chirikure, S. 2020. *Great Zimbabwe: Reclaiming a 'confiscated' past*. London: Routledge.
Chirikure, S., and G. Pwiti. 2008. Community involvement in archaeology and cultural heritage management: An assessment from case studies in southern Africa and elsewhere. *Current Anthropology* 49 (3): 467–485.
Clist, B.-O., P. Béarez, C. Mougne, J. Lesur, W. Hubau, and K. Bostoen. 2023. First archaeological excavations along the Atlantic Ocean coastline of the Democratic Republic of Congo: The Iron Age sites at Muanda. *African Archaeological Review* 40:711–739.
Coccia, M. 2008. Science, funding and economic growth: Analysis and science policy implications. *World Review of Science, Technology and Sustainable Development* 5:1–27.
Colwell, C. 2019. Can repatriation heal the wounds of history? *Public Historian* 41 (1): 90–110.
Connah, G. 2004. *Forgotten Africa: An introduction to its archaeology*. London: Routledge.
Culotta, E., S. Chakradhar, and R. P. Ortega. 2025. How scientists are confronting the lingering imprint of colonialism [online]. *Science*. Available from https://www.science.org/content/article/scientists-confronting-lingering-imprint-colonialism. Accessed on 17 March 2025.
Darvill, T. C., and B. Russell. 2002. *Archaeology after PPG16: Archaeological investigations in England 1990–1999*. Bournemouth: University of Bournemouth.
Davis, D. S., and K. Douglass. 2020. Aerial and spaceborne remote sensing in African archaeology: A review of current research and potential future avenues. *African Archaeological Review* 37 (1): 9–24.
Day, J. C., S. F. Heron, I. Odiaua, J. Downes, E. Itua, A. L. Abdu, B. Ekwurzel, A. Sham, and W. Megarry. 2022. *An application of the climate vulnerability index for the Sukur Cultural Landscape, Nigeria*. Abuja: ICOMOS-Nigeria.

De Matos, D., A. C. Martins, J. C. Senna-Martinez, I. Pinto, A. G. Coelho, S. S. Ferreira, and L. Oosterbeek. 2021. Review of archaeological research in Angola. *African Archaeological Review* 38 (2): 319–344.

Deacon, H., L. Dondolo, M. Mruba, and S. Prosalendis. 2004. *The subtle power of intangible heritage: Legal and financial instruments for safeguarding intangible heritage.* Cape Town: Human Sciences Research Council.

Delius, P., L. Chewins, and T. Forssman. 2024. Turning South African history upside down: Ivory and gold production, the Indian Ocean trading system and the shaping of southern African society, 600–1900 AD. *Journal of Southern African Studies* 50 (3): 499–520.

Dewar, G., S. Badenhorst, C. Arthur, and P. Mitchell. 2018. After the silt: Middle and late Holocene hunter-gatherer archaeology of the Metolong Dam, Lesotho. *Southern African Humanities* 31 (1): 129–179.

Duarte, R. T. 2012. Maritime history in Mozambique and East Africa: The urgent need for the proper study and preservation of endangered underwater cultural heritage. *Journal of Maritime Archaeology* 7:63–86.

Ekblom, A. 2024. Paul Sinclair (1949–2023)—In memoriam. *Azania: Archaeological Research in Africa* 59 (1): 173–178.

Esterhuysen, A., and P. J. Lane. 2013. Archaeology and education. In *The Oxford handbook of African archaeology*, ed. P. J. Mitchell and P. J. Lane, 239–252. Oxford: Oxford University Press.

Fagan, B. 2018. *A little history of archaeology*. New Haven: Yale University Press.

Fongwa, S. 2018. Diaspora collaboration and knowledge production in Africa: Reflections on caveats and opportunities. *Journal of Higher Education in Africa/Revue de l'enseignement supérieur en Afrique* 16 (1/2): 115–134.

Fontein, J. 2006. *The silence of great Zimbabwe: Contested landscapes and the power of heritage.* London: Routledge.

Forssman, T., and J. Van Heerden. 2025. The design and implementation of a new travelling museum initiative to bring heritage to people in Southern Africa. *Journal of Community Archaeology & Heritage* 12: 1–15.

Gabel, C. 1985. Archaeology in sub-Saharan Africa. *International Journal of African Historical Studies* 18 (2): 241–264.

Gibbon, V. E. 2020. African ancient DNA research requires robust ethics and permission protocols. *Nature Reviews Genetics*21 (11): 645–647.

Gokee, C. D., and A. Ogundiran. 2023. The African archaeological review turns forty: Some reflections on the past, present, and future. *African Archaeological Review* 40 (1): 1–19.

González-Ruibal, A. 2014. An archaeology of predation, capitalism and the coloniality of power in Equatorial Guinea (Central Africa). In *Historical archaeologies of capitalism*, ed. M. Leone and J. Knauf, 421–444. Cham: Springer International Publishing.

González-Ruibal, A. 2020. Colonies, missions, violence and trade: The historical archaeology of northeast Africa. In *Routledge handbook of global historical archaeology*, ed. C. E. Orset, A. Zarankin, P. Funari, S. Lawrence, and J. Symonds, 660–680. Abingdon: Routledge.

Govender, L., and D. Naidoo. 2023. Decolonial insights for transforming the higher education curriculum in South Africa. *Curriculum Perspectives* 43:S59–S71.

Hatton, A., B. Collins, B. J. Schoville, and J. Wilkins. 2022. Ostrich eggshell beads from Ga-Mohana Hill North Rockshelter, southern Kalahari, and the implications for understanding social networks during Marine Isotope Stage 2. *PLoS One* 17 (6): e0268943.

Heleta, S. 2016. Decolonisation of higher education: Dismantling epistemic violence and Eurocentrism in South Africa. *Transformation in Higher Education* 1 (1): 1–8.

Hitchner, R. B. 2022. The historiography of North Africa in antiquity: An overview. In *A companion to North Africa in antiquity*, ed. R. B. Hitchner, 3–8. Wiley Blackwell: Hoboken.

Holl, A. F. C. 1990. West African archaeology: Colonialism and nationalism. In *A history of African archaeology*, ed. P. Robertshaw, 296–308. Oxford: James Currey Ltd.

Horsburgh, K. A. 2020. Genetics and domestic fauna in southern Africa. In *Oxford Research Encyclopedia of Anthropology*, ed. M. Aldenderfer, Oxford University Press. https://doi.org/10.1093/acrefore/9780190854584.013.247

Huffman, T. N. 2004. Beyond data: The aim and practice of archaeology. *South African Archaeological Bulletin* 59:66–69.

Humphreys, R., J. Bam-Hutchison, and R. Ackermann. 2020. Archaeology is changing, slowly. But it's still too tied up in colonial practices. *The Conversation*. Available from http://theconversation.com/archaeology-is-changing-slowly-but-its-still-too-tied-up-in-colonial-practices-133243. 20 March 2025.

Ibanga, D.-A. 2020. Paths to African personhood and identity in the diasporas: The case for reburial of African enslaved ancestors. *Journal of Contemporary African Philosophy* 1:8–27.

Ichumbaki, E. B. 2023. Training and collaboration in African archaeology. *African Archaeological Review* 40:785–788.

Ioannidis, J. P. A., J. Baas, R. Klavans, and K. W. Boyack. 2019. A standardized citation metrics author database annotated for scientific field. *PLoS Biology* 17 (8): e3000384.

King, D. A. 2004. The scientific impact of nations. *Nature* 430:311–316.

King, R., and L. N. Eoin. 2014. Before the flood: Loss of place, mnemonics, and 'resources' ahead of the Metolong Dam, Lesotho. *Journal of Social Archaeology* 14 (2): 196–223.

Laguna-Palma, D., M. Toscana, and C. Rodrígues-Rellán. 2023. Building and integrated database of north-eastern African archaeological and heritage sites for mapping complex social landscape. *Journal of Open Archaeology Data* 11:5.

Lane, P. J. 2021. Archaeology, hybrid knowledge, and community engagement in Africa: Thoughts on decolonising practice. In *The Routledge companion to global indigenous history*, ed. A. McGrath and L. Russell, 603–628. London: Routledge.

Lewis-Williams, J. D. 2006. The Evolution of theory, method and technique in southern African rock art research. *Journal of Archaeological Method and Theory* 13 (4): 341–375.

Luckett, K. 2001. Responding to equity and development imperatives: Conceptualizing a structurally and epistemically diverse undergraduate curriculum in post-apartheid South Africa. *Equity & Excellence in Education* 34 (3): 26–35.

Luckett, K. 2016. Curriculum contestation in a post-colonial context: A view from the South. *Teaching in Higher Education* 21 (4): 415–428.

Luckett, K., S. Morreira, and M. Baijnath. 2019. Decolonising the curriculum: Recontextualisation, identity and self-critique in a post-apartheid university. In *Re-imagining curriculum: Spaces for disruption*, ed. L. Quinn, 23–44. Cape Town: Sun Press.

MacEachern, S. 2000. Genes, tribes, and African history. *Current Anthropology*41 (3): 357–384.

MacEachern, S. 2013. Genetics and archaeology. In *The Oxford Handbook of African Archaeology*, eds. P. J. Mitchell and P. J. Lane, 65–76. Oxford: Oxford University Press.

Meirmans, S., R. K. Butlin, A. Charmantier, J. Engelstädter, A. T. Groot, K. C. King, H. Kokko, J. M. Reid, and M. Neiman. 2019. Science policies: How should science funding be allocated? An evolutionary biologists' perspective. *Journal of Evolutionary Biology* 32 (8): 754–768.

Mitchell, P. J. 2005. Why hunter-gatherer archaeology matters: A personal perspective on renaissance and renewal in southern African Later Stone Age research. *South African Archaeological Bulletin* 60 (182): 64–71.

Mitchell, P. J., and J. Seneši. 2023. Trends in southern African archaeology 1980–2019: Changing publication patterns in the 'South African Archaeological Bulletin'. *South African Archaeological Bulletin* 77:127–139.

Moser, S., D. Glazier, J. E. Phillips, L. N. El Nemr, M. S. Mousa, R. N. Aiesh, S. Richardson, A. Conner, and M. Seymour. 2002. Transforming archaeology through practice: Strategies for collaborative archaeology and the Community Archaeology Project at Quseir. *Egypt. World Archaeology* 34 (2): 220–248.

Murimbika, M., and B. Moyo. 2008. Archaeology and donor aid in the 'developing world': The case for local heritage in Zimbabwe. In *Managing archaeological resources*, ed. F. P. McManamon, A. Stout, and J. A. Barnes, 87–105. London: Routledge.

Ndlovu, N. 2009. Decolonizing the mind-set: South African archaeology in a postcolonial, post-apartheid era. In *Postcolonial Archaeologies in Africa*, ed. P. Schmidt, 177–192. New York: Springer.

Ndlovu, N., and B. W. Smith. 2019. The past is a divided country: Transforming archaeology in South Africa. *African Archaeological Review* 36:172–192.

Ndoro, W., and G. Pwiti. 2001. Heritage management in southern Africa: Local, national and international discourse. *Public Archaeology* 2 (1): 21–34.

North, M. A., W. W. Hastie, and L. Hoyer. 2020. Out of Africa: The underrepresentation of African authors in high-impact geoscience literature. *Earth-Science Reviews* 208:103262.

Northedge, A. 2003. Rethinking teaching in the context of diversity. *Teaching in Higher Education* 8 (1): 17–32.

Nyamnjoh, A. 2017. The phenomenology of Rhodes Must Fall: Student activism and the experience of alienation at the University of Cape Town. *Strategic Review for Southern Africa* 39:256–277.

Odeny, B., and R. Bosurgi. 2022. Time to end parachute science. *PLoS Medicine* 19 (9): 1004099.

Ogundiran, A. 2016. A continental vision for African archaeology. In *African archaeology without fontiers: Papers from the 2014 PanAfrican Archaeological Association Congress*, ed. K. Sadr, A. Esterhuysen, and C. Sievers, xxix–xliii. Johannesburg: Wits University Press.

Petersen, O. H. 2021. Inequality of research funding between different countries and regions is a serious problem for global science. *Function* 2 (6): zqab060.

Pikirayi, I. 2009. What can archaeology do for society in southern Africa? *Historical Archaeology* 43 (4): 125–127.

Pikirayi, I. 2014. Sharing the past: Archaeology and community engagement in southern Africa. In *Sharing archaeology*, ed. P. Stone and Z. Hui, 150–166. London: Routledge.

Pikirayi, I. 2015. The future of archaeology in Africa. *Antiquity* 89 (345): 531–541.

Posnansky, M. 1959. Progress and prospects in historical archaeology in Uganda. In *Discovering Africa's past*, ed. M. Posnansky, vol. 4, 31–39. Kampala: Uganda Museum Occasional Paper.

Posnansky, M. 1982. African archaeology comes of age. *World Archaeology* 13:345–358.

Posnansky, M. 2017. Archaeology and the local community in Africa: A retrospective. *Journal of Community Archaeology & Heritage* 4 (2): 77–84.

Powell, K. 2016. Young, talented and fed-up: Young scientists tell their stories. *Nature* 538:446–449.

Prendergast, M. E. 2023. Genetics and archaeology. *African Archaeological Review*40 (4): 805–809.

Prendergast, M. E. M. Buckley, A. Crowther, L. Frantz, H. Eager, O. Lebrasseur, R. Hutterer, A. Hulme-Beaman, W. Van Neer, and K. Douka. 2017. Reconstructing Asian faunal introductions to eastern Africa from multi-proxy biomolecular and archaeological datasets. *PloS one* 12 (8): e0182565.

Prendergast, M. E. and E. Sawchuk. 2018. Boots on the ground in Africa's ancient DNA 'revolution': Archaeological perspectives on ethics and best practices. *Antiquity* 92 (363): 803–815

Pwiti, G. 1996. Let the ancestors rest in peace? New challenges for cultural heritage management in Zimbabwe. *Conservation and Management of Archaeological Sites* 1 (3): 151–160.

Rajan, R. S., and H. Rüther. 2007. Building a digital library of scholarly resources from the developing world: An introduction to Aluka. *African Arts* 40 (2): 1–7.

Reilly, M. C. 2019. Futurity, time, and archaeology. *Journal of Contemporary Archaeology* 6:1–15.

Reilly, M. C. 2022. Archaeologies of whiteness. *Archaeological Dialogues* 29:51–66.

Robertshaw, P., M. Wood, E. Melchiorre, R. S. Popelka-Filcoff, and M. D. Glascock. 2010. Southern African glass beads: Chemistry, glass sources and patterns of trade. *Journal of Archaeological Science* 37 (8): 1898–1912.

Rødland, H. 2023. Crafting Swahili beads: Exploring a new glass bead assemblage from northern Zanzibar, Tanzania. *African Archaeological Review* 40:335–356.

Rüther, H., C. Held, R. Bhurtha, R. Schroeder, and S. Wessels. 2012a. From point cloud to textured model, the Zamani laser scanning pipeline in heritage documentation. *South African Journal of Geomatics* 1 (1): 44–59.

Rüther, H., C. Held, R. Bhurtha, R. Schroeder, and S. Wessels. 2012b. Challenges in heritage documentation with terrestrial laser scanning. In *Proceedings of AfricaGeo 2011*. Presented at the AfricaGeo Conference, AfricaGeo, Cape Town.

Rüther, H., and G. Palumbo. 2012. 3D laser scanning for site monitoring and conservation in Lalibela World Heritage Site, Ethiopia. *International Journal of Heritage in the Digital Era* 1:217–232.

Sacko, O. 2021. The involvement of local communities in the conservation process of earthen architecture in the Sahel-Sahara region—The case of Djenné. *Mali. Built Heritage* 5 (1): 26.

Sadr, K. 2019. Kweneng: A newly discovered pre-colonial capital near Johannesburg. *Journal of African Archaeology* 17 (1): 1–22.

Said, E. 1983. *The world, the text, and the critic*. Cambridge: Harvard University Press.

Schmidt, P. 2005. Teaching revolutionary archaeology: African experiments in history making and heritage management. *Archaeologies* 1:46–59.

Schmidt, P. R. 1995. Using archaeology to remake history. In *Making alternative histories: The practice of archaeology and history in non-western settings*, ed. P. R. Schmidt and T. C. Patterson, 119–147. Santa Fe: School for Advanced Research Press.

Schmidt, P. R., and T. C. Patterson. 1995. *Making alternative histories: The practice of archaeology and history in non-western settings*. Santa Fe: School for Advanced Research Press.

Schneider, T. D., and K. Hayes. 2020. Epistemic colonialism: Is it possible to decolonize archaeology? *American Indian Quarterly* 44:127–148.

Shaw, T. 1963. Field research in Nigerian archaeology: A brief survey and discussion of policy. *Journal of the Historical Society of Nigeria* 2 (4): 449–464.

Shaw, T. 1977. *Unearthing Igbo-Ukwu*. Ibandan: Oxford University Press.

Shepherd, N. 2002. The politics of archaeology in Africa. *Annual Review of Anthropology* 31:189–209.

Shepherd, N. 2007. Archaeology dreaming: Post-apartheid urban imaginaries and the bones of the Prestwich Street dead. *Journal of Social Archaeology* 7:3–28.

Simpson, M. G. 2008. Indigenous heritage and repatriation: A stimulus for cultural renewal. In *Utimut: Past heritage—Future partnerships: Discussions on repatriation in the 21st century*, ed. M. Gabriel and J. Dahl, 64–77. Copenhagen: Greenland National Museum & Archives.

Sinclair, P. J. J., and C. Bendegard. 2004. *Urban origins follow up*. Uppsala: Department of Archaeology and Ancient History, Uppsala University.

Sinclair, P. J. J., J. M. F. Morais, L. Adamowicz, and R. T. Duarte. 1993. A perspective on archaeological research in Mozambique. In *The archaeology of Africa: Food, metals and towns*, ed. T. Shaw, P. J. J. Sinclair, B. Andah, and A. Okpoko, 409–431. London: Routledge.

Sooryamoorthy, R. 2018. The production of science in Africa: An analysis of publications in the science disciplines, 2000–2015. *Scientometrics* 115:317–349.

Spivak, G. 1988. Can the subaltern speak? In *Marxism and the interpretation of culture*, ed. C. Nelson and L. Grossberg, 271–313. Urbana-Champaign: University of Illinois Press.

Stone, A., G. Leader, D. Stratford, T. Marks, K. Efraim, R. Bynoe, R. Smedley, A. Gunn, and E. Marais. 2024. Landscape evolution and hydrology at the Late Pleistocene archaeological site of Narabeb in the Namib Sand Sea, Namibia. *Quaternary Science Advances* 14:100190.

Thondhlana, T. P., E. C. Lyaya, and E. Mtetwa. 2022. The politics of knowledge production: Training and practice of archaeological science in Africa. *African Archaeological Review* 39:461–477.

UNESCO, 2012. Reconstructing and Restoring Timbuktu's Mosques and Mausoleums [online]. *Google Arts & Culture*. Available from https://artsandculture.google.com/story/reconstructing-and-restoring-timbuktu-s-mosques-and-mausoleums/pwWBjgmaagX5JA. Accessed on 19 March 2025.

Waast, R. 2002. *The state of science in Africa: An overview*. Paris: L'Institut de Recherches pour le Développement.

Wood, M., S. Panighello, E. F. Orsega, P. Robertshaw, J. T. Van Elteren, A. Crowther, M. C. Horton, and N. Boivin. 2017. Zanzibar and Indian Ocean trade in the first millennium CE: The glass bead evidence. *Archaeological and Anthropological Sciences* 9 (5): 879–901.

Wynne-Jones, S., and J. Fleisher, eds. 2015. *Theory in Africa, Africa in theory: Locating meaning in archaeology*. London: Routledge.
Wynne-Jones, S., and A. J. LaViolette, eds. 2018. *The Swahili world*. London: Routledge.

Index

T. Forssman, *Archaeology in Africa: Why the Past Matters*, Archaeology of Africa, https://doi.org/10.1007/978-3-032-13365-6

I

J

T